CONTENTS

Part Three: Social and Peer Issues

Part Four: School Issues

Part Five: Anxiety Issues

CONTRIBUTORS

Anne Marie Albano, PhD, ABPP
Columbia University Clinic for Anxiety
and Related Disorders

Keith D. Allen, PhD, BCBA
Munroe Meyer Institute for Genetics and
Rehabilitation
University of Nebraska Medical Center

Barry S. Anton, PhD, ABPP
University of Puget Sound
Rainier Behavioral Health

Sasha G. Aschenbrand, PhD
Columbia University Clinic for Anxiety
and Related Disorders

Deborah C. Beidel, PhD, ABPP
University of Central Florida

Courtney L. Benjamin, MA
Temple University

James H. Bray, PhD
Baylor College of Medicine

Brandon G. Briery, PhD
Children's Association for Maximum
Potential

Robert B. Brooks, PhD, ABPP
McLean Hospital
Harvard Medical School

Jeffrey L. Brown, PsyD, ABPP
McLean Hospital
Harvard Medical School

Sarah A. Crawley, MA
Temple University

Kevin M. David, PhD
Northeastern State University, Oklahoma

Joanne Davila, PhD
Stony Brook University

Robin M. Deutsch, PhD
Children and the Law Program,
Massachusetts General Hospital
Harvard Medical School

Nathan D. Doty, PhD
Children's Hospital of Philadelphia

Sheila M. Eyberg, PhD, ABPP
University of Florida

Patrick C. Friman, PhD
Boy's Town
University of Nebraska School of
Medicine

Julie A. Fulton
Mosaic College Prep

Deborah R. Glasofer, PhD
Columbia University Medical Center
New York State Psychiatric Institute

Tracy R. Gleason, PhD
Wellesley College
Wellesley College Child Study Center

Sam Goldstein, PhD
George Mason University
University of Utah School of Medicine

Amanda Gordon, BA (Hons Psyc)
Fellow Australian Psychological Society

Linda Sayler Gudas, PhD
Needham Psychotherapy Associates
Harvard Medical School

Robin H. Gurwitch, PhD
Cincinnati Children's Hospital Medical
Center
National Center for School Crisis and
Bereavement

David A. F. Haaga, PhD
American University

Courtney Haight
University of Nevada, Las Vegas

Jeanne Swickard Hoffman, PhD, ABPP
Department of Pediatrics Tripler Army
Medical Center

Shelley J. Hosterman, PhD
Lehigh University
Munroe-Meyer Institute

Yo Jackson, PhD, ABPP
University of Kansas

Elissa Jelalian, PhD
Alpert Medical School of Brown
University

Rebecca A. Jones, PhD
American Schools of Professional
Psychology
Argosy University Atlanta

Michael H. Joseph, MD
Center for Pediatric and Adolescent Pain
Care

Anne E. Kazak, PhD, ABPP
The Children's Hospital of Philadelphia
The University of Pennsylvania

Christopher A. Kearney, PhD
University of Nevada, Las Vegas

Philip C. Kendall, PhD, ABPP
Temple University

Gerald P. Koocher, PhD, ABPP
Simmons College
Harvard Medical School

Annette M. LaGreca, PhD, ABPP
University of Miami

Gary X. Lancelotta, PhD
Baptist Children's Hospital, Miami, FL.
Child Psychology Associates, P.A., South
Miami, FL

Kathleen L. Lemanek, PhD
Nationwide Children's Hospital
Ohio State University College of Medicine

Kristin M. Lindahl, PhD
University of Miami

Meghan McAuliffe Lines, PhD
DuPont Hospital for Children

Thomas R. Linscheid
Ohio State University

Neena M. Malik, PhD
University of Miami Miller School of
Medicine

Teresa Marino-Carper, MS
University of Central Florida

Casey J. Moser, PsyD
Private Practice Winter Park, Florida
Private

Timothy D. Nelson, PhD
University of Nebraska, Lincoln

Kelly A. O'Neil, MA
Temple University

Tonya M. Palermo, PhD
Seattle Children's Hospital

Jennifer Shroff Pendley, PhD
A.I. duPont Hospital for Children and
Jefferson Medical College

William S. Pollack, PhD, ABPP
Harvard Medical School Center for
Men and Young Men
McLean Hospital

Sanford M. Portnoy, PhD
Independent Practice, Waban, MA

Joan F. Portnoy
Independent Practice, Waban, MA

Mitchell J. Prinstein, PhD, ABPP
University of North Carolina at
Chapel Hill

Nadja N. Reilly, PhD
Children's Hospital Boston
Harvard Medical School

Anna S. Romanoff
UCLA School of Medicine

Amy F. Sato, PhD
Alpert Medical School of Brown
University

Karen J. Saywitz, PhD
UCLA School of Medicine
Center for Healthier Children, Families,
and Communities

Lindsay Scharfstein, MD
University of Central Florida

Merritt Schreiber, PhD
Center for Public Health and Disasters
UCLA Center for the Health Sciences

Heather Shaw, PhD
Oregon Research Institute

Barbara J. Siegel, MA
Parents in a Pinch, Inc.

Wendy K. Silverman, PhD, ABPP
Florida International University,
Miami

Ric G. Steele, PhD, ABPP
Clinical Child Psychology Program,
University of Kansas

Sara J. Steinberg, PhD
Cognitive & Behavioral Consultants of
Westchester, LLP

Monica L. Stevens, MS
University of Florida

Eric Stice, PhD
Oregon Research Institute

Susan M. Swearer, PhD
University of Nebraska, Lincoln

W. Douglas Tynan, PhD, ABPP
Nemours Health & Prevention Services
Jefferson Medical College

Alison R. Zisser, MS
University of Florida

INTRODUCTION

Every child will encounter bumps, scrapes, infections, and similar misadventures as part of growing up. Similarly, many psychological crises arise that are akin to these physical events and that will predictably challenge the emotional resilience of children and their caregivers. This practical guide brings together expert advice on promoting coping, resilience, and recovery when such events occur.

Each chapter covers a different "predictable crisis" that can challenge parents' and children's coping skills (and patience!), and includes pragmatic advice on how parents might deal with such situations. The advice provided is also appropriately tailored toward children's developmental level. We also suggest relevant books and websites for those seeking more information.

The chapters were prepared by expert professionals in mental health and education who not only work with parents and children in these problem areas, but who also conduct research to better understand the bases of child and adolescent problems and how best to prevent or treat them. Thus, the advice provided within each chapter draws on the "best evidence" we currently have on how to deal with the "normal" emotional crises of growing up.

You may find that we have omitted some topic of importance or have suggestions about how we might improve the next edition of this guide. If you do, please contact us by sending an electronic message to Koocher@gmail.com. If we use your idea, we will send you a free copy of the next edition.

Gerald P. Koocher and Annette M. La Greca
Boston, Massachusetts and Miami, Florida

In this book, authors strived to use gender-neutral language whenever possible, and refrained from referring to a child or adolescent as "he" or "she." However, on occasion, this was not possible without creating an awkward or complicated sentence. Thus, on such occasions, authors refer to a child or adolescent as "he" or "she" with the understanding that they intend for the statements to be applicable to all children, regardless of whether they are male or female.

The Parents'
Guide to Psychological
First Aid

PART ONE

Health Issues

CHAPTER 1

Toilet Training

Patrick C. Friman

The phone rang at 8:30 A.M. and on the line a small voice reported a successful poop in the potty. The voice belonged to Ted, a 3 1/2-year-old boy, who had previously resisted toilet training. After a short program, however, he quickly began urinating in the toilet. Defecation took a bit longer, but when told he could call his grandmother if he had a success, he agreed to try harder, and the result: a poop in the potty and a happy phone call to grandma.

Full toilet training marks a critical developmental milestone. In some agrarian cultures, children actually achieve full training before their first birthday. Unfortunately for children and parents in fully industrialized cultures like the United States, complete continence before age 1 requires intensive daily training that takes months to complete. Few parents in the United States have that kind of time. Historically, children in the United States completed their training by an average age of 2 1/2 years. Currently, however, full training has become more delayed, and many children do not accomplish full success until the middle of their third year. We do not know all of the reasons for this shifted pattern, but changing cultural practices, parental attitudes, and the availability of highly absorptive underclothing (e.g., pull-up training pants) all partly contribute. Folklore about toilet training can also create an impediment to its progress. For example, parents may hear stories about children who virtually train themselves and think of this as normal. Such stories can lead parents to forestall training until their children initiate it themselves and/or terminate it prematurely if their children exhibit any resistance at all. Although some children may successfully self-initiate and complete training, they are few and very far between. For most children, toilet training requires good timing, proper planning, and concentrated child and parental efforts. This chapter provides some general information about how to proceed.

WHEN SHOULD TRAINING BEGIN?

First and foremost, parents need to feel ready. Has the crisis at work passed? Does the household seem relatively stable now, and likely to continue without unusual disruptions in routine for a few weeks? Having other parts of life running smoothly eases the chore of toilet training. The child also needs to feel ready for training, and several clues can help you identify your child's readiness. For example, prior to starting potty training, your child should:

- Have reached the age of at least 20 months; preferably 2 years old or older
- Have the ability to pick up objects, lower and raise pants or clothing, and walk from room to room easily
- Have the ability to stay dry for several hours at a time, urinating about five to six times a day, and completely emptying the bladder
- Understand household toileting words, words like "wet," "dry," "pants," "bathroom"
- Understand simple instructions, such as "Come here, please" and "Sit down"
- Follow reasonable instructions without raising a big fuss
- Show some awareness of the need to urinate or defecate

HOW DO I BEGIN?

Parents should announce the beginning of training in a way that makes the event seem important and fun for their child. In terms of equipment, a potty chair should suffice. You will need to allow plenty of time. Ideally, set aside at least two full days to start training. Starting on a weekend free of any of out-of-home obligations provides an ideal situation. You should also prepare to set aside personal modesty, because parent modeling plays an important role in effective toilet training.

HOW DO I TEACH MY CHILD TO USE THE TOILET?

Once you have determined that your child is ready, you may begin the toilet training process. Follow these steps:

1. Warm the house. A cold bathroom can feel very unwelcoming. Also, dressing and undressing, an important part of training, feels more comfortable in a warm environment.
2. Remove your child's disposable training pants or other absorptive undergarments.
3. Have your child bare to the waist. This way you can tell from watching your child's belly whether elimination seems imminent. If household standards allow for complete undress, having your child free of clothing can prove even more helpful. Some sensibility about toileting privacy emerges early, and most children prefer to eliminate in their diaper or clothes and become reluctant to do so when fully unclothed.

4. Allow your child to drink as much as possible. Increased fluid intake means increased urine output and thus increased learning opportunities for your child.

5. Schedule regular toilet or potty chair sits. If a weekend has been set aside, toilet sits should occur at least every 2 hours. Additionally, if your child exhibits any indication of toileting urgency, call for an immediate toilet sit.

6. Take your child to the bathroom; do not ask, "do you need to go?" Most children would prefer not to go the bathroom and thus asking them may not yield useful answers.

7. Ensure that your child's feet rest upon a firm surface. This may require a stool. Stability optimizes comfort and performance, especially with bowel movements.

8. Read to your child during extended toilet sits; doing so makes the sit more tolerable and possibly even fun.

9. Point out, but do not criticize or punish accidents. Say, for example, "Honey you've had an accident, let's get you cleaned up."

10. Praise all successes. In the early stages, it may be helpful to supply small rewards for success (e.g., sticker, a small toy, a piece of candy).

Try to make the entire affair unhurried, relaxed, and fun. Children love games, and toilet training can be structured like one. Try keeping score: hits go in the toilet and deposits everywhere else count as misses. Parents should do everything they can to have their child "win." If your child does not win immediately, it is okay to express disappointment, but not in your child, merely in the outcome. Say, for example, "Oh, too bad, maybe you can get it in the toilet next time."

WHAT DO I DO IF MY CHILD INITIALLY FAILS?

Avoid using the word "failure" in a toilet training program. Delays can happen, however. If 2 or 3 weeks of trying produce no consistent progress, and you and your child are beginning to feel frustrated, it is best to declare a full moratorium on toilet training for a month. During that time, allow your child to resume using disposable training pants. Let your child know that he/she may use the toilet, but only if he/she specifically asks to. At the end of the month, the program can begin anew.

SUMMARY

Unfortunately, parents cannot escape this task. Full toilet training remains one of the primary criteria for civilized, independent, socially engaged living. It has increasingly become a criterion for entry into preschool and even into some daycare settings. Fortunately, although the task can require a lot of time, it does not involve a lot of complexity, and it can provide a fun parent–child learning opportunity and sense of accomplishment.

WHERE TO FIND OUT MORE

Books

Fifteen favorite potty training books:
http://www.parents.com/toddlers-preschoolers/potty-training/gear/
    15-favorite-potty-training-books/

Websites

American Academy of Family Physicians
Toilet training
    http://familydoctor.org/online/famdocen/home/children/parents/toilet/179.html
Parenting.org
Starting Toilet Training: The 7 P Plan
    http://www.parenting.org/precious-beginnings/life-lessons/starting-toilet-training-7-p-plan
Intensive Toilet Training
    http://www.parenting.org/precious-beginnings/life-lessons/intensive-toilet-training

CHAPTER 2

Bed Wetting

Patrick C. Friman

Tom, an 8-year-old otherwise completely healthy boy, woke up this morning in urine-soaked pajamas and bedclothes, just as he has nearly every day since he stopped wearing diapers. Fortunately for Tom, his parents consulted their pediatrician when they realized that the success of his early toilet training did not extend to nighttime. He told them that Tom did not wet the bed because of laziness, stubbornness, or emotional disturbance, but because he suffered from a condition called enuresis.

Enuresis is the technical term used for chronic urinary accidents that occur after the age of 5 years. Historically, professionals as well as parents tended to treat afflicted children harshly. Today, however, the situation for these children has improved considerably. Professional and parental science-based knowledge of enuresis has expanded steadily over the past 40 years, and afflicted children have benefitted tremendously. Where professionals formerly interpreted enuresis as a sign of serious psychiatric disturbance, they now recognize it as a largely inherited condition, much more likely caused by an overly sensitive bladder or very deep sleep than a disturbed psyche. They also know it has a time-limited course and usually proves highly responsive to appropriate treatment. However, although most cases do not give parents reason for serious worry, some medical conditions can also cause wetting accidents, most notably diabetes and urinary tract infections. Therefore, the first professional a parent should consult is a medical doctor, preferably the child's primary care provider.

WHAT CAUSES BED WETTING?

There are two types of enuresis—*nocturnal* (accidents occur only during night time sleep) and *diurnal* (accidents occur only during waking hours). The best-known and best-documented cause of both types of enuresis involves family history; the probability of enuresis increases with the number and closeness of blood relatives who have a history of wetting. Children with enuresis also often have bladders that are overly sensitive to filling. This causes them to urinate more frequently throughout the day and night than do children who do not suffer from the condition. Afflicted children are often slow to mature physiologically, especially in the areas of bone growth, secondary sexual characteristics, and height, each of which catches up to normal levels over time. Scientific evidence indicates that bedwetting children often prove more difficult to awaken than their non-bedwetting peers. Some evidence, mostly but not entirely anecdotal, suggests that increased stressors (e.g., birth of a sibling, family disruption) can cause continent children to become temporarily incontinent.

IS ENURESIS A MENTAL HEALTH PROBLEM?

Scientific studies do not support the view that chronic bed wetting is a psychological problem. Children with enuresis do exhibit a slight increase in psychological problems, but the increase seldom signals something serious. More likely, the enuresis itself, as well as the reaction of others, causes the increase in emotional problems.

HOW IS ENURESIS TREATED?

The need for treatment of enuresis predates modern civilization, and the variety of techniques used in antiquity appear to have been limited only by the imagination of the ancient therapists and their tolerance for inflicting unpleasantness on young children in order to eliminate urinary accidents. Some of the noxious treatments reported in a review of ancient approaches to enuresis included binding the penis, burning the buttock and lower back, and forcing children to wear urine-soaked pajamas. In fairness to the ancient therapists, the health consequences of prolonged enuresis during their era became quite serious, due to the limited means for cleaning bedding and ineffective methods for managing infections.

The evolution of treatment for enuresis that began in earnest early in the 20th century abandoned the physically harsh treatments in favor of far more humane and highly effective approaches. The initial breakthrough involved use of an alarm that parents could place on the bed. The alarm, attached to a sensor pad, would emit a loud buzzing sound almost instantly after urine moistened the pad. The child would then awaken (independently or in concert with a parent), clean up the accident, use the toilet appropriately, and return to bed. Published reports of successful alarm treatment for bedwetting appeared in the early 1930s and have steadily continued since then. Alarm-based treatment for bedwetting provides one of the best scientifically supported treatments for child behavior problems of any kind. Between the time of those early reports and now, scientific investigators have modified alarm treatment and supplied a variety of supplemental strategies that increase the odds of success by using multipart treatment packages. For example:

- *The pajama alarm.* Most therapists now use an alarm that attaches to the pajamas instead of the bed. These employ smaller, easier-to-use sensors, and work just as effectively. When attached to clothing during the day, they also help treat daytime accidents.

- *The silent vibrating pajama alarm.* An alarm that vibrates after accidents is available, and it too works as effectively as the bed-based alarms. Parents find it particularly useful for situations in which more than one child sleeps in the same room and for treatment of daytime accidents.
- *Retention control training.* This frequently used supplemental treatment involves teaching children to keep themselves from urinating when they get the urge to go. This allows children to learn to expand the time between trips to the bathroom and produce greater volumes of urine during at each toilet stop.
- *Over-learning.* During the early stages of treatment, some therapists encourage children to drink large amounts of fluid before bed in order to increase the number of accidents and thus the number of times the child can learn from reacting to the alarm.
- *Scheduled toilet visits.* All bedtime programs should include at least one and prefer-ably two scheduled toilet visits: one before the child's bedtime and again before the parent's bedtime. If your child has already wet before your bedtime, begin waking him or her a bit earlier. For daytime wetting, multiple bathroom visits are needed, and should be scheduled when the probability of urination is high or instructed whenever a child's physical movements indicate urination is imminent (e.g., grabbing pants, shifting weight from foot to foot).
- *Kegel exercises.* These involve starting and stopping urine flow three or four times during the course of a urination (wet practice) or exercising the muscles used to do so (dry practice). These exercises work for a broad range of wetting in children and adults, including postpartum and geriatric patients.
- *Self-monitoring.* Requiring children to record any behavior they are trying to reduce typically results in at least a small reduction in that behavior. Asking the child to chart his or her progress during treatment for enuresis is a strategic part of many programs.
- *Incentive systems.* Enuresis treatment requires effort on a child's part, sometimes a lot of it, and incentives for small amounts of progress can sustain the child's moti-vation to continue. At a minimum, offer your child praise for an accident-free day or night. You may even reward your child with a small gift such as a coloring book, some stickers, or a small toy. In particularly stubborn cases, a decrease in the size of the accident (i.e., urine spot) might provide a reason for an incentive.

The preceding strategies and treatments can be used to help you manage and ulti-mately eliminate your child's wetting problems. It is important to note that there is one particular strategy that many parents use, but that is not at all effective. Do not limit or prohibit your child from drinking before bed. Many parents try this strategy before they seek professional help. It does not work and, in fact, can take an already unpleasant situ-ation and make it worse for the child. Enuretic children should be allowed to drink a reasonable amount of fluid before bed if they feel thirsty.

WHAT ABOUT MEDICATION?

An additional option for both nocturnal and diurnal enuresis involves medication. Unfortunately, the only two medications that have been shown to effectively reduce urinary accidents, imipramine (brand name: Tofranil) and desmopressin (brand name: DDAVP), can have some serious side effects such as nervousness, sleep disorders, stomach and intestinal problems, and tiredness. These drugs should be used with caution. Additionally, neither drug cures enuresis. Typically, accidents resume when the use of the medication stops. Thus, medicines make the most sense in situations where an accident-free night is truly needed, such as a sleep-over or at camp, rather than as a primary treatment.

SUMMARY

Enuresis or bed wetting is a common childhood problem that has a long history of misunderstanding and of ineffective approaches to, and mistreatment of, afflicted children. Scientific research, however, has led to much more accurate and benign understanding of the problem, as well as highly effective forms of treatment. In fact, the breakthroughs in treatment over the past several decades represent one of the most significant achievements in clinical child and pediatric psychology.

WHERE TO FIND OUT MORE

Books

Mills, J.C. & Crowley, R. (2005). *Sammy the Elephant and Mr. Camel: A story to help children overcome bedwetting*, 2nd ed. Washington, DC: Magination Press.

Websites

American Academy of Child and Adolescent Psychiatry
    http://www.aacap.org/cs/root/facts_for_families/bedwetting
American Academy of Family Physicians
    http://familydoctor.org/online/famdocen/home/children/parents/toilet/366.html

CHAPTER 3

Fecal Soiling

Patrick C. Friman

Poor Tim—at 6 years old, he has few friends, often seems distracted or unhappy, and occasionally exudes an odor not unlike a soiled diaper. In fact, he frequently soils his underwear and often hides it, only to have it discovered as the odor intensifies. His increasingly frustrated parents view Tim as stubborn or lazy, as well as sneaky. They scold him frequently for the accidents and punish him for the hidden underwear. Tim's parents feel somewhat embarrassed and have not consulted a doctor for this problem.

Tim isn't stubborn or lazy; he has a condition called *encopresis*. Encopresis is the medical term for fecal soiling by a child who has already been toilet trained. Unfortunately, such problems are common, often underreported, undertreated, and overinterpreted. Because of underreporting, this condition can actually go untreated for extended periods of time (as in Tim's case), which can result in frustrating, serious, and potentially life-threatening medical problems. It can also cause problems with the child's social relationships and emotional development. Early detection and treatment is also important because the primary causes of encopresis can include physical diseases. For example:

- *Hirschsprung's disease,* in which a person's colon lacks certain nerve cells, leading to constipation
- Diseases of the spine that affect healthy colon function
- Some forms of developmental disability

Social problems can result from encopresis because soiling evokes more revulsion from peers, parents, and important others than almost any other child behavior problem. Fecal accidents are a major contributor to child abuse, and children who soil themselves still frequently suffer shame, blame, and punishment for a condition almost totally beyond their control. When children hide their underwear, as Tim does, it usually happens because some form of punishment has occurred, either verbal or physical or both.

WHAT CAUSES ENCOPRESIS?

There are two types of encopresis: *retentive* and *nonretentive*. Retentive encopresis is the most common. Approximately 85%–90% of children with encopresis have the retentive type, the most fundamental cause of which is constipation. For children, a combination of factors can trigger the process including: family history (i.e., genetics), dietary factors (e.g., insufficient roughage or bulk in the diet, irregular eating habits), difficulties with toilet training (e.g., punitive or unstructured approaches), and toileting avoidance by the child. Any of these factors, alone or in combination, puts the child at risk for slowed movement of fecal matter through the colon and the uncomfortable and often painful bowel movements that result. Uncomfortable or painful bowel movements, in turn, motivate afflicted children to retain feces, and this leads to a range of problems including fecal accidents. When severe retention occurs and the problems become chronic, the child may develop *fecal impaction*, a large blockage caused by the collection of hard dry stool. When this occurs, liquid feces will seep around the hard mass, producing what some call *paradoxical diarrhea*. Although the child actually has serious constipation, he or she appears to have diarrhea. Some parents try to "treat" this condition with the over-the-counter antidiarrheal agents, which only makes the problem worse.

IS ENCOPRESIS A MENTAL HEALTH PROBLEM?

In short, retentive encopresis is not a psychological disorder. A small number of studies have detected an increase in psychological problems among children with encopresis, but the increase is seldom clinically significant. It is more likely that the encopresis, and social reactions to it, cause the mental health issues than it is that mental health issues cause the encopresis.

An important exception regarding mental health problems as a cause of soiling does exist. As mentioned, a small percentage of children with encopresis (5%–20%) have the nonretentive type. These cases involve children who have regular, well-formed, soft bowel movements somewhere other than the toilet, usually but not always in the clothing. We do not have a good understanding of the causes of these cases; we do know that they are routinely difficult to treat. And, it does seem very likely that mental health problems play a significant role in nonretentive encopresis.

HOW IS ENCOPRESIS TREATED?

Treatment for the two subtypes of encopresis (retentive and nonretentive) differs. Treating the retentive type involves a combination of psychological, behavioral, and biological components typically referred to as the *biobehavioral approach*. This treatment has proven successful in a number of scientific studies and involves the following steps:

1. Seek a medical evaluation to rule out specific illnesses and any secondary medical concerns.
2. Eliminate all sources of punishment for bowel accidents.

3. Undertake a "cleaning out" of the colon (initiated by medical personnel and transferred to parents on an as needed basis).

4. Use stool softeners as prescribed by your family physician or treatment provider. The most frequently used softener is oral polyethylene glycol 3350 (MiraLax), an over-the-counter, tasteless white powder that softens stools through fluid retention.

5. Establish a consistent toileting schedule, one that requires one or two toilet sits a day that should last at least 5 minutes but no longer than 10 and that are timed to correspond with times when your child typically has a bowel movement.

6. Make sure your child's feet are supported by a firm surface (this may require a step or stool) whenever he or she sits for a bowel movement. The support makes it easier for your child to exert the push necessary for a bowel movement.

7. Establish dietary changes as prescribed by your family physician or other health-care professional.

8. Ensure that your child drinks enough fluids (e.g., six to eight 8-oz glasses of fluid a day).

9. Reward your child for successful bowel movements—at a minimum, give your child praise.

In contrast to treatment for retentive encopresis, no treatment has become widely accepted or even well defined for the nonretentive type. In very general terms, treatment for nonretentive encopresis appears to involve a combination of problem solving, toilet scheduling, psychotherapy, and elements of the biobehavioral approach based on a sound diagnostic process. If you think your child may be suffering from nonretentive encopresis, you should seek professional advice.

SUMMARY

Fecal soiling is a common childhood problem that has been misunderstood for centuries, and the result has been a long history of ineffective approaches to, and mistreatment of, afflicted children. Scientific research, however, has led to a biobehavioral approach to assessment and treatment, and it has consistently proven effective. Nonretentive encopresis will prove more difficult to treat because its causes differ. But the breakthroughs over the past 30 years have proven significant, and professional psychotherapeutic intervention can help in such cases.

WHERE TO FIND OUT MORE

Books

Bennett, H. J. (2007). *It hurts when I poop!: A story for children who are scared to use the potty.* Washington, DC: Magination Press.

Cohn, A. (2007). *Constipation, withholding and your child: A family guide to soiling and wetting.* Philadelphia, PA: Jessica Kingsley Publishers.

Reiner, A. (1991). *The potty chronicles: A story to help children adjust to toilet training.* Washington, DC: Magination Press.

Websites

American Academy of Family Physicians
   http://familydoctor.org/online/famdocen/home/children/parents/toilet/166.html
Soiling Solutions
   http://www.soilingsolutions.com/index.htm

CHAPTER 4

Sleep Problems

Tonya M. Palermo

Four-year-old Becky's mother wakes up to see her daughter at her bedside and hears, "Mommy, I'm lonely. I want to sleep in your bed." This has been happening quite frequently and Becky's mother always pulls her daughter into bed with her. She wonders however, if this is the right thing to do.

Nine-year-old Fred has recently had nightmares that wake him up. He dreams about ninjas stalking him. After awakening, he has trouble getting back to sleep without checking under his bed and in the closet. He wants to keep a flashlight and baseball bat near his bed, just in case he needs them for self-defense.

Childhood sleep problems are common. Approximately 25%–40% of children experience problems such as taking a long time to fall asleep, refusing to settle to sleep, sleepwalking, nightmares, or waking during the night. Although parents may expect that young children will demonstrate some difficulties with sleep, it may not feel like a problem until the sleep difficulties become frequent, prolonged, and require a substantial amount of parent time during the night. One common misperception holds that children will grow out of sleep problems. Some children will spontaneously improve their abilities to settle to sleep as they age; however, sleep problems often extend past early childhood and many children have sleep problems at different developmental stages. Problems related to falling asleep or maintaining sleep during the night also come up in middle-childhood and adolescence. However, parents may or may not recognize problems during these developmental stages as children become more independent in their sleep patterns. In older children, feeling excessively sleepy during the day often may offer the only visible clue that the child has a sleep problem.

COMMON SLEEP PROBLEMS FROM INFANCY TO ADOLESCENCE

Infants and Young Children

In infancy, the most common problems with sleep involve settling to sleep and waking during the night. Many infants seem unable to settle to sleep on their own and may require parents to help out by rocking, feeding, or holding them. Quite often, the same behaviors used to settle the infant to sleep at bedtime bear repeating during the night when the baby awakens. Studies of normal sleep show that people experience multiple arousals during the night as they make transitions between light and deep sleep states. Most individuals won't remember waking during the night because routine behaviors, such as turning over or repositioning one's pillow, typically allow them to return to sleep almost immediately. However, when infants or young children have this normal transition between sleep states they may become alert, and cry out for the parent. We call this a problem of *sleep onset associations.* This refers to the comforting experience that the baby or young child had at bedtime (e.g., being rocked or fed) and their wanting to recreate this experience during the night.

It is not always easy to tell whether your child is waking up for a "good reason." Parents often try to discern a specific problem that may be keeping their child awake, such as hunger, teething, illness, or feeling uncomfortable. Often, problems go on for many months before parents consider other explanations. While sleep onset association problems occur more commonly in infants, they may also come up in older children. An older child may require that his parent lie with him at bedtime and later seek out his parent in the middle of the night after a normal arousal. Typically, the parent needs to lie with the child again for the child to return to sleep.

There are other types of problematic sleep behaviors that children may exhibit. Children may demonstrate repetitive body movements during the night or may get out of bed in a confused state. Sleepwalking occurs fairly commonly in childhood. This problem worsens with sleep deprivation, so it can often intensify when children sleep in other settings, such as at a friend's house or while on vacation. During sleepwalking episodes, some children may rock back and forth, bang their heads, or engage in repeated leg movements. This can be alarming, so it is helpful to take certain safety precautions. Keeping your front door locked so that your child doesn't sleepwalk out of the house and removing dangerous objects so that your child doesn't hurt himself can provide some sense of security.

Parents often ask about the difference between nighttime fears, nightmares, and night terrors. *Nighttime fears* are typically normal and harmless. Such fears peak at ages 5–6 years and again at ages 9–11 years. Some very common fears include fear of killers or intruders, being left alone, hearing noises, thinking there is someone else in the room, and monsters. These fears typically come up at bedtime or in the middle of the night and make it hard for children to settle to sleep. *Nightmares,* on the other hand, are frightening dreams that usually awaken a child. Many children feel afraid to return to sleep and go to their parents seeking comfort. Nightmares usually occur during the latter half of the night and differ from night terrors because the child remembers the event, does not seem confused or disoriented, and will typically feel soothed by his parent's presence and reassurance. Sleep or *night terrors* typically occur in the first third of the night and involve sudden arousals, often with a piercing cry or scream. The child looks extremely fearful and usually seems unresponsive and cannot be soothed. Children do not remember night terrors. During a night terror, the best strategy may involve standing back and watching your child to make sure your child is safe, but waiting to comfort him until after the night terror ends.

Older Children and Adolescents

In later childhood and adolescence, children may develop problems with *insomnia*, meaning difficulty with settling to sleep quickly or waking during the night and having difficulty falling back to sleep. Similar to adults with insomnia, children typically have negative thoughts about their ability to fall asleep and may worry about how they will function the next day. Unfortunately, these worries often increase problems with settling to sleep. Insomnia seems to affect about 12% of adolescents, a rate similar to the adult population. Parents may have gone to sleep long after their teen but notice problems with getting the teen out of bed in the morning to go to school. Daytime sleepiness can become a serious problem for the sleep-deprived teen, who may be unable to concentrate and function optimally during the school day. A significant number of drowsy driving accidents also occur among teenagers, creating an important public health issue.

Another related problem affecting teenagers involves *delayed sleep phase*. This refers to a sleep cycle that shifts toward later bedtimes and later wake times. A normal phase delay does occur during puberty. This problem usually intensifies over weekends, summer vacations, and other breaks from school, when the teen can revert back to late bedtimes and wake times. The major problem usually identified with delayed sleep phase is that the child's internal clock conflicts with expectations set by peers, society, or family. Late bedtimes make it difficult for the teen to receive enough sleep, given that the high school day begins quite early. This can lead to a pattern of the teen receiving insufficient sleep during the school week. Often, the teen will "crash" and try to catch up on sleep on the weekends. Because social activities often keep teens up late at night, parents may need to set firm rules about when such activities are to occur, in order to help protect their teens' sleep time during the school week.

Children and teens may also experience temporary disruptions in their sleep in response to a stressful event (e.g., family move, death of a loved one). These sleep disruptions may flow from anxiety at bedtime, difficulty settling, and night wakings. Typically, these disruptions pass as more time elapses from the stressful event.

IS MY CHILD GETTING ENOUGH SLEEP?

Separate from sleep problems, parents often wonder if their children get enough sleep. Several useful resources listed at the end of this chapter can provide information concerning sleep requirements across childhood. While people do vary in their sleep needs, some estimates can provide useful guides.

- By age 1, most children typically sleep about 9–12 hours at night and nap 2–4 hours during the day.
- Toddlers and preschoolers typically sleep 11– 12 hours, and may split those hours between night and daytime sleep.

- School age children typically require about 10–11 hours of sleep.
- Adolescents usually need about 9–9.5 hours of sleep, but most adolescents get only about 7 hours and 15 minutes of sleep.

These sleep needs may surprise parents, who have come to believe that 8 hours of sleep will prove sufficient; adult sleep requirements differ significantly.

The amount of sleep that children receive has important implications for many aspects of their health and well-being. Children who receive less sleep tend to have worse academic performance, more problems with inattention, worse mood, and more aches and pains in comparison to children who sleep longer. Another common misconception holds that people can recover or make up for lost sleep, but sleep deprivation actually has lasting effects that extend over multiple days, even after obtaining periods of adequate sleep. This makes it even more important to ensure that children get an adequate amount of sleep.

WHY DO CHILDREN DEVELOP SLEEP PROBLEMS?

Sleep professionals believe that many factors may contribute to the development of sleep problems in children, including the child's biology, development, environment, and behavior. For example, early on in life, important differences occur in how parents put infants to sleep. While some parents put their infant in the crib slightly awake, other parents may rock or nurse the infant to sleep. Babies also have individual differences in their responses and behaviors that may increase or decrease the likelihood of parents using good sleep practices early on. Good evidence shows that parents can train their infants to fall asleep on their own. Practices that promote good sleep for infants are listed here. Description of specific techniques such as the cry-it-out approach can be found in many of the resources listed in the reading list at the end of this chapter.

- Develop a positive and calming bedtime routine. This routine may involve a bath, feeding, or singing a song. Do everything in the same order and with the same timing, so that your baby knows when it is time to fall asleep.
- Keep the bedroom dark, quiet, and not too warm. Avoid using devices that need to be turned on and off such as playing music from a CD player. Create an environment that helps your baby develop his own ability to soothe himself to sleep.
- If your baby becomes very sleepy with bottle feeding or nursing, gently arouse your baby to make sure he enters the crib slightly awake.
- Put your baby in the crib slightly awake, say goodnight, and leave the room. If your baby begins to cry, allow her to try to settle on her own for 5–10 minutes.

Certain types of sleep problems, such as rhythmic movement disorders and sleep walking, tend to run in families. Stressors in the child's life may trigger temporary problems with sleep. In addition, habits that children develop pertaining to bedtime and sleep may place them at risk for developing sleep problems. For example, children who never develop a consistent bedtime routine and who have irregular night-to-night sleep patterns seem more likely to develop sleep problems. Illnesses, as well as chronic health conditions such as headaches, asthma, and belly aches, or depression, can also impact sleep. Sometimes the treatments for medical conditions are part of the problem, and expert advice from a physician is needed. For example, medicines used to treat attention-deficit hyperactivity disorder (ADHD) can make it difficult for children to settle to sleep. If your child takes medication for ADHD and is experiencing sleep problems, talk to your physician. He or she can make some adjustments to help reduce the impact on your child's sleep.

TREATMENTS FOR SLEEP PROBLEMS

Treatments for sleep problems in infants, toddlers, and preschoolers focus mostly on changing behavior, and very rarely require medication. Education about proper sleep environments often focuses on the presence of electronic devices that are known to contribute to sleep problems in the bedrooms of children. For example, televisions, video games, computers, and cell phones in the bedroom can decrease protected sleep time. Children with televisions in the bedroom tend to sleep less than children without televisions in the bedroom. In older children and teens, parents may not know about use of electronics late at night, such as text messaging that occurs in the wee hours of the night, which can disrupt sleep. Table 4.1 includes suggestions for good sleep practices for children and adolescents.

Behavioral interventions are the most effective form of treatment for bedtime problems and night wakings in infants and young children. Not only do they improve children's sleep, but they also promote parent and family well-being. The two types of behavioral techniques recommended for infants who have difficulties with settling and night waking include *unmodified extinction* and *extinction with parental presence*. Extinction means not rewarding a child with attention. Some call this *planned parental ignoring*, or the "cry-it-out approach." The strategy involves establishing a regular bedtime routine and bedtime and wake time, and avoiding any response to the child after the child goes to bed (e.g., a response to crying). In the modified version, the parents remain in the child's room but still avoid responding to the child. Dr. Richard Ferber popularized this technique in his 1986 book called *Solve Your Child's Sleep Problems*. In addition, popular media, such as television sitcoms, have demonstrated this technique and pointed out aspects of the challenge that parents face in carrying it out.

Listening to your infant or young child cry and not responding can create a lot of distress, and parents often worry that they may cause psychological harm or trauma by not responding to their child's cries. There is no evidence that ignoring a child's cries during such preparation for sleep leads to any negative psychological consequences. Fortunately, this technique usually works within a few days, so most parents can tolerate following through.

Various forms of positive reinforcement can help toddlers or preschoolers develop new behaviors around sleep. Similar to reward systems that parents may have used to develop other behaviors such as potty training, reward systems can also apply to developing good sleep behaviors. For example, a child might earn small tokens or prizes in the

TABLE 4.1. Good sleep practices from infancy to adolescence

Good Sleep Preparation

Infants and Toddlers

- *Always follow the same routine.*   Do everything in the same order and with the same timing (e.g., snack, bath, etc.), so that your child knows when it is time to fall asleep.
- Calm down exciting games and turn off the television. Close the curtains and dim the lights.
- Encourage toddlers to pick up toys as a winding-down process.
- If your child is used to having a drink of water by his or her bedside, make sure it is in place ahead of time. Do not allow your child to hop out of bed again while you are getting it.
- Encourage an older child (2 years and older) to look at the clock. Help your child read the time and then reinforce it with, "Yes, it's 8 P.M. Bedtime!" This makes the *clock* the "bad guy," instead of you. The *clock* decides it is time to turn out the light and go to sleep.
- Tuck a favorite doll or toy into a doll's bed. Say, "See time for doll's bed. Time for you to go to bed, too." Make sure your child has his or her special bedtime toy or stuffed animal.
- Say your special goodnight phrase. Keep it the same every time.
- Keep the time you spend with your child when he or she is in bed to a minimum. The longer you stay, the more likely your child will protest when you leave, and cry during the night.
- Turn off the bedroom light. Leave the hallway light on if necessary. Leave the room and shut the door. Remember that you have already made sure the room is safe.

Older Children

- Keep the same sleep schedule every day of the week. In general, there should not be more than an hour difference in bedtime and wake-up time between school nights and non-school nights.
- Make sure your child's bedroom is comfortable, quiet, and dark. A night light is okay, as completely dark rooms can be scary for some children.
- Keep your child's bedroom at a comfortable temperature during the night (cooler than 75 degrees).
- Your child should not go to bed hungry. A light snack (like milk or crackers) before bed can be a good idea.
- Your child should avoid products containing caffeine for at least several hours before bed. These include caffeinated sodas, coffee, tea, and chocolate.
- Make the hour before bed a quiet time for your child. Your child should not get involved in high-energy activities like rough play, playing outside, or watching exciting TV shows or movies.
- Your child should spend some time outside everyday and be involved in regular exercise.
- Avoid using your child's bedroom for time-out or punishment.
- Avoid putting a TV in your child's bedroom.

Continued

TABLE 4.1. Continued

Teens

- Your teen should wake up and go to bed at approximately the same time every day of the week. Do not go off schedule for two or more nights in a row. Encourage your teen to wake up no more than 2 hours later than his normal schedule on weekends (for example, if normal wake time is 6 A.M., weekend sleep should be no later than 8 A.M.).
- Make sure your teen's sleep environment is comfortable. A cool, dark, quiet room is best.
- Avoid having your teen take naps during the day. Too much daytime sleep will cut into your teen's sleep at night.
- Try to make the hour before bedtime a quiet time. Finishing homework earlier in the evening will allow for more "wind-down" time at bedtime.
- Avoid stimulating television, music, videogames, or phone conversations right before your teen is trying to settle down to sleep.
- Avoid caffeine for at least several hours before bed including caffeinated sodas, coffee, tea, and chocolate. It interferes with falling asleep.
- Establish consistent daytime routines, including eating regular meals and participating in regular activities.
- Make the bed a sleep-only zone. Have your teen do homework at a desk or table, and play games, watch television, and use the computer *outside* of the bedroom.
- If your teen has difficulty settling to sleep, encourage him to get out of bed and do a quiet activity like reading, organizing his desk, etc., and return to his bed when he feels sleepy again.

morning for reaching a goal, such as staying in bed all night. It is important to let your child know very specifically what behavior goals apply and to make sure that she can actually achieve the goal with a little effort. Reward systems only work if children actually receive the rewards! Developing new, more advanced goals can help your child remain motivated.

Certain sleep problems may require professional assistance, either because of their persistence or the distress they cause. For example, professional help will often prove necessary for treatment of insomnia. Treatment may involve helping the child or teen to develop better sleep habits, use strategies to reduce the amount of time he lies in bed awake, and to think differently about sleep. Sometimes teaching relaxation strategies can help children who have a lot of tension at bedtime. One strategy called *stimulus control* (also used for treatment of adult insomnia) involves instructing the child to get out of bed if she has not fallen asleep quickly to engage in a boring activity. Selected boring activities, such as reading a math book or a phone book, are intended to make the child sleepy again. The goal is to decrease the amount of time that the child spends just lying in bed (and not sleeping). Once the child starts to fall asleep faster, she can usually develop a good positive routine and learn to incorporate the right amount of sleep.

SUMMARY

Children may have temporary disruptions to their sleep or show patterns of more persistent sleep problems related to how they fall asleep, what happens during sleep, or how they wake up in the morning. Different types of problems may be present across infancy to adolescence. Treatments for children's sleep problems most typically involve education and behavioral strategies. Ensuring protected sleep time is an important goal for parents, so that they can promote an environment that is conducive to the child receiving enough sleep. Many resources are available to help parents learn more about children's sleep and to provide instruction in behavioral strategies that can be carried out at home.

WHERE TO FIND OUT MORE

Books

American Academy of Pediatrics. (1999). *Guide to your child's sleep.* New York: Villard Books.

Ferber, R. (1986). *Solve your child's sleep problems.* New York: Simon and Schuster.

Durand, V.M. (1997). *Sleep better: A guide to improving sleep for children with special needs.* Baltimore: Brookes.

Mindell, J.A. (2005). *Sleeping through the night, revised edition: How infants, toddlers, and their parents can get a good night's sleep.* New York: Harper Perennial.

Websites

The American Academy of Sleep Medicine
www.aasmnet.org
National Sleep Foundation
www.sleepfoundation.org

CHAPTER 5

Overeating and Obesity

Elissa Jelalian and Amy F. Sato

Ben is a 6-year-old boy who has always been a "normal" weight. Recently, Ben's mother has noticed that he asks for more food at mealtimes and has begun gaining excess weight. He likes to eat while watching television or playing on the computer, which are his favorite activities. He is also reluctant to go outside and play with children in the neighborhood. Ben's mother shares her observations with a close friend who reassures her that she has nothing to worry about and that Ben is experiencing a normal "growth spurt" and will "grow into his weight." However, Ben's mother isn't sure how to gauge what qualifies as normal development and what types of weight gain warrant further attention.

Childhood obesity has become a common concern for families and healthcare providers. Over the past 30 years there has been a dramatic, three-fold rise in the prevalence of obesity among children and adolescents. A recent national survey found that between 24% and 34% of children and adolescents in the United States qualify as overweight (defined by a body mass index or BMI above the 85th percentile), with another 12%–18% categorized as obese (a BMI above the 95th percentile). The rates of obesity climb higher among older children and those from some ethnic minority groups, with Mexican American children and Non-Hispanic Black children at particularly high risk.

HOW DO I KNOW IF MY CHILD IS OVERWEIGHT?

A number of terms describe weight concerns in children and adolescents, including "overweight," "obese," and "at risk of overweight." These terms can be confusing. Obesity has a very specific definition involving the amount of excess body fat, called *adiposity*, in relation to overall body weight when compared against a given weight standard.

The most widely accepted measure for determining weight status is BMI, a measure of weight adjusted for height (kg/meters²). Among adults, absolute BMI values can be used to define obesity (i.e., BMI greater than 30). However, because a child's body composition changes with age and differs between boys and girls, BMI percentile scores are used among children and adolescents. The Centers for Disease Control and Prevention (CDC) has an online BMI calculator that you can use to determine your child's BMI (http://www.cdc.gov/obesity/childhood/defining.html). This calculator uses information about a child's exact age, sex, height, and weight.

Typically, a child's primary care physician will plot the BMI value on a CDC growth chart to determine the BMI-for-age percentile. Children qualify as overweight when their BMIs fall between the 85th and 94th percentiles for gender and age; they qualify as obese when their BMI value reaches the 95th percentile or higher.

WHY IS THIS IMPORTANT?

Although people widely recognize that being overweight is "not healthy," they may have less appreciation for the extent to which obesity can negatively affect a child's health. Childhood obesity can lead to health problems such as asthma, sleep apnea, liver disease, high blood pressure, type 2 diabetes, and other medical conditions. Not only may overweight youth experience these immediate health consequences, but they stand at risk for significant long-term consequences as well. Specifically, obese children and adolescents have a risk for obesity into adulthood, when it becomes harder to treat and is associated with increased risk of illness and death.

In addition to the negative effects on physical health, many overweight children and adolescents experience negative emotional consequences, such as dissatisfaction with their bodies and lower self-esteem. In comparison to kids who are normal weight, overweight children and adolescents have poorer health-related quality of life, which includes areas such as physical, social, emotional, and academic functioning. In general, the more overweight the child is, the more significant the negative impact on quality of life. Concerns about physical appearance and body image also become significant for adolescents.

With respect to social relationships, overweight school-age children describe more social problems than non-overweight children, and overweight adolescents are more likely to be bullied by their peers. They are also more likely to find it harder to make friends. Unfortunately, many adolescents with a BMI in the obese range experience weight-related teasing by family members as well as peers. This is particularly important given that parental criticism of weight and weight-based teasing by peers predicts poorer self-esteem among overweight children. Overweight children and adolescents are at risk for psychological distress, such as anxiety and depressive symptoms, although it appears that the child's body satisfaction and experience of weight-related teasing and stigma are important factors influencing their level of distress.

HOW DO CHILDREN BECOME OVERWEIGHT?

At the most basic level, weight gain is the result of taking in more calories than needed for normal growth and development. But, a complex host of genetic, behavioral, and environmental factors work together to lead a child to become overweight. While certain genes may increase the chances of becoming overweight, the dramatic rise in obesity over the past three decades cannot be attributed to genetics alone.

In recent years, the U.S. population has become less physically active, more sedentary, and more likely to consume diets high in calories and fat, but low in nutrient-dense foods, such as fruits and vegetables. Along with adults, children consume more calories while the quality of their diets has steadily declined. Many children fail to meet current dietary recommendations of the U.S. Department of Agriculture (USDA). For example, more than 85% of adolescents do not eat the recommended five or more servings of fruit and vegetables per day and nearly a third of the daily energy intake for children and adolescents comes from sweeteners/sweetened drinks and snack foods (e.g., salty snacks and desserts). Consumption of food produced outside the home has also increased over the past 20–30 years, accounting for up to 40% of children's meals. Since foods prepared at restaurants and fast-food establishments often have substantially more calories than the same foods prepared at home, a pattern of "eating out" has become associated with greater calorie intake and increased chances of becoming overweight.

While the quality of children's diets has worsened and the amount of calories consumed increased, the average child in the United States spends less time engaged in physical activity and more time involved with "sedentary behaviors" or screen time. Increases in physical activity lead to decreases in BMI in children and adolescents; however, most youth do not meet current recommendations from the USDA and the U.S. Department of Health and Human Services for physical activity. Indeed, more than half (55%–66%) of adolescents do not satisfy the recommended 1 hour of moderate to vigorous physical activity per day. At the same time, children spend greater than a 1/4 of their waking hours watching television. Greater television viewing is linked to an increased risk for obesity among children. One reason for this is that children tend to snack on high-calorie foods while watching television.

HOW CAN I HELP MY CHILD?

Parents may wonder what they can do to support their child in managing his or her weight with all of the challenges related to living in an "obesogenic" society—one that encourages obesity-related behaviors. Preventing obesity in your children should be a priority. Parents can provide an environment that encourages healthy eating and activity choices regardless of weight status. Addressing eating and activity habits, as well as factors in the home environment, can help your child maintain or achieve a healthy weight.

Regardless of which healthy habits you try to support, an important guideline involves changes at the level of the family. While it may initially seem "unfair" to other family members to remove snack foods from the home and cut down on television time, even normal-weight siblings benefit from a healthy diet and less time spent in sedentary behaviors.

Parents can do several things to support children in decreasing their overall calorie intake, increasing their physical activity, and decreasing sedentary behavior (also see the CDC website for a review). With regard to eating, cutting down on access to high-calorie/high-fat snacks and sugar-sweetened beverages, while at the same time providing more opportunities to consume fruits and vegetables, will help. Gradually introducing new foods, such as fruits and vegetables, and presenting them several times will also help. Research has shown that food familiarity becomes important in developing taste preferences, so we recommend multiple exposures to new foods.

With regard to activity, parents can help children increase physical activity and decrease sedentary behavior. Encourage your school-age children and adolescents to participate in regular physical activity through involvement with athletics or organized exercise programs (e.g., dance, basketball, swimming) as well as "lifestyle" activities such as walking to school, taking stairs rather than the elevator, or biking to a friend's house on the weekend. Encourage young children to participate in fun physical activity (e.g., playing catch, jumping rope, playing hopscotch, climbing on a jungle gym). Try to make physical activity enjoyable and supported by an environment that encourages a developing sense of self-confidence. To reduce sedentary behavior, set limits on the amount of time your family spends watching television, limit your child's total amount of "screen time" (including television, video, and leisure-time computer use), and support involvement with alternative activities (e.g., craft projects, hobbies, clubs such as Girl or Boy Scouts, etc.). Ben's mother could help him by setting healthy limits (e.g., 2 hours per day) on the amount of time he watches television and plays on the computer each day, while encouraging him to be more physically active. For example, she could help him to sign up for a sport that he enjoys (e.g., t-ball) or encourage healthy family activities (e.g., bike rides). For more ideas, she could visit her local YMCA center, which may provide programs Ben could participate in (see http://www.ymca.net/ to find the YMCA branch in your area).

In summary, here are several key points:

- Increase fruit and vegetable servings, with the goal of reaching a minimum of five servings per day.
- Decrease or eliminate consumption of sugar-sweetened beverages such as soda and fruit drinks.
- Decrease the frequency of eating out and fast-food consumption, limiting it to a maximum of one time per week.
- Increase participation in physical activity to a goal of 60 minutes per day. This need not involve continuous activity. Younger children, for example, will engage in short "bouts" of play that can accumulate throughout the day.
- Limit "screen time" unrelated to homework assignments to a maximum of 2 hours per day.

Children will have better success in achieving changes in eating and activity habits if they live in a supportive environment that includes many "cues" for healthy behaviors and few "cues" for unhealthy choices. While parents may not want to entirely eliminate the availability of high-calorie/high-fat foods, reducing access to these foods in the home becomes an important way to decrease them from a child's diet.

At the same time, parents can increase cues for healthy behaviors, such as by keeping fruits and vegetables accessible and visible, and keeping exercise equipment in places where it may be safely and easily used. Parents can also help their child or adolescent by establishing structure through family eating patterns and rules. Having a designated location for eating (e.g., kitchen or dining room) and avoiding other activities, such as television viewing, during meals or snacks also becomes important. Increased structure at mealtime will decrease the likelihood of "mindless" eating and also limit cues for eating to one location in the house. With younger children, parents should decide where their child will eat, as well as how many meals per day to prepare, and what types and how much of each food is presented. Children, as well as adults, tend to consume more when presented with larger portions. Therefore, parents should strive to present portion sizes appropriate to the child's age. Ben's mother could help him to break the unhealthy habit of eating while watching television or playing on the computer by establishing a new family rule that *everyone* eats meals and snacks only at the kitchen table.

In summary, key points include the following:

- Decrease/limit the number of high-calorie/high-fat foods in the home.
- Increase availability of healthy food choices (e.g., fruits and vegetables, low fat dairy).
- Discourage eating in places other than the kitchen or dining room.
- Serve age-appropriate portion sizes.
- Provide structure related to meal-time.

Finally, parents can play an important role by modeling healthy eating and exercise behaviors and maintaining a positive, supportive attitude. Children learn healthy eating behaviors both through their own experience and by observing others. You can model healthy eating by consuming the recommended allowance of fruits and vegetables per day, while showing your child that these foods are enjoyable. Similarly, you can have a positive influence on your child's weight status by modeling regular involvement in physical activity. Another key to supporting healthy choices involves acknowledging positive behaviors. Positive reinforcement for healthy behaviors (e.g., praising your child for eating fruit) leads to greater intake of healthier foods, increased physical activity, and decreased intake of sweetened beverages and snacks. At the same time, avoid criticizing or teasing your child about his or her weight. Remember to listen to your child's concerns about weight. Also remember that overweight youth often experience weight-related teasing or social stigma. Ben's mother may not have guessed that his reluctance to play with other children could be related to his weight gain. Since many overweight children experience weight-related teasing, she could be proactive by talking with him about whether he has been having trouble with other kids in the neighborhood or at school.

- Act as a positive role model for healthy eating and physical activity.
- Reinforce a child's healthy choices instead of criticizing less healthy ones.
- Avoid teasing, and encourage family members to do the same.
- Listen and offer support to help cope with stigma and teasing.

WHAT KINDS OF HELP ARE AVAILABLE AND WHAT SHOULD I LOOK FOR?

Different kinds of help are available for overweight children and their families. Recent research involving collaboration among several key medical agencies suggests a tiered approach to overweight and obesity, with recommendations about which step is appropriate according to a child or adolescent's age, BMI percentile, and medical risk. This tiered approach suggests increasingly intensive stages of intervention based on a child's level of overweight and coexisting health concerns. Although the first stage can be a good starting place for all overweight children, more intensive interventions are appropriate for children who are very obese or have co-occurring medical problems (e.g., high blood pressure or cholesterol, diabetes). Children may also be advanced to more intensive interventions if they are not making progress toward their weight goals, their BMI increases, or co-occurring medical conditions develop or worsen.

The first stage, "prevention plus," is appropriate for obesity prevention in normal-weight children and as a starting place for helping overweight children. Ben's mother may start here even, though she is not sure whether his increased weight and appetite reflects that of a "growing child" or an eating problem that could lead to obesity. The prevention plus stage involves the whole family and includes several eating and behavioral recommendations, such as increased consumption of fruits and vegetables, limiting screen time to 2 hours or less per day, ensuring daily physical activity, and addressing eating behaviors (e.g., daily breakfast). You may want to look for a health promotion or prevention program that you can implement yourself. These programs typically focus on ways for the whole family to develop healthy habits. For example, the We Can!™ program provides a host of resources designed for families, such as ways to make healthy food choices and encourage your family to become more physically active (see http://www.nhlbi.nih.gov/health/public/heart/obesity/wecan/index.htm). Another resource is the My Pyramid website (http://www.mypyramid.gov/kids/), which provides tools for families, such as an interactive menu planner and tips for developing healthy eating habits depending upon your child's age (preschooler ages 2–5, or child ages 6–11).

Changing the eating and activity patterns within a family may be enough to positively influence a child's weight. However, children may continue to gain excess weight even after taking these steps. The next recommended stages are more intensive and should be considered only after consulting with your child's primary care physician. A primary care physician, such as a pediatrician, can provide you with guidance regarding whether your child has a healthy weight status. A doctor also can help determine the level of help your child needs.

The second stage, "structured weight management," involves developing a plan for a balanced diet (emphasizing small amounts of calorie-dense food), further limiting screen time and increasing physical activity, implementing child and/or parent monitoring (e.g., of dietary intake), and performing medical screening (e.g., checking vital signs such as blood pressure). At this stage, parents may want to look for a dietician or other health professional (for example a physician or nurse practitioner) to provide guidance about specific recommendations. In addition, some commercial weight-loss programs allow adolescents to participate, although a doctor's referral may be required. Commercial weight loss programs may involve attending groups with other people who are trying to lose weight, keeping a journal of what you are eating and the amount of exercise you get, or tracking food through the use of a point-based system. Parents could also look for a structured physical activity program (e.g., team sports, program through a fitness center) for their child to participate in. For example, you could contact your local YMCA branch about programs for children and teens in your area.

The third stage involves "comprehensive multidisciplinary intervention," which includes parental involvement (especially for younger children); ongoing assessment of diet, physical activity, and weight; structured behavioral programming (e.g., monitoring, goal setting); parent/caregiver training; and structured interventions for dietary and physical activity. This stage of intervention is typically more appropriate for children with higher BMI or children who have not been successful with less intensive approaches. Comprehensive multidisciplinary programs are often affiliated with a hospital or medical center, and your child's pediatrician may be able to help you find one in your area. At this level, parents should look for the ability to work with a team that has expertise in childhood obesity, ideally including a registered dietician, exercise specialist, and behavioral counselor such as a social worker or psychologist.

Finally, more intensive options are available for children who are already experiencing medical complications related to obesity and need additional help. This includes continued diet and activity counseling plus consideration of meal replacement, medication, very-low-energy diet, and surgery, and would only be delivered within a pediatric weight management center or residential setting with medical supervision.

SUMMARY

Parents today face a society in which children and adolescents commonly lead a sedentary lifestyle and consume diets that are high in fat and calories. These societal trends have contributed to the substantial number of children and adolescents who become overweight or obese, and who are thus at risk for serious physical health complications and emotional and social consequences. Still, parents should not give up hope. There are many ways in which parents can help an overweight child to achieve a healthier weight. Given that it is vital for change to occur at the family level, many of the recommendations in this and other resources can be considered steps for improving the healthy of the entire family.

WHERE TO FIND OUT MORE

Books

Jelalian, E., & Steele, R.J. (Eds.). (2008). *Handbook of childhood and adolescent obesity.* New York: Springer.
Rao, G. (2006). *Child obesity: A parent's guide to a fit, trim and happy child.* New York: Prometheus Books.

Websites

American Academy of Pediatrics
    http://www.aap.org/healthtopics/overweight.cfmbarnes
Centers for Disease Control and Prevention
    http://www.cdc.gov/obesity/childhood/defining.html
Kidnetic
    http://www.kidnetic.com

MyPyramid
  http://www.mypyramid.gov/kids/
U.S. Department of Agriculture and U.S. Department of Health and Human Services
  Dietary Guidelines for Americans
  http://www.health.gov/dietaryguidelines/dga2005/document/default.htm
WeCan!™ Ways to Enhance Children's Activity and Nutrition
  http://www.nhlbi.nih.gov/health/public/heart/obesity/wecan/index.htm
Weight-Control Information Network
  http://win.niddk.nih.gov/publications/over_child.htm
YMCA
  http://www.ymca.net/

CHAPTER 6

Picky Eating and Concerns about Anorexia

Gary X. Lancelotta and Thomas R. Linscheid

Manny is a charming and engaging 7-year-old boy who is slightly overweight, yet average height for his age. His parents are concerned about his eating patterns. Manny will only eat at a certain McDonald's near his grandparents' home. His parents are at odds over how to address their son's growing eating problem. They have two other children and want to prevent them from exhibiting this same picky eating behavior.

Maria is a 12-year-old girl who has always had a normal weight, even though she had demonstrated a bit of picky eating behavior all her life, with a definite preference for fast-food and deserts, as opposed to vegetables and fruits. She had always been a happy child with many friends, who performed well academically. When Maria entered middle school, her peers started to tease her for being "fat." This, along with the fact that Maria had entered puberty, contributed to her distress about her weight. To avoid being teased and to fit in with the other girls at school, Maria began engaging in unhealthy habits such as reading diet books, skipping meals, and over-exercising. She became so preoccupied with her weight that she lost interest in friends and her usual hobbies and activities. In only a few months, Maria went from 110 lbs. to 75 lbs. and ended up in the hospital due to malnutrition and electrolyte imbalance.

"My child doesn't eat anything!" is a common complaint among parents. What it usually means is that the child isn't eating the variety of foods that parents want the child to eat. This chapter's focus is on eating habits in children and covers not only "picky eating," but the more severe problem of disordered eating (e.g., anorexia and bulimia). We offer tips for improving your child's eating habits and suggestions for what to do if you think your child may have an eating disorder.

SELECTIVE FOOD REFUSAL

Selective food refusal is a common concern for parents of pre-school age children. By the time their children reach 24 months of age, 50% of parents describe their child as a picky eater. This common concern raises the issue of what is perceived versus what is reality. Are you overly concerned about your child's eating, or does your child truly have a problem with nutritional intake that may contribute to growth or cognitive problems in the future?

Studies of picky eaters' habits contrasted with children with normal diets found that the picky eaters did differ on variety of foods eaten, but did not differ from non-picky eaters on nutritional status. Thus, picky eating does not automatically equal poor nutrition. Only a nutritional analysis of a child's intake and an assessment of growth parameters can establish whether a child with limited variety has actually become nutritionally or medically compromised.

A second conclusion from the research suggests that often there is no reason to worry about most picky eaters. Of course, if you are concerned about your child's eating habits, there are many safe and effective strategies you can use. We do not condone force feeding or other feeding strategies that can create more serious and longstanding feeding problems.

HOW DO I RECOGNIZE MY CHILD'S RISK FACTORS FOR EATING AND FEEDING PROBLEMS AND HOW DO I HANDLE THEM?

It is important to understand the risk factors associated with parental feeding practices that lead to more serious eating difficulties. The first involves parental overconcern with their child's growth. Parents may think that any variation from their perceptions of an ideal diet can lead to health and developmental problems.

Additional risk factors for problem eating and feeding behaviors in children include developmentally appropriate and normal phenomena that serve to change a child's natural approach to eating. Sometimes parents do not understand these phenomena, which may lead to misperceptions about eating habit changes. It can be helpful for you to be aware of these developmentally appropriate changes, so that you can better judge your child's eating habits. For example, there is something called *food neophobia*. This arises from the natural tendency to feel somewhat anxious when presented with a new and unfamiliar food. Imagine how you would feel if you were served a plate of raw beetles during a formal meal at a business associate's house. We are not suggesting that you're trying to get your child to eat beetles, but your child may think about eating salad in the same way you think about eating bugs.

Neophobia begins near the first year of life and reaches its peak during the toddler and preschool years. Parents who try to force a child to eat a new food or exhibit extreme anxiety over the child's refusal of a new food may increase the child's natural anxiety or neophobia, resulting in increased anxiety associated with that food. This decreases the chances a child will accept that food when it is next presented. Over time, this process can result in a full-blown phobia of that food, and lead to extreme resistance to eating the food in the future.

Introduction of a new food should flow in a way that does not increase your child's natural anxiety, and this may require many presentations, often as many as 10 to 15, before your child accepts it. Many parents give up after only 3–5 attempts. You must be persistent.

One casual and "low stress" way to introduce a new food might involve modeling, by placing the item on your plate during family mealtime. When your child sees you eating and enjoying the new food, he or she may become interested and ask for a taste. Allow your child to take a bite from your plate. Another strategy might involve renaming the food to take advantage of known preferences. For example, when a 4-year-child who enjoyed eating tuna salad saw her parents eating salmon, she asked for the name of the food. One parent said "salmon," and the child replied, "Yuk!" Thinking quickly, the other parent said, "Another name for that is pink tuna." The child tried a bite from her parent's plate and pronounced it "delicious."

Another naturally occurring phenomenon relates to the dramatic slowing of a child's growth rate during the second year of life. Infants generally triple their birth weight by 12 months of age, but then the rate of growth slows dramatically, with a normal weight gain of only 4–6 pounds during the second year of life. Due to this slowed growth rate, young children may not feel hungry at meal times, have variable taste preferences, and have an increasing interest in their environment and autonomy that competes with their interest in eating. Put this together with food neophobia and you get a child who seems fearful of new foods, is often not hungry when presented with food, and thus is picky about what and how much he or she will eat at mealtimes. This can cause concern in parents, who may be well-intentioned, but misinformed, and can lead to coercive practices or to offering their child only those foods that they know their child likes. Often, these foods are not healthy or nutritious (e.g., ice cream, fast-food, etc.) and can disrupt the child's balanced diet and regular mealtimes. It is important to understand that most toddlers will self-regulate their intake to produce normal growth and consume a variety of foods, if they are consistently offered a balanced diet at scheduled mealtimes.

With knowledge of the risk factors for the development of picky eating, it is easy to understand how Manny (at the beginning of the chapter) came to feel that he could only eat at McDonalds. He was the first-born child of Cuban immigrant parents, who, along with Manny's grandparents, had excessive concerns about his nutrition. At 13 months of age, Manny began to show the classic signs of reduced appetite and variable food preferences, which led to near panic by his parents that he would become malnourished. On a visit to McDonalds, his parents were thrilled that Manny enthusiastically ate most of his father's French fries, sampled chicken nuggets, and drank a small amount of a chocolate milkshake. This sealed the deal, and Manny's parents began taking him to their local McDonalds whenever they felt he hadn't eaten well for a meal or two. Manny quickly learned that food refusal at home led to a trip to McDonalds. He felt happy as he enjoyed the food and playground there, and his parents felt relieved that at least he had eaten something.

HOW DO I HANDLE MY CHILD'S SEVERE PICKY EATING?

Severe picky eating that can lead to growth and nutritional problems can be very difficult to correct. It is likely that your child will not willingly participate in the rehabilitation process and will steadfastly resist your efforts to introduce new foods. The process requires denying your child access to preferred foods in order to produce the motivation for your child to accept a few bites of a new food. This is tough for many parents to do; no parent likes to deny their child his or her favorite foods. There is also concern about malnutrition, if your child won't eat. This makes it very hard for parents to hold out until their child accepts a new food.

It may be helpful for you to imagine you are stranded on a small desert island and are convinced that you will not be saved for months. The island has plenty of water, but no food except worms and caterpillars. Picture yourself in this situation and think about how many days it would take before you decided you will have to eat the worms and caterpillars. How would you feel taking that first bite? Probably not very good, but over time you would get used to it. You may even end up liking worms!

This scenario is meant to help you understand why your child feels so resistant to new foods and how important it is to allow your child's hunger to become a strong motivator to eat; one that outweighs the fear of new food. If you can picture yourself eating insects, you can be confident that your child will eventually eat the new foods you offer.

The point is this—you can get anyone to eat anything, if you can create a situation in which extreme hunger exists and the person becomes convinced that there is no other food available. Unfortunately, many times parents try to change their child's eating habits but allow their child to fill up on favorite foods. Even if children don't fill up on favorite foods, they consume sufficient calories that they can withstand mild hunger for days. It is akin to the desert island scenario, with your favorite food delivered to you each day but only enough to meet half of your caloric needs. While you would feel hungry, the hunger would not likely prove sufficient to motivate you to eat worms.

Extreme selectivity has as its core a phobia of new foods, much as we have a phobia of eating worms. You have to feel confident that you can follow through, as the problem will only get worse if you start this approach but then give in to your child's demands for a favorite food. Implementing this plan takes a lot of preparation, discussion of "what-ifs," and reassurance that this approach will work with no long-term physical or psychological damage to your child.

When using the "food restriction" approach just described, be sure to provide your child with access to water throughout the treatment in order to prevent dehydration. It will be more difficult to implement this approach with older children, as they can find ways to gain access to their favorite foods. Implementing this approach may require coordinating with your child's school, informing neighbors and relatives, and devising ways to prevent your child from "sneaking" into the pantry at night or when you and your spouse or partner are occupied. Be sure to discuss this approach with your child's pediatrician, who can provide reassurance that short-term weight loss will not harm your child physically and who can offer daily office visits to weigh your child and assess his or her medical condition if you are highly concerned.

Following are some summary points to remember if you are concerned about your child's picky eating habits:

- Selective food refusal and picky eating starts very early, in the first 2 years of a child's life.
- The development of poor eating habits often becomes shaped by behavioral, developmental, emotional, cultural, and family dynamics.
- Breaking the cycle of selective food refusal and picky eating patterns requires you to control your child's access to preferred foods and liquids, so that your child becomes hungry enough to want to eat what you are offering.
- Always allow your child access to water and other zero-calorie, sugar-free beverages to decrease the potential for dehydration during an intervention.
- Whatever intervention you choose to implement, be sure to elicit the help of your pediatrician. He or she can monitor your child's medical status throughout the program. You also may need to engage the support of a pediatric psychologist to address the behavioral, emotional, and psychological aspects of treatment needs.
- Once you've begun the intervention, make sure to follow through until the end. Stopping the intervention too early can make your child's food refusal behaviors even stronger and more difficult to change.

ANOREXIA, BULIMIA, AND OTHER EATING/WEIGHT CONCERNS

According to the National Eating Disorders Association, as many as 10 million females and 1 million males in the United States suffer with some form of eating disorder, such as anorexia nervosa or bulimia nervosa. *Anorexia nervosa* is a serious, potentially life-threatening condition characterized by restriction of nutritional intake, body image disturbance, excessive exercise, and excessive weight loss. Anorexia often begins in adolescence, when teens become preoccupied with their weight and with their body in general. Media glamorization of thinness (for girls) or muscularity (for boys) also contributes to adolescents' weight and body concerns. For example, many girls feel a strong need to lose weight and thus they avoid eating or eat very little in order to lose weight.

Bulimia nervosa also has potentially life-threatening consequences. It typically involves a cycle of bingeing, eating excessive quantities in a short period of time, and then purging the extra calories. Purging may include behaviors such as self-induced vomiting, laxative abuse, or extended periods of calorie deprivation, designed to compensate for the binge eating. Unlike anorexia nervosa, where the goal involves losing weight, bulimia involves preventing weight gain from the bingeing.

Parents of children who become picky eaters often worry that this pattern will lead to an eating disorder, such as anorexia nervosa, later on. Only one study has suggested that individuals with anorexia nervosa were picky eaters when younger. However, the connection is not very strong, and it seems likely that many other factors, such as social pressures and a child's personality and family dynamics, are better predictors of the onset of anorexia nervosa than picky eating.

Children and adolescents at risk for anorexia nervosa generally come from high-achieving families who value appearance and accomplishment. These girls (only one in 20 is a boy) often present as high achievers with admirable self-control and self-management attributes. Despite having many accomplishments and many friends (like Maria at the beginning of the chapter), they do not seem to develop strong self-confidence. Rather, they often believe that they are really not as smart or as good as their peers and that their achievements are only due to their extra efforts. Such youth often have a rigid personality characterized by concrete thinking patterns. As weight loss progresses, these feelings accelerate, and they become more rigid and compulsive, to the point that fear of weight gain (i.e., losing control) can render them incapable of abstract and rational thinking.

In the description of Maria, we see how personality, normal developmental stages (puberty), peer pressure, and media glamorization of thinness all came together in the onset of her eating disorder. While her developmental history included mild picky eating that may have led to becoming mildly overweight, it did not become the sole determinant of her condition.

WHAT DO I DO IF MY CHILD HAS AN EATING DISORDER?

It is important to recognize that eating disorders can pose serious and potentially life-threatening problems. While picky eating may play a minor role in the development of an eating disorder, the greatest risk factors lie in family dynamics, the child's personality and developmental stage, and media and peer pressure. Early identification and intervention are crucially important in anorexia nervosa because the more weight your child loses and the longer your child stays at a low weight, the worse the prognosis.

Here are some tips for helping your eating disordered child:

- Educate yourself. Become aware of the risk factors for eating disorders. Consult legitimate medical resources for the facts about eating disorders in children (see Where to Find Out More).
- Note any changes in your child's eating habits and eating-related behaviors, especially those that are unhealthy, such as unnecessarily reducing caloric intake, increased focus on weight and appearance, escalating self-derogatory statements, and signs of social withdrawal.
- If you notice any of these changes in your child, immediately begin monitoring your child's weight loss through weekly weigh-ins. If your child's weight loss is too rapid or extreme, contact a professional. Early intervention is key.
- Enlist the help of your pediatrician to monitor the medical and physical aspects of your child's condition.
- Consult other professionals, including a psychologist, to address the behavioral, emotional, and psychological aspects of your child's condition, as well as a nutritionist and physical therapist to address your child's food intake and exercise.

SUMMARY

Eating and feeding problems are a common source of concern for parents of young children. Parents of adolescents may have questions or concerns about whether their child has an eating disorder or is excessively preoccupied with their weight and shape. This chapter focused on eating habits in children, including "picky eating," and offered tips for improving child's eating habits and reception of new foods. The chapter also reviewed adolescent eating problems, such as anorexia and bulimia, and provided strategies for recognizing and dealing with a child's potential eating disorder.

WHERE TO FIND OUT MORE

Books

Ernsperger, L., Stegen-Hanson, T., & Gradin, T. (2005). *Finicky eaters: What to do when kids won't eat.* New York: Future Horizons, Inc.

Ernsperger, L., Stegen-Hanson, T., & Gradin, T. (2004). *Just take a bite: Easy, effective answers to food aversions and eating challenges.* New York: Ingram Pub Services.

Websites

American Academy of Pediatrics

Anorexia. http://www.healthychildren.org/English/health-issues/conditions/emotional-problems/pages/Anorexia.aspx

Bulimia: http://www.healthychildren.org/English/health-issues/conditions/emotional-problems/pages/Bulimia.aspx

Picky eating and related topics: http://www.healthychildren.org/english/search/pages/results.aspx?Type=Keyword&Keyword=picky+eating

Contemporary Pediatrics–Guide for Parents (2005). Strategies to reduce picky eating. http://contemporarypediatrics.modernmedicine.com/contpeds/data/articlestandard/contpeds/122005/151500/article.pdf.

National Eating Disorders Association. (2008). Learn basic terms and information on a variety of eating disorder topics. http://www.nationaleatingdisorders.org/information-resources/general-information.php.

CHAPTER 7

Hygiene Problems

Monica L. Stevens and Sheila M. Eyberg

Harris's parents are at their wit's end. Harris had mastered self-help skills before his third birthday, and now at age 4, he is "forgetting" and resisting reminders for tasks from washing up before dinner to brushing his teeth before bed. His parents work long days and have felt too exhausted to stick with any consistent routine, although they both know doing so would help. Harris sometimes brushes his teeth on his own, but his parents are so irritated with his seemingly intentional forgetting that they don't feel he deserves to be rewarded for doing what should be a routine behavior only when he feels like it.

"Hygiene" refers to cleanliness behaviors or habits that promote health (e.g., brushing teeth regularly, washing hands before eating, etc.). Expectations for good hygiene behaviors increase throughout development, although most basic hygiene behaviors are learned during the preschool years. Young children need lots of assistance with health behaviors like teeth-brushing, whereas older children are expected to manage basic self-help skills independently. Although adolescents are largely independent in managing personal hygiene, they face new challenges to maintaining good hygiene, such as practicing safe sex. Teaching positive hygiene behaviors and attitudes to preschoolers when they are first able to understand and perform them establishes a strong foundation for future health behaviors. The preschool years are also when children typically experience most behavior problems related to good hygiene. As with other behavior problems that arise early in development, dealing effectively with hygiene problems when they first arise is the best solution for future hygiene problems. This chapter outlines a number of strategies that work for teaching healthy hygiene practices from the beginning and for dealing with hygiene problems when they first arise. However, the basic principles for dealing with hygiene problems apply to older children and adolescents as well.

WHAT SHOULD I EXPECT FROM MY CHILD?

There is great individual variation in how children grow and learn, and it is important to remember that developmental expectations are *just that*—estimates of when a child is ready to learn new skills. Readiness to master new skills is determined by a number of factors, including the child's development of cognitive and motor skills. This means that you need to be flexible in setting expectations for your children.

Ages 9–12 Months

By the time children reach their first birthday, they have made great advances in their fine and gross motor skills, cognitive and emotional development, and communication skills. They can typically grasp small objects, such as child-sized cups and small food items, which means that this is a good time to begin shaping healthy eating habits in your children. Even though communication in the first year is largely nonverbal, children are learning to recognize language (e.g., "no" and their name), and often are speaking their first words. If your children are very young, it is important to talk about what you are doing in their presence, even though they cannot yet contribute to the conversation. Children also learn a great deal by observing and imitating their parents' behaviors. Begin teaching good health behaviors in your child's first year by modeling them, such as by covering your mouth when you cough or sneeze. Your child will notice these behaviors and imitate them.

Ages 1–2 Years

Between their first and second year, children are busy learning to walk and talk, which means their motor and communication skills are developing dramatically. By about 18 months, children are able to brush their teeth with water and a child-sized toothbrush with some help from parents. Children's communication has progressed to the point that they often point to objects of interest, say familiar words or names and, by about 2 years, begin to put together short sentences (e.g., "icky hands"). Because of children's advanced cognitive, motor, and communication skills, this is the ideal time for parents to label hygiene-related behaviors and objects to build a vocabulary for future routines.

Ages 2–3 Years

Between the ages of 2 and 3, children begin to eat more independently, and with their greater coordination of motor skills they can be expected to wash their hands before meals as well. They are now also ready to use small amounts of toothpaste with brushing, and this is the time to help your children establish a routine of brushing at least twice a day. With their increasing communication skills, children can now understand simple directions (even though they may not follow them) and can clearly communicate in short sentences.

Ages 3–5 Years

These are years of quickly growing independence. At meal time, preschoolers are now able to use utensils, and because of their improved language comprehension, are able to understand and demonstrate table manners. They are also capable of following daily bathing routines with supervision. However, it is not uncommon for children to resist day-to-day self-care activities during these years, making it especially important for parents to set clear expectations and maintain consistent routines to establish good hygiene habits early in development.

If you are concerned that your child is not meeting developmental milestones as expected, you should consult your family pediatrician. The National Center on Birth Defects and Developmental Disabilities provides comprehensive resources on developmental delay at http://www.cdc.gov/ncbddd/autism/actearly/.

HOW DO I MANAGE MY CHILD'S RESISTANCE TO GOOD HYGIENE HABITS?

Having accurate developmental expectations for your child's self-care is important. Yet, as every parent knows, even though children are *capable* of certain behaviors, they do not always do them! Patience and consistency are key when teaching your child proper hygiene. This process can be exhausting at first, but the investment of time and energy will have long-term benefits for both you and your children.

Provide Positive Reinforcement

The most powerful technique for changing the behavior of young children and adolescents is positive reinforcement. Positive reinforcement involves giving your child something pleasant or rewarding following a desired behavior, which then increases the frequency of that behavior in the future. Have you ever noticed that when you laugh at something your child has done, your child repeats that behavior? That's because smiling and laughter serve as positive reinforcement for children—to them, it means you are happy with what they have done. Laughter is not the only form of reinforcement, and finding effective and suitable rewards for your child is essential to making positive change. Because behavior change requires consistent positive reinforcement initially, an appropriate reward would not be something extravagant or expensive. Appropriate rewards include things like stickers, small treats, and not surprisingly, parents' positive attention! The types of rewards that motivate children vary, and you may need to try several options to find the best source of reinforcement for your child.

Once you have identified several appropriate rewards for the desired behavior, reward your children each time they exhibit that behavior. Consistency is very important, particularly for young children learning to do something new or different. But what about more complicated behaviors like those involved in toilet training? You can *shape* children's behavior by rewarding them each time they take steps toward performing that behavior. In potty training, for example, you should reward children first simply for telling you that they need to "go potty" regardless of whether they "make it" to the bathroom. The reward expresses your appreciation for your child's effort and increases the likelihood that your child will repeat that behavior. Once your child has mastered one step in the process (in this case, identifying the urge), you can then provide rewards for further steps toward the goal (e.g., sitting on the potty chair). It is important to remember that behavior change takes time, especially when your child has become accustomed to a particular way of doing things.

Create Behavior Charts

Behavior charts are an easy and effective way to reward young children for hygiene behaviors. For a preschooler, a behavior chart typically starts with just one or two very specific behaviors you would like your child to do routinely (e.g., "brushing my teeth in the morning," "washing my hands before dinner"). Once your child has mastered the first behaviors (i.e., does them every day without fuss), you can gradually add two or three more specific behaviors, one at a time. On the chart, list the behaviors on the left, with each one on a separate row. Across the top, mark the time points (e.g., each day of the week) when your child needs to complete the behavior. With older children, behavior charts can start with as many as five specific tasks, but you should keep the list no longer than seven tasks at a time (see http://www.freeprintablebehaviorcharts.com for sample charts that you can download at no cost).

When your preschooler performs a behavior listed on the chart, draw a star or use a sticker to indicate successful completion of that behavior on that day, so that your child sees the progress and is rewarded by the positive attention. It is especially important with preschoolers to praise the child enthusiastically for completing the task and for earning a star or sticker. With older children, charts are more effective if you add a tangible reward that your child can earn for getting a certain number of marks or stickers (*e.g.,* a trip to the amusement park with you for earning 30% of the possible stickers during the first week). The number of marks needed to earn a reward should start at a level the child can easily achieve. You can gradually increase the level each week or two.

SPECIFIC HYGIENE ROUTINES

Positive reinforcement and the use of behavior charts are general techniques that can be applied to many behaviors. When making any behavior change, the use of consistent reinforcement is essential. For young children, there are several common milestones related to hygiene that parents find challenging. For example, many children fight bath time, and you may find yourself struggling to get your child to bathe. You can use the tips described earlier to help manage this behavior, such as rewarding your child for getting in the bath tub or helping with the soap. Additionally, you can try some of these tricks:

- Make bath time fun by using this time to praise your child and play with him or her, using toys that are special, like waterproof books and bath crayons. This will help your child learn to think of bathing as pleasant and relaxing, and affords you the opportunity to spend one-on-one time with your child while taking care of a chore.
- For children who fear the drain, put them in the tub after it is full and take them out before you let the water drain.
- Be sure the water is warm, not hot. Children tolerate temperature differently, so pay attention to their reaction to the water so that you can be sure they are comfortable.

- Use bubbles! Most children enjoy bubble baths, and you can use the bubbles to show them how to wash their body.
- Model how to wash using toys (e.g., baby dolls, toy animals). Your child will likely want to help or even show you how to do it. This will give you a chance to praise your child for being a great bather!

Another important hygiene milestone is toilet training. Because toilet training is often the most difficult, we will discuss it in most detail (see Chapter 1 on toilet training for more information).

TOILET TRAINING AS AN ILLUSTRATIVE EXAMPLE

A common battle between children and parents is the one over toilet training. There is considerable variability in when children are ready to be toilet trained. The average child in the United States is trained between 24 and 36 months of age, and by 48 months (age 4) most children have been trained. Most parents and professionals find that focusing on the child's *readiness* to begin toilet training is more useful than considering a particular age.

To decide whether your child is ready to begin toilet training, consider whether your child (a) is physically capable of controlling the muscles needed to urinate and defecate (e.g., she or he goes several hours in between wetting a diaper), (b) is able to communicate the need to use the bathroom, and (c) has a desire to use the restroom. Once you have determined your child is ready, you should spend about a week regularly checking your child's diaper and commenting if it is dry, wet, or soiled. This procedure helps your child become more aware of the condition of his or her diaper and also helps you both become more aware of the schedule you will likely follow during toilet training.

The next step involves using the diaper only at nap time and during the night, when it would be especially difficult for your child to verbalize the need to use the bathroom. Although training pants can be convenient for you during this period, you may wish to transition your child right into regular underpants to help your child more quickly notice when he or she is wet or soiled. Wet or soiled underpants are typically quite unpleasant to children, which can motivate them to use the toilet.

Once your child can easily identify and verbalize the urge to urinate or defecate, you should gradually introduce your child to sitting on the toilet. It is not uncommon for children to be fearful of the toilet, and it may be useful to start with a potty seat. At every step, provide consistent praise for all your child's appropriate efforts toward using the toilet.

Your child will likely have accidents when learning to use the toilet. It is best to respond to these incidents calmly and engage your child in helping to clean up the mess. It is also important for you to seat your child on the toilet for a short amount of time after an accident, to give your child ample time to finish and to remind your child to sit on the toilet when he or she needs to use the bathroom. Occasional accidents are to be expected even after your child has been toilet trained, but persistent accidents may be cause for concern. If this is the case, consult a healthcare professional.

Teeth Brushing and Oral Health

You will care for your child's teeth until about 2 years of age. Between 12 months and 2 years, it is important to establish the routine of brushing twice a day. You can begin encouraging your child to brush independently at about 2 years old. The most important goal at this time is to make brushing a positive experience. You can (and need to) brush your child's teeth again after your child has finished to be sure they are clean. However, the most important goal at this time is to make brushing a positive experience for your child—more important than your child's skills in polishing every tooth.

To begin, show your child how to brush and plan on brushing right along side your child during this learning process. Doing this gives you a chance to be sure your child is using the right amount of toothpaste, brushing and rinsing for the right amount of time, and learning that tooth brushing can be fun.

Letting your child play an active role in planning for tooth brushing will increase the chances that your child will enjoy brushing. For example, you can allow your child to choose a favorite toothbrush and toothpaste. You can also make dental care fun by designating a song to hum or making silly faces while brushing and flossing.

When your child is learning to brush his or her own teeth, it is important to praise every effort and every new step in the learning process. Young children are still developing their fine motor skills, which means that your child's attempts at brushing will likely be far from perfect initially. Brace yourself for stray toothpaste and sloppy rinsing, and be extra supportive during this time so as to set a positive tone for brushing. Using a behavior chart will help maintain teeth brushing until your child is skilled at remembering to brush as well as the brushing itself. You may find it helpful to place the behavior chart right in the bathroom. You can add pictures of teeth or toothbrushes to help your child remember at first.

If you have tried these strategies and still face problems with routine brushing, study the situation to understand the cause. It may be that there is some kind of reinforcement your child is getting inadvertently for resisting regular brushing. For example, an 8-year-old might refuse to brush her teeth before bed because doing so means bedtime may be delayed for 15 extra minutes while her mother tries to coax her into brushing. Once you understand what is contributing to negative behavior, then you can change the situation. Perhaps in this example, the mother could change the child's bedtime to 20 minutes earlier until she is able to demonstrate consistent brushing for a certain number of days. At that point, the child could be rewarded for "remembering" with a later bedtime. With older children, it helps to remove privileges for disobeying routine hygiene behaviors, combined with praise or other reinforcement for correct hygiene behavior.

SUMMARY

Children vary in their development and mastery of self-care skills. Be sure to consider your child's physical and emotional readiness rather than age when introducing new hygiene routines. Consistent use of reinforcement is essential to implementing and maintaining behavior change. It is important to remember that children need reminders, and parents can pair verbal reminders with visual cues like behavior charts to help their children be successful. With the investment of time and patience, you can help your children become independent, healthy individuals!

WHERE TO FIND OUT MORE

Books

Pantley, E., (2007). *The no-cry potty training solution: Gentle ways to help your child say goodbye to diapers.* New York: McGraw-Hill.

Turner, K. (2007). *H is for hygiene.* St. Louis, MO: Trurngroup Technologies.

Manning, M. (1999). *Wash, scrub, brush.* London: Franklin Watts.

Websites

Free Printable Behavior Charts.com
   http://www.freeprintablebehaviorcharts.com/
KidsHealth
   http://kidshealth.org/
American Academy of Pediatrics
   http://www.aap.org/healthtopics/oralhealth.cfm
BabyCenter
   http://parentcenter.babycenter.com/

CHAPTER 8

Pain and Medical Procedures

Kathleen L. Lemanek and Michael Joseph

Your 5-year-old daughter Emma's routine pediatric check-up is coming up. You know this check-up will include all her pre-kindergarten immunizations. You feel a wave of anxiety, and decide the best plan is not to say anything to Emma and to ignore it yourself. The day arrives soon enough and your daughter asks, while eating breakfast, about the plans for the day. You feel a cold sweat rising from the base of your neck and stammer out the words, "We are going to your doctor dear." As she slowly looks up from her corn flakes, you can see her pupils dilate and she asks in a barely audible voice, "Will I have to get a shot?" You tell her that she will get her immunizations and how sorry you feel. You add, "It won't hurt as much as it did last time, and you really don't have to do anything you don't want to do." At the office, the doctor completes an interview and an examination. He steps out of the room stating, "Please wait. Susan will be in soon." Five minutes later Susan comes in, carrying a tray of syringes and needles with various amounts of fluid inside them. Emma starts to scream. Susan asks you to lie Emma down and says, "OK, here we go." Needle after needle, scream after scream, pleading after pleading, and then it is done. While sobbing, you help your daughter dress and say "See honey, that wasn't so bad." Neither of you believe it.

The ear nose and throat surgeon tells you that your 3-year-old son Jake's sleep study indicates he has sleep apnea and will need his tonsils out. You are not surprised. Before you have a chance to worry, you and Jake are scheduled for a presurgical visit to the hospital. Three days before the procedure you get a tour, watch a video, and have your questions answered in language you and Jake understand. You learn all the steps of the procedure in detail, what it might feel like, and what each of you are supposed to do. During the next 2 days, you and Jake talk about what you have learned and you answer his questions as best you can. You and Jake practice the breathing and relaxation exercises that you were given. On the day of the surgery, you remember to bring his favorite book and stuffed animal.

In the preoperative area, they put a cream on Jake's arm to numb the area for his IV, and he is given an oral medication to help him relax. While you are sitting with Jake, giving him a big hug, and talking to him about his day at preschool, the nurse places the IV after explaining each step of what she is going to do. As the anesthesiologist delivers the anesthesia, you hold Jake's hand and tell him how proud you are of him. After a nurse walks you back to the waiting area, it seems only a short time when you are told that Jake is headed to the recovery area. You meet him there and are present when his wakes.

WHAT IS PAIN?

To better understand how to help children through painful procedures, whether needle sticks or surgery, we need to start with a basic understanding of pain. We all have a basic understanding of pain because of our own experiences, but pain is quite complex. Pain is the perception of tissue damage. How much attention you pay to the pain, how aroused (upset) you are by the pain, what the pain means to you, how much control you have over it, how others (e.g., parents) have reacted to pain, the number and type of previous painful experiences, the age of the child, and cultural experiences all play a roll in pain perception. For example, the amount of attention children pay to a particular sensation, painful or otherwise, increases the intensity of that sensation. In addition, children's level of arousal directly impacts the intensity of pain, such that calm children will perceive less pain than those who are anxious or afraid.

HOW DO I HELP MY CHILD MANAGE PAIN?

Before the Procedure

Preparing your child before any procedure that may cause pain is the first and essential step to good pain management. "When" and "how" are the two main considerations when preparing your child for a painful procedure.

The *timing* of the preparation depends on both on your child's age and the perceived severity of the procedure. For young children, a short lead time is best. If your child is an infant, preparation does not need to begin until immediately before the procedure. Preschool children need slightly more planning. You want to provide your preschoolers enough time to inform them of what is going to happen, but not so much time that they worry and start to believe that it is going to be much worse than it really is. The greater the perceived risk of the procedure, the longer children should have to ask questions and manage their fears. For minor procedures, such as a blood draw or single injection, providing information the same day is often adequate. If the procedure is more intensive, and your child is age 6 or older, it is best to begin preparation 5–7 days in advance.

The *content* of the preparation also is very important. When preparing your child for a painful procedure, be sure to:

- Use language that your child will understand.
- Include specific information about what will happen during the procedure.
- Let your child know what to expect in terms of sensory experiences, such as taste, smells, and touch.

- Outline the expectations for your child.
- Provide your child with ways to cope.

Although it may seem counterintuitive, too much empathy, reassurance, apologies, and relinquishing control to children can increase their anxiety. Vague or veiled information also is counterproductive. For example, Emma's mother used language that Emma did not understand, tried to minimize the sensory information, and gave Emma the control to say she did not want any shots even though the immunizations were essential for her to start school. In addition, the medical assistant, Susan, was very unclear about the procedures. It would have been better for Susan to say, "You will feel cold when I clean your skin. After that it is very important you don't move. You may feel a pinch with each shot." In contrast, Jake's mother and hospital did an excellent job of providing him with positive coping skills to prepare him for his surgical procedure. Coaching in distraction and relaxation techniques is beneficial for both children and parents. Table 8.1 provides a list of techniques that can be practiced well before the procedure, so that children and parents can use them when needed.

When preparing your children for an upcoming medical procedure, be sure to take into account their physical comfort and discomfort. Needle sticks are an integral part of almost any medical procedure and can be very traumatic to all involved. However, topical anesthetic cream may help greatly. Either lidocaine cream (available over the counter), or prilocaine and lidocaine combination cream (available by prescription) can be effective in reducing the pain of needle sticks. These medications are easy to apply, but they take 30–60 minutes for adequate effectiveness. Simply place a dollop of cream on uncleaned skin over the site of the intended needle stick and cover with a plastic dressing. These dressings usually come with the topical cream but, if not, clear food-grade plastic wrap works well.

In addition to topical anesthetic creams, the position of children during a medical procedure greatly affects their anxiety level and, therefore, their pain. Lying on your back is a position of submission and may increase anxiety. Many procedures can be done with children sitting on parents' laps, either facing forward or facing the parent, and parents providing a "big hug." In this position, children's arms and legs can be accessible for injections or IV starts, and parents are able to distract them (e.g., count out loud) and to coach them to breath.

In addition to preparing your child, you should prepare yourself as well. Have a conversation with your child's healthcare provider in advance of the procedure. It is important to know what the expectations are for you. Where will the procedure take place? What time should you be there? When do you have to be apart from your child? When can you and your child be together? Following are some questions that may not be addressed by your child's healthcare provider, so we recommend that you specifically ask:

- Do you routinely use topical anesthesia? If not, are you adverse to its use?
- What is available to keep my child distracted during the procedure?
- Can my child bring a favorite toy and book to the procedure?
- Can my child be in a secure sitting position rather than lying down?
- If anesthesia is necessary, can I be present at the time of induction?

TABLE 8.1. Recommended comforting techniques by child age

Technique	Age-level examples
TOUCH — soothing and provides physical distraction	**Infant** – Pat, rock, or let suck on pacifier **Toddler** – Rock, stroke, use attachment object **Preschooler** – Pat, stroke, give a bath **School-age** – Stroke arms, back, face, or brush hair in continuous motion **Adolescent** – Massage, ice packs/heating pads (depends on procedure)
DISTRACTION — shifts attention to more pleasant objects or activities	**Infant** – Show squeaky, bright, or movable toy/object, play lullaby music **Toddler** – Use puppet play, read favorite or new book, play favorite music tape or DVD **Preschooler** – Count out loud, play "I Spy" games, talk about favorite story/movie **School-age** – Play electronic game, play name games, talk about favorite hobby or activity **Adolescent** – Play electronic game, listen to CD player or iPod, play guessing game
BREATHING — increases oxygen and refocuses attention using slow, steady breaths	**Infant** – Blow bubbles to touch or see them **Toddler** – Blow bubbles, pinwheels, or party blowers **Preschooler** – Blow bubbles or pinwheels **School-age** – Breathe in, hold, exhale for counts of 2–3; exhale party blower or pinwheel **Adolescent** – Breathe in, hold, exhale for counts of 4
RELAXATION — increases feelings of comfort and releases tension by imagining pleasant experiences or tensing and relaxing muscles	**School-age** – Talk about feeling heavy, limp, and warm with images of Raggedy Ann or pleasant, relaxed places **Adolescent** – Tense/release major muscle groups; images of pleasant, relaxed places

During the Procedure

Cognitive behavioral therapy (CBT) is a "well-established treatment" for medical procedure-related pain in children and adolescents. CBT is a group of techniques designed to change faulty thinking patterns, attitudes, attributions, and behaviors. CBT has been used to decrease procedure-related pain and distress in children and adolescents, by using the following techniques: distraction, relaxation, imagery, breathing exercises, preparation, hypnosis, modeling, and coaching. Table 8.1 provides age-related examples of these strategies. It is essential that you, the medical staff, or a psychologist actively coach your child to use the strategies during the actual medical procedure. Reinforcement or some type of reward or incentive for using these coping strategies, or for lying still, also is important following the medical procedure.

Active Coaching

Active coaching involves several steps before, during, and after the medical procedure. *Before the procedure*, give your child information about the procedure itself and also instruct your child in the different coping strategies. The specific strategies you will use will depend on the age of your child, the medical procedure, and your child's temperament. Either you or the clinician should demonstrate and model the procedure for your child. Following this demonstration, have your child practice the strategy and reward her for practicing and learning it. *During the procedure*, either you or the clinician should prompt your child to use the strategy. You can also continue to demonstrate the strategy during the procedure. For example, in Emma's case, her mother should have informed her about the timing of her injections, what she was expected to do, and instructed her to practice deep breathing, as she has a tendency to scream or hold her breath. During her procedure, both Emma and her mother would have benefitted from practicing deep breathing. Jake, on the other hand, does better with his mother using his I-Spy book for distraction. He is younger and not able to master more complex coping strategies like deep breathing.

Distraction Techniques

Anything that shifts children's attention away from the procedure can decrease their perception of pain. Some research indicates that children under the age of 6 have problems learning the skills involved in progressive muscle relaxation, imagery, and deep breathing. Distraction is the technique most used for decreasing procedure-related distress in such young children. Overt forms of distraction, such as reading a picture book or watching TV may be beneficial in younger children versus more covert forms (such as mental imagery), which can be used in older children, especially adolescents. You can help to distract your child or young adult during painful medical procedures by engaging in "non–procedure-related talk" (i.e.,, talking about something *other than* the procedure the child is going through) or by using humor.

Imagery

Imagery is a specific cognitive technique that teaches the child to cope with the distress of the procedure by imagining a pleasant experience, such as a calm day at the beach or in the woods. Children also can be taught to use positive coping statements during the procedure (e.g., "I can do this"). However, it is important that these coping statements be developed in advance and placed on cards to have on hand during the procedure. Here is an example of a brief visual imagery script that can be used during a medical procedure to distract and relax your child. You may even find it helpful yourself:

> Sit comfortably or lie down, with your eyes closed or open. Take a deep breathe in. Then let it out slowly. Breathe in and out, not too fast or too slow. With each breath, you feel

more and more relaxed and calm. Picture yourself standing on a rainbow high in the sky. You feel a cool breeze all around you. See the color red under your feet. Say the word red to yourself and then picture a delicious apple. As you take a step down, you are now on the color orange. Picture a bright organ sunset in the sky. As you step down think yellow. Take a slow breath as the sunlight falls on your face. You are becoming calmer as you walk down the rainbow. Now step to green, feeling cool green grass between your toes. Your next step is blue. Think blue and hear cool blue water gurgling around you. Take your next step, think violet, and picture rich violet flowers growing around you. You are completely relaxed and calm. Take a slow breath. You can picture the rainbow whenever you want.
(Adapted from *Ready, Set, R.E.L.A.X.* by Allen and Klein, 1996)

Parental Coaching

You can benefit from coaching on how to handle not only your child's medical distress, but your own feelings as well. Children's distress is directly related to parents' anxiety and fear. These same techniques of relaxation, imagery, and breathing can help you relax and remain calm. A calm demeanor will allow you to coach and model relaxation for your child. The importance of a calm parent being present at the time of the procedure cannot be underestimated.

After the Procedure

The procedure is over, but it is time to prepare for the next one since there will be another shot, blood draw, stitches, or even possibly surgery. Changing the experience from one of punishment to one of achievement is important for managing and coping with future procedures. Simple praise such as "I am so proud of you" is effective but targeted praise such as "I am so proud of you for holding still, you are so brave" both increases children's confidence and reinforces their use of coping skills. Rewards should be linked to coping behaviors, and need not be material or monetary in nature to be effective. For example, extra time with a parent or special privileges can be more reinforcing than a toy that only lasts for 5 minutes out of the box. "You did such a great job with your breathing. Why don't you and mommy go home and work on that puzzle you wanted to put together?" Last, it is important not to make false promises, such as "I will never let this happen to you again!" Your children will eventually lose trust in you if you make these kinds of statements.

SUMMARY

The bottom line is that there are many things that you can do to reduce your child's suffering before, during, and after medical procedures. Preparation, coaching in coping behaviors, proper positioning, topical anesthetics, and positive reinforcement are critical elements for decreasing emotional upset and pain in children undergoing medical procedures. When these relatively simple tools are employed in a calm and timely fashion, everyone benefits. Parents can, therefore, be instrumental in ensuring that best practice guidelines to reduce procedure-related pain are developed and implemented for their children.

WHERE TO FIND OUT MORE

Books

Allen, J.S., & Klein, R.J. (1996). *Ready, set, relax. A research-based program for relaxation, learning, and self-esteem for children.* Watertown, WI: Inner Coaching.

Culbert, T., & Kajander, R. (2007). *Be the boss of your pain: Self-care for kids.* Minneapolis, MN: Free Spirit Publishing.

Kuttner, L. (1996). *A child in pain. How to help. What to do.* Vancouver, BC: Hartley & Marks Publishers.

Zeltzer, L., & Schlank, C.B. (2005). *Conquering your child's chronic pain. A pediatrician's guide for reclaiming a normal childhood.* New York: Harper Collins Pub., Inc.

Websites

American Academy of Pain Management
    http://www.aapainmanage.org
American Pain Society
    http://www.ampainsoc.org
Beth Israel Medical Center
    http://www.stoppain.org
Centre for Pediatric Pain Research
    http://pediatricpain.ca/
Pediatric Pain Sourcebook
    http://www.painsourcebook.ca

CHAPTER 9

Medical Adherence

Ric G. Steele and Timothy D. Nelson

Phil and Violet just learned that their 4-year-old son Zach has asthma. His treatment regimen includes oral medication and a steroid inhaler, as well as regular use of a peak flow meter to evaluate how well air moves out of his lungs. Zach's parents worry about what the diagnosis means for their son, and about keeping him well. To make matters worse, Zach throws a fit every time either of his parents tries to administer the pills, the inhaler, or test his peak air flow. His parents usually win these battles, but Violet is concerned that the resulting fights and tension are having a negative effect on her relationship with her son.

Cammy's 8-year-old daughter Grace has taken oral antibiotics for strep throat for the past week. Her doctor said to stay on the medication for a full 2 weeks, but Grace says her throat feels fine, and her fever broke several days ago. Grace also says that the medicine makes her stomach hurt, especially in the mornings before school. Cammy feels unsure of whether to discontinue the medication or to follow through with the doctor's orders. She doesn't like the thought of her daughter taking medicines for longer than needed, but the doctor insisted that Grace finish the whole prescription.

In healthcare, we define *adherence* as the degree to which a person's health-related behavior coincides with medical or health advice. Medical adherence might include taking medications, following dietary recommendations, engaging in preventative behaviors like exercise, or obtaining recommended services (e.g., eyeglasses or physical therapy). Conversely, medical *nonadherence* refers to behavior that does *not* align with prescribed behaviors. This might include taking more or less medication than prescribed, not following the prescribed medication schedule, failing to engage in prescribed behaviors, or not following through in getting recommended services. Simply put, adherence refers to how closely one "follows the doctor's orders."

Considerable research and clinical work with children and adolescents has focused on adherence issues. Many people don't realize that rates of adherence to medical advice range from 18% to 95%, with most estimates between 50% and 66%. This means that, depending on the medical condition, between one-half and one-third of patients do not adequately follow through on the recommendations given by their healthcare providers.

WHY IS IT IMPORTANT FOR MY CHILD TO FOLLOW DOCTOR'S ORDERS?

The consequences of nonadherence or inadequate adherence vary widely across situations and circumstances. At the individual level, nonadherence to medical treatment can translate into wasted healthcare dollars, increased suffering (due to disease progression), lost days of work productivity, lost school days, and increased risk of contagion. Surprisingly, individual nonadherence can also lead to *over-prescription* of medications. For example, healthcare providers may prescribe stronger medications or higher doses to a person who does not seem to recover well, when, in fact, the poor outcome resulted from non- or incomplete adherence rather than drug failure. At the community level, nonadherence has been linked to increased healthcare costs, increased costs of drug research and development (because of nonadherence during drug testing), decreased cost-efficacy of healthcare, and increased risk of resistant bacterial strains (i.e., bacterial infections that do not respond to some antibiotics; see, for example, http://www.cdc.gov/Features/MRSAInfections/).

WHAT MAKES ADHERENCE DIFFICULT?

Families routinely face a number of issues that may make adherence to their child's prescribed medical regimen difficult. Just as adherence is not an all-or-nothing proposition (that is, there are degrees of adherence), it is also rarely determined by a single factor. Rather, many factors may influence the degree to which families and individuals adhere to medical recommendations. These factors include the complexity of the medical regimen, misunderstanding of the prescription, behavioral or emotional issues (such as child noncompliance, or difficulty with pill-swallowing), peer-related factors (such as the perceived stigma associated with the medical regimen), and instrumental barriers (such as the financial cost). Several of these issues deserve special attention.

Complexity of the Medical Regimen

Most research suggests that parents have more difficulty correctly following complicated prescriptions, particularly when families face a number of life stresses or complicated personal schedules. For any medication, a range of blood concentrations (i.e., plasma levels) exists within which the drug will have a maximum safe effect. To ensure the balance of efficacy and safety, prescriptions are written with a range of complexities for how and when to take the medication. For example, some medications work well when taken once daily. Others require three doses per day, or involve other special instructions (e.g., take on an empty stomach or take with food). While the complexity of the prescription increases the chances of a favorable outcome and decreases negative side effects, it also *decreases* the likelihood of taking the medication *as prescribed*. This may happen because the parent or patient misunderstands the prescription or because of scheduling problems (e.g., having to take medications while at school or away from home). It is important that parents (or adolescents who are responsible for their own dosing) make sure that they fully understand both *what* the prescription requires of them, *why* it is required, and *how* they are to go about following the prescription.

Behavioral Issues

Depending on the child's age, a range of behavioral issues may play a role in families' struggles to maintain good adherence. Zach's parents apparently understand both what they should do and how to complete their son's treatment regimen. However, their struggle with Zack's opposition to the treatment represents a significant issue that could undermine their adherence and, ultimately, Zach's health. Often, nonadherence to medical treatments occurs against a backdrop of child noncompliance with other parental directives (see Chapter 23). Noncompliance with health behaviors should be addressed in much the same way as noncompliance with other caregiver directions (e.g., by using time-outs, removing privileges, etc.). This can present a challenge for parents of children struggling with significant illnesses, and support from health or mental health professionals will sometimes help ensure that the child's behavior does not compromise his or her physical health.

In addition to oppositional behavior, many children also have difficulty with the mechanics of completing their prescribed medical regimen (e.g., difficulty swallowing pills or correctly using inhalers). Sometimes these mechanical difficulties result in oppositional behavior, avoidance, or anxiety and, ultimately, nonadherence. Thus, making sure that your child can perform the tasks central to his or her medical regimen is an essential part of successful adherence, and may result in fewer battles like those just described.

Emotional Problems

Adherence can also suffer because of children's anxiety and/or feelings of depression. Children with chronic or very serious medical conditions may become discouraged at the prospect of long-term medication use, or may feel hopeless about their health. Such feelings may give rise to an "It's just not worth it . . . " mentality. Adolescents, in particular, may have a greater likelihood of noncompliance with their medications or treatments, given their increased risk for depression, their increased capacity for risk-taking behaviors, and their increasing need for independence.

Peer-related Issues

Children and adolescents who must adhere to medical regimens in public places (e.g., at school) sometimes report stigma related to a treatment, the condition that necessitates the treatment, or an outcome associated with the treatment. For example, concerns such as "I do not want other people to notice me taking the medicine" and "I don't like what the medication does to my appearance" can be associated with lower adherence among adolescents. Similarly, children with diabetes who must check blood sugar levels or children who must take regular preventative treatments for asthma may attempt to "normalize" their appearance by avoiding these tasks. In some cases, you can work with your child's healthcare provider to arrange your child's medication schedules so that he or she does not have to perform the health behavior in public. In other cases, the appropriate action may be to help your child or adolescent overcome the anxiety associated with performing the medical regimen in relatively public places or in front of peers. It is important to remember that children and adolescents do not always have an adult perspective on the relevant issues. Considering how the illness or the treatment might seem from the child's perspective may help you understand why adherence can be challenging.

Volitional Nonadherence

Sometimes children or families make conscious decisions to alter their medication dosing schedules. This may occur as a means of avoiding conflict (i.e., to avoid a fight with a child), as a means of protecting privacy or keeping a normal appearance, as a means of stretching healthcare dollars, or as a means of reducing unwanted side effects of the medication. For example, Grace indicated that her antibiotic caused stomach upset, prompting her mother to consider discontinuing the medication. We refer to such choices as *volitional nonadherence*. While good intentions underlie the decision to change dosing schedule, the consequences of these actions can prove very harmful. Parents who find themselves wanting to change their child's medical regimen or those who suspect that their adolescent may be avoiding their recommended health behaviors (e.g., checking blood sugar less frequently than recommended) should contact their healthcare provider to talk about whether alternative treatments are available. If not, your healthcare provider may be able to recommend strategies to make the necessary health behavior easier to live with.

HOW CAN I IMPROVE MY CHILD'S ADHERENCE?

A number of steps can help improve a child's adherence to a medical plan. In general, interventions fall into one of four broad categories: (1) educational, (2) organizational, (3) behavioral, and (4) problem-solving interventions. The most effective strategy, or combination of strategies, depends on the nature of your child's medical condition, the complexity of the treatment plan, and your child's age or developmental level. Promoting good adherence usually requires ongoing monitoring and flexibility to adapt as your child's needs change.

Educational Interventions

Educational interventions are the most fundamental methods of improving adherence. Simply put, the better you understand the reasons for your child's medical regimens, the more likely you are to follow through with them. Information can be provided by physicians, nurses, pediatric psychologists, or other healthcare professionals and can be delivered in a variety of forms, including handouts, videos, website links, or discussions with your family. This information can be tremendously beneficial in helping your family to understand why you need to follow a specific regimen. Cammy's reluctance to complete Grace's full course of antibiotics may have resulted from incomplete understanding of how the medication works, or from not understanding the consequences of failing to take the full supply as prescribed. Further, ongoing communication can help you and your child's healthcare provider minimize unpleasant side effects, such as the stomach upset reported by Cammy.

Organizational/Structural Interventions

Organizational strategies for promoting adherence help families make treatment components fit into their everyday routines, and reduce adherence problems related to keeping track of medicines or other treatment requirements. For example, pillboxes organize medications by time of day, or day of the week; calendars can help coordinate multi-part treatment plans or treatments that do not come up every day; and reminder notes (for example, on the bathroom mirror or in a lunchbox) and electronic medicine bottle caps (with timers) can remind families of specific dosing times. These organizational strategies are especially important with complex regimens, such as those with many parts that must be carried out in a particular sequence on a regular schedule.

However, in addition to these organizational methods, your family should talk with your healthcare providers about any special challenges you encounter. Perhaps there is an alternative medication available that is easier to use. For example, sometimes a medication that must be given three times a day can be replaced by an equally effective medication that only has to be given twice a day. When faced with decisions about which of two similar medications to use, healthcare providers and parents should consider the complexity of the dosing schedule in their decision making. Be sure to talk with your child's healthcare provider if you feel concerned about a particularly complex medicine or regimen—a simpler prescription may be available.

Behavioral Interventions

Behavioral interventions apply basic learning principles to encourage adherence and reduce oppositional behaviors that come along with treatments that seem unpleasant to the child. Positive reinforcement techniques (that is, giving small rewards or praise for "good behavior") encourage adherence by teaching the child that "good things happen when I follow my parents' directions." Such interventions can also help the family make the necessary medical regimen more fun for the child. For example, Zach's parents might reserve a special DVD for him to watch *only* when he uses his peak flow meter without complaining.

One common example of a positive reinforcement intervention involves the "point system" or "token economy," in which the child earns rewards for adherence. For example, Zach might earn tokens or chips each time he cooperates with his parents by taking his pills or using his inhaler. The tokens could be exchanged later in the day or week for a special privilege. The parents' expectations, the rewards chosen for adherence, and schedules of reinforcement (that is, how often rewards are given), should match the developmental level of the child. Young children will require more frequent rewards to encourage positive behaviors. Over time, expectations can gradually increase, so that a higher level of adherence is necessary to earn a reward. As with any behavioral reward system, the key involves finding rewards that will motivate your child and adjusting rewards as needed to maintain enthusiasm.

Other behavioral strategies focus on teaching the mechanics of good adherence. For example, younger children may have difficulty correctly using an asthma inhaler or correctly reading and coding their blood sugar monitor. Similarly, children transitioning from liquid to solid-form medications frequently have trouble swallowing pills or capsules. Failure to perform these behaviors correctly can negatively impact adherence and child health, and can create unnecessary frustration among all family members. A number of online resources offer help for parents and practitioners to teach children to take their medications or perform necessary health behaviors (a list of recommended websites can be found in *Where to Find Out More*, at the end of this chapter).

Problem-Solving Interventions

Problem-solving interventions help families identify and overcome specific challenges or barriers related to adherence. As with many interventions, these efforts may involve the family, with both you and your child learning creative ways to work around obstacles to adherence. Problem-solving activities can focus on issues that have already come up or on developing skills to manage future issues. Rather than merely telling families what to do, healthcare providers can teach children and parents a process for identifying challenges, generating ideas to address them, and implementing plans to maintain high adherence even under difficult circumstances. Such interventions can prove especially helpful for children with chronic illnesses who repeatedly face obstacles to ideal adherence due to intensive treatment demands or a variety of life stresses.

DEVELOPMENTAL CONSIDERATIONS

Regardless of the intervention chosen, tailoring these efforts to the developmental level of the child or adolescent is critical for success. What works for a young child may not work for an older child or adolescent and vice versa. This is especially true when choosing rewards for adherence and when developing expectations about the child's responsibility for adherence. You and your family's healthcare providers should continually evaluate your expectations and interventions to ensure that they are appropriately matched to your child's developmental level.

One of the most difficult issues for parents with regard to medical adherence is deciding when and how to transition the responsibility for a treatment regimen from the parent to the child. While parental involvement may continue throughout adolescence, transitioning to greater child independence can be advantageous *when developmentally appropriate*. There is no recommended cutoff age for determining the optimal timing of such transitions. The gradual shift to increased child responsibility should occur within the broader context of the child or adolescent taking on responsibility in other areas (e.g., academics, chores).

Adolescence is often an appropriate time for increasing these responsibilities, but teens differ considerably on maturity and readiness. If you are the parent of an adolescent, it is important that you closely monitor your teen's handling of new responsibilities and look for opportunities to promote independence whenever possible. This may require some trial-and-error in determining the amount of responsibility that your adolescent can accept. If questions arise, consult a healthcare professional familiar with adherence issues to obtain recommendations about responsibilities and transitions from parent to child responsibility.

WHEN TO SEEK PROFESSIONAL HELP

Most of the time, parents can make the necessary modifications to routines or contingencies to ensure that their children maintain good adherence to health behaviors. However, if your family is still experiencing problems, we encourage you to talk to your healthcare provider to determine whether a referral to a mental health professional seems appropriate. A referral to a mental health professional is particularly important if adherence issues are causing relationship problems between you and your spouse or partner, or you and your child. A mental health professional can also be helpful if your child or adolescent begins showing symptoms of depression or withdrawal (see the topic triggering the behavior), anxiety (see Chapters 26, 29, 30 or 31), peer victimization (see Chapter 40), or oppositional behavior (see Chapter 23). In addition, you may wish to consult with your healthcare provider about whether alternative dosing schedules (e.g., twice a day instead of three times a day) or alternative medication delivery systems (e.g., insulin pumps instead of injections) seem appropriate.

SUMMARY

Although necessary for ensuring optimal health, adherence to medical regimens can present challenges for many families. A number of issues may prevent a family from maintaining good adherence, including child noncompliance or emotional problems, pressure to appear "normal," misunderstanding of healthcare provider instructions, and organizational/structural problems. Fortunately, a number of effective intervention strategies exist to help caregivers address these problems. The following list summarizes our recommendations:

- *Communicate with your child's healthcare provider.*   Keep asking questions until you fully understand the recommended medical regimen.
- *Consider whether a medication or regimen schedule will pose problems for your family.*   Your prescriber may have simpler alternative treatments, or may recommend organizational interventions to help you overcome these challenges.
- *Develop a routine.*   Health behaviors that are part of the family's normal day are more likely to be completed. Consider using reminder notes for new health behaviors.
- *Make the health behavior as fun as possible for your child.*   Special rewards for a job well done will help your child make the most of a difficult situation.

- *Make sure your child is capable of doing what is being asked.* Training videos and online resources are available for most medial regimens.
- *Keep an eye out for emotional or behavioral problems that may impact your child's health.* Consult a mental health professional if symptoms begin to impact the child's health or relationships.
- *Think outside of the box.* Creative problem-solving strategies that get input from all family members can produce outstanding results.

WHERE TO FIND OUT MORE

Books

Rapoff, M.A. (2010). *Adherence to pediatric medical regimens* (2nd edition). New York: Springer.

Websites

Pediatric Oncology Resource Center
  http://www.acor.org/ped-onc/treatment/Pills/pills.html (for help with pill swallowing)
American Diabetes Association
  http://www.diabetes.org/living-with-diabetes/parents-and-kids/
Mayo Clinic
  http://www.mayoclinic.com/health/asthma-inhalers/HQ01081 (for help with inhaler use)

CHAPTER 10

Helping Children Cope with a Visit to the Dentist

Keith D. Allen and Shelley J. Hosterman

Tim, a 3-year-old boy, arrives for his first dental visit. He sits next to his mother while she reads a magazine. When the dentist enters the waiting room, Tim whines and hides behind his mom. He refuses to take the dentist's hand or walk to the exam room, and his mother must eventually carry Tim to the exam area. The dentist attempts to engage Tim in playful banter, with no success. Instead, Tim pleads desperately with his mother, who reassures him that everything will be okay. The dentist finally suggests that Tim's mother leave and then resorts to gentle but firm commands for Tim to lie back in the chair and open his mouth. Tim screams, kicks, and later vomits when the dentist places a finger in his mouth attempting to exam his teeth. Tim's mother feels mortified at the intensity of Tim's thrashing and screaming, and later learns that the dentist restrained Tim to complete the exam.

Kelsey, a 4-year-old girl, arrives for her first dental exam. Racing into the waiting room ahead of her mother, Kelsey heads immediately to the large playhouse she enjoyed during her "getting to know you visit" last week. As the dentist arrives, Kelsey plays busily at the Lego table in the middle of the room. She jumps up, takes the hands of the dentist and her mother, and asks if they can make the chair move up and down like they did last week. The dentist praises Kelsey each step of the way and lets her choose a DVD to watch during the exam. The dentist easily looks around in Kelsey's mouth, conducts an exam, and cleans her teeth. Her mother seems pleased and wonders if the dentist could manage her husband that well.

Perhaps the biggest surprise is not so much Tim's dramatic emotional reaction to his first dental visit, as the fact that more children don't respond exactly the same way.

Despite the largely painless nature of pediatric dentistry today, one in four children becomes so distressed and/or disruptive as to require special management procedures. Given the nature of dental exams, it should come as no surprise that some children find a trip to the dentist a traumatic event.

WHY DO CHILDREN FEAR THE DENTIST?

To understand why Tim reacted so strongly during his visit to the dentist, it helps to consider what children are typically afraid of. The most common triggers of fear for young children ages 2 to 5 include loss of emotional support, loud noises, separation from parents, exposure to strangers, novel stimuli, and masks. Now consider that during a typical visit to the dentist, a child must lie on his back, open his mouth, and allow an unfamiliar adult wearing a mask and gloves to insert multiple foreign instruments into his mouth; instruments that make unusual noises, create unfamiliar sensations, and sometimes inflict discomfort or even pain. Given these types of experiences common to many dental visits, it should prove no surprise that some children feel fearful, anxious, or become disruptive. Furthermore, the likelihood of disruptive problem behaviors correlates strongly with age. Younger, preschool-aged children pose more challenges than do school-aged children.

In addition to the problems presented by the presence of many fear triggers, young children do not yet possess the reason and logic necessary to understand that caring for teeth today brings significant benefits later in life. Indeed, children and adolescents regularly choose immediate pleasures over delayed ones. Even adults struggle to tolerate minor discomfort now for improved health later, despite knowing the importance of, for example, flossing, exercising, and eating better. Why expect more from children?

Consider also that parents often display anxiety about their own trips to the dentist. Think about your last visit and how you felt and what you might have said in the presence of your children. Did you make any comments about not wanting to go? Or, did you wonder aloud if it would hurt? Sometimes parents unintentionally convey that fear, anxiety, pain, and avoidance are to be expected at the dentist.

Finally, despite great strides toward eliminating discomfort, dental care can at times involve pain. Shots can hurt, especially in the gums and roof of the mouth where tightly packed tissues have many nerve endings. Even a general cleaning can be uncomfortable, and the seemingly harmless act of spraying water into one's mouth can elicit an unpleasant gag reflex in some children. And, sadly, dentists sometimes can exacerbate an already unpleasant experience by resorting to threats, coercion, and restraint to control behavior.

Thus, within the context of a visit to the dentist, children encounter potentially unpleasant, fearful, and painful stimuli without the ability to appreciate the benefit of good dental care. Predictably, unprepared children will likely attempt to escape or avoid the experience. Tim's actions make sense in that context. If screaming and flailing make the dentist stop, even briefly, then who can blame him?

So, what's a parent to do?

HOW CAN I HELP EASE MY CHILD'S FEAR OF THE DENTIST?

The Five E model described in the sections that follow can help you reduce your child's fear of the dentist.

Expectations: Build Positive Ones

We can expect children to respond better to visits to the dentist when they have preparation that leads to positive expectations about the visit. You can create positive expectations in several ways.

First, it is important to model teeth-brushing and flossing as fun and productive tasks, rather than chores. For example, you might brush and floss in front of your children while saying, "I love to brush my teeth and floss; it makes my mouth feel so clean."

Second, use enthusiastic, labeled praise and rewards to encourage and support your child's attempts at imitation. *Labeled praise* describes specific desired actions such as, "Oh look, you are brushing your teeth like such a big girl. The dentist (or 'tooth doctor') is going to be so impressed!" Children also respond well to public posting of feedback about their performance in the form of stickers, prizes, or even their own photographs.

Third, build positive expectations by avoiding threats that associate dental experiences with fear, pain, or unpleasantness. For example, avoid statements such as, "The dentist isn't going to like that," or threats of the sort, "If you don't brush, your teeth will get cavities and the dentist will have to pull them out."

Finally, be sure to speak positively about your own visits to the dentist. This includes talking optimistically about your own upcoming appointments, (e.g., "I get to go to the dentist today, and I feel happy about getting my teeth cleaned"), as well as reflecting positively on recent dental visits (e.g., "My teeth feel so clean, and I got a new toothbrush and a cool little tube of toothpaste!").

Experiences: Arrange Early Good Ones

One of the best ways to reduce the potential for trauma at the dentist involves creating positive early experiences. Children who show up for the first time at the dentist and must undergo extensive procedures will be more likely to find the experience unpleasant and stressful. Furthermore, children who have had negative initial experiences have a greater risk for emotional distress and disruptive behavior problems at future visits. Instead, you can help create positive early experiences for your children by arranging for a fun, exploratory visit to the dentist before any dental work becomes necessary.

A good first visit includes opportunities for your child to engage in fun activities in the waiting room and to explore the treatment rooms. It will be more enjoyable for your child if the adults involved (you, the dentist, the dental assistant, etc.) empower your child to make choices. For example, a young child might explore the treatment room, taking turns with his mother riding up and down in the chair and perhaps even operating the chair. The visit might also include squirting the water, switching the lights off and on, or looking at his teeth in a mirror. Since evidence suggests that young children may find masks and loss of support (i.e., lying back in the chair) as potentially threatening, a relaxed first visit could offer gentle exposure to these experiences in a nonthreatening way.

For example, the child might be offered the chance to hold a mask in her hand and put it on her parent or to watch her parent lie back in the chair. At the end of the visit, offering the child an opportunity to select a favorite toothbrush or tube of paste and choose a sticker or trinket from a prize chest can help make the first visit a rewarding experience.

These types of visits also allow children to become familiar with the dentist and staff and to associate them with positive experiences. This requires a dentist and staff who appreciate the importance of a visit free from demands and required dental procedures. The dentist and clinic staff can strengthen these positive associations by following the child throughout the visit and acting as the person who permits each activity, offers choices, and delivers prizes.

For many children with developmental disabilities, creating positive early experiences can prove particularly important. Unfamiliar stimuli can cause fear and distress in developmentally disabled children. Intense and unfamiliar sensory experiences, like those experienced at the dentist, can heighten this fear and anxiety. As a result, some children may require more gradual exposure, sometimes warranting more than one "getting to know you" visit to build familiarity with staff before attempting an exam or treatment.

Effective Models: Provide One

Children from ages 3 to13 can benefit from watching peers show the calm, coping behaviors desired while undergoing dental treatment. Peer models need not appear calm the entire time, as long as they model "learning to cope." Studies have repeatedly shown better coping by children who had an opportunity to observe peers or older siblings demonstrating "how it's done." Some dentists accomplish this through an "open bay" concept, in which children entering the treatment area readily see peers participating in dental exams. Other dentists schedule visits for entire preschool classes, where children can not only explore the environment, but also observe peer models who *volunteer* to sit in the chair, lie back, and allow the dentist to look in their mouths.

Expert Provider: Choose One

It seems obvious that selecting the right provider will prove paramount to building positive expectations and experiences. Parents must first find a dentist who is experienced with children. Pediatric dentists (called *pedodontists*) have at least 2 years of additional, specialized training in work with infants, children, teens, and children with special needs. The American Academy of Pediatric Dentistry (AAPD) website at www.aapd.org provides a list of qualified pediatric dentists. However, training alone does not necessarily assure that the dentist will understand the importance of creating positive initial experiences for young patients. Thus, you should search for a dentist willing to plan individual or group visits solely for this purpose.

It can be helpful to assemble a list of screening questions to aid you in choosing a dentist. Important questions might include:

• Can my child come for a pre-appointment visit?
• What would happen during the visit?

- What policies do you have regarding parental presence in the treatment room; permitted, encouraged, or discouraged?
- What strategies do you use to make dental visits pleasant for children?
- How do you handle children who feel anxious or fearful?

Ideally, you will find a dentist who relies on positive strategies for managing children. Providing information about what to expect demonstrates one simple example of a positive approach for improving child responses. Studies show that even preschool children benefit from receiving information about what will happen and how it will feel. Many dentists use the popular "Tell-Show-Do" technique for this purpose and incorporate "kid friendly" terminology. For example, a dentist might describe an injection of pain medication as putting "sleepy water" around the tooth to numb it and tell children to expect a pinch followed by warmth. Such explanations help children feel less anxious and act more cooperatively.

A second positive means of managing children involves giving them a sense of control. Dentists have long understood that children feel more positive and comfortable when they feel able to influence what happens. As a result, many dentists allow children to use a signal, such as a raised finger, to request a break. However, dentists can also offer both predictability and control by building in frequent breaks for children who exhibit calm, coping behavior. Interestingly, allowing children to have predictable breaks from treatment, regardless of how they cope, also seems a powerful way to reduce distress and disruptive behavior.

Providing children with a variety of distractions during dental work represents a third positive approach. Common sources of distraction include televisions, videogames, and/or CDs of music or popular stories. Such distractions may prove more effective if they actively engage the child during dental treatment by allowing them to make choices. For example, children might be allowed to select and change the music or the television show that is playing during the visit. The availability of distractions appears to create a more enjoyable dental experience for many children.

Finally, referrals from friends and family may assist in the pursuit of a good dentist, but an adult-only visit may provide the best solution. Considerable evidence supports the notion that specific characteristics of the dental staff, office, and clinic have potential to affect the fear, anxiety, and even the pain experienced by patients. If you are able to visit potential dental offices, you can evaluate whether the environment seems pleasant and inviting for children. In-person office visits also allow you to directly question office staff and get first impressions of these professionals. You should also request a tour of both the waiting room and treatment areas. Tours offer opportunities to explore whether there are distracting activities available to children during exams and treatment.

Emphasize Coping

On the day of an actual exam, you can promote success by emphasizing coping and a calm manner. Of course, this requires that you remain calm yourself. Although no particular parenting style predicts which children will act calmly at the dentist, parents who cope poorly with their own anticipation, anxiety, or distress about the impending visit will increase the probability of child distress. Using pleasant imagery, practicing calming self-talk, and taking slow deep breaths can help you manage your own anxiety.

Interestingly, the same coping skills suggested for parents who are anxious prove effective when used by children who feel distressed or anxious about a dental visit. Children who are taught to think about a favorite place, say the words *calm* or *relax* to themselves, or use slow, regular breathing act less anxious and more cooperative. If your child seems particularly distressed, encourage active coping by modeling and practicing coping skills.

If the dentist allows parents in the treatment room, which they *should* in the case of children from 2 to 3 years of age, parents can support coping best by allowing the dentist to direct the child's activities. Although parental presence provides familiarity and comfort, some parents may also introduce elements of distress and disruption for both the child and the dentist. For example, efforts by parents to reassure a child with statements such as "you're okay," or "just a little while longer" can be counterproductive. Alternatively, children appear to benefit most when a parent says very little or limits their comments to distracting, non-dental topics, such as talking about a pet, the weather, or future plans.

Finally, following through with scheduled visits regardless of the distress a child may exhibit will prove important. Any kind of fear and anxiety can become strengthened by avoidance. Scheduling a special activity for after a dental visit may not diminish the distress or fear a child experiences, but it may help motivate the child to cooperate in spite of that fear.

SUMMARY

Numerous elements of dental settings generate developmentally appropriate fear and avoidance in children. If not addressed during younger years, dental anxiety can develop into severe dental phobia as one gets older. To prevent bad oral hygiene later in life, the Five E Model can work to calm your child's fear of dentists.

WHERE TO FIND OUT MORE

Books

Preparation for first dental visit
Berenstain, S. & Berenstain, J. (1981). *The Berenstain Bears Visit the Dentist*. New York: Random House.
Mayer, M. (2001). *Just Going to the Dentist*. New York: Golden Books.
Keller, L. (2000). *Open Wide: Tooth School Inside*. New York: Henry Holt & Co.
Reader's Digest (1993). *Brush Your Teeth Please Pop-Up*. New York: Simon & Schuster. Websites
American Academy Pediatric Dentistry – Find a Dentist
    http://www.aapd.org/finddentist/
American Dental Association – Games for Kids
    http://www.ada.org/public/games/games.asp
Motivational charts for rewarding good dental hygiene
    http://www.dentists4kids.com/parents/Motivational_Charts.html

PART TWO

Family Issues

---------- **CHAPTER 11** ----------

Conversing with Your Uncommunicative Child

Robin M. Deutsch

Jackie seemed to have friends, eagerly attended gymnastics three times a week, and her teachers said she performed well in school. But she shared nothing with her parents. At the dinner table, she said nothing, and answered questions in monosyllables. In the car, it was difficult to get beyond the iPod, but if you did get her attention she often just stared ahead.

Carlos was a sweet little boy but very insular. He spent a lot of time playing with his dog. His parents were frustrated that they could not get a sense of what he was thinking or feeling as he often responded to questions with a shrug or "I don't know."

Parents have many reasons to worry when their child doesn't communicate. Suddenly, the little child you used to be able to read and understand has been replaced by a person unfamiliar to you. You mourn the loss of a connection that was so important. You feel as if you have lost control, you fear that your child is involved in something risky, or that he or she is depressed. In this chapter, we explore some of the reasons why children may be uncommunicative and describe techniques for improving communication.

WHY WON'T MY CHILD TALK TO ME?

Some children are born wired to respond to the environment in certain ways. The way your child organizes herself in the world is shaped by her inborn temperament. Some children with difficult or slow-to-warm temperaments tend to withdraw in the presence of new situations, they may not adapt well to change or transitions, and they tend to react in a generally negative way. Such children can also prove difficult to communicate with and may withdraw in response to stimulation.

A child's physical characteristics and abilities may also influence how other people interact with him or her. Children who are unattractive, clumsy, or poorly coordinated tend to receive more negative responses from others than attractive, well-coordinated children. These negative responses can negatively affect children's self-esteem. When children receive negative feedback and experience negative interactions with others, they may learn to withdraw from others or respond in difficult ways. This response ties directly to the way children feel about themselves and their expectations for how others in the world will respond to them.

Children who have anger issues or impulse control problems may communicate behaviorally and aggressively. While they may recognize their feelings, they do not express them in acceptable ways. As parents, we may not accurately read our children's nonverbal communications. These children do not say aloud what they think or feel, but instead may lash out physically or yell inappropriate things.

Children may not talk to their parents because they don't believe that their parents listen to them. Perhaps some parents have become so intent on having their children listen to what they have to say, that they have stopped listening to their children.

CONVERSATION STARTERS

Critical or judgmental statements will not facilitate conversation with your child. Saying something like, "I can't believe you did that" will only lead your child to feel misunderstood, ashamed, or irritated, and your child will likely respond with withdrawal or anger. Saying something like, "Can you think of another way to handle that?" or "How was that for you?" or "Let's think of another way to respond," will reduce the likelihood of defensive response, provide a model for decision making, and connect you with your child as an ally, not critical other.

General questions such as, "How was school?" or "Did you have fun?" will generally elicit one-word answers such as "Fine" or "Yes," without any detail. For children of all ages, questions that begin with who, what, or where are likely to elicit more detailed responses. The more specific the question, for example, "What did you discuss in science class?" or "Sorry I could not make it to the basketball game. Can you walk me through it?" or "Will you give me a preview of your part in the play?" the more likely your child will give you more than a one-word answer. Follow-up questions such as, "What was that like for you?" or "Where do you see this going?" may also prompt more detail or elaboration.

Parents often have a specific issue that they want to discuss with their child. Carlos's parents had reason to believe that some of the boys in his class were teasing him quite a bit. However, Carlos would not talk about it and spent increasing amounts of time in his room. One day, as his father drove Carlos to school, he told Carlos a story from his own childhood about how he always seemed chosen last for the sports teams. Feeling more understood, Carlos began to talk about being teased at school by some of the boys. Sharing your own stories can prove a very effective strategy in getting your child to open up about what is going on in his or her life. For example, if you tell your child about a conflict at work, your child may respond with an account of his or her own conflict at school.

One strategy that can also prove effective involves using another child (real or made-up) to introduce conversation or initiate problem solving about something specific. In our family, we used "Judy stories" to prompt conversations about risks and moral lessons for our toddler and preschool children. For older children, relying on another, such as a cousin or friend's story, whether real or embellished, can help get to the issue.

For children of all ages, the quickest way to engage them in conversation is through their interests. Spending time learning everything you can about your child's interests, whether they be videogames, sports, cars, fashion, or books, will help you connect with your child. You may get extra points for being "cool" or knowledgeable but most important, you have found a way to start and maintain an ongoing conversation.

SCHOOL-AGED CHILDREN

If children spend most of their free time in front of a TV or computer screen, there will not be much opportunity for conversation. Allowing your child to have a television in his or her bedroom opens up the possibility for your child to withdraw and isolate him- or herself. It may seem radical, but limiting TV and computer time each day and placing the television in a family area, such as the den or living room, can go a long way toward creating an environment in which better communication with your child is possible.

Changing the environment can also open children up to conversation. Leaving the house and spending time with your child in a different environment can alter patterns and perspectives. We know that by changing our landscape we can change the lens through which we view things. Taking a walk outside, going out for a meal, or having a picnic lunch on the living room floor creates a new setting for conversation. Of course, car rides can often prove effective, as no one can leave the car to isolate themselves. You can learn much by listening carefully if another child is in the car and picking up any clues about conversation topics for use in later communication.

Engaging in an activity together, such as playing a board game, doing an art project, or reading together about a specific interest, provides a way to keep the focus on something else while finding opportunities for both observation and communication. Noticing how your child engages in the activity can provide insight into your child, as well as conversational topics. Negotiating the rules of the game or the goals for the project also offers a template that your child can apply to other life situations.

Sometimes children need other ways to communicate, other than conversation. Writing notes and putting them in your child's backpack, lunch box, on the bed, or on the bathroom mirror can begin a dialog or at least a protocol for communication. Notes can include humor, encouragement, or plans. After a time, you can ask your child a question in the note hoping for a response that does not require further prompting.

Probably the most important strategy for communicating with an uncommunicative child is to spend time together. Developing a predictable routine of time together, even 15 minutes, will help your child feel valued, and your child will notice that you are reliably available. That time can involve any of the suggestions just noted or can focus on bedtime.

ADOLESCENTS

The chief developmental task of adolescence involves separating from parents and becoming independent. Even though an adolescent may not have the actual cognitive and neurological maturity to consistently make good independent decisions, they practice these decision-making skills daily. "You don't understand" is a common refrain teenagers give their parents and any other adult authority figures in their lives (e.g., teachers). So, while adolescents attempt to develop as free and separate beings, they also keep their worlds private. They act this way because they think they are capable of making their own decisions, and also because they don't believe that adults would understand. In the service of these normal aspects of growing up, and most basically, to get what they want, adolescents are prone to lie. Whether the lies involve omission of relevant details or active fabrication, adolescents *do* lie if it can help them get what they want.

How can you get access to your teenager's private world? Listening—really listening—without giving advice is the first step in communicating with an adolescent. You can listen even if your teen isn't actually talking. Teenagers often express their feelings and emotions nonverbally. Regardless, you cannot communicate with your teen, verbally or nonverbally, if he or she is otherwise engaged. The popularity of iPods and cell phones can make communication with your teenager impossible. Instituting earphone-free and cell phone–free "zones" in your home can go a long way. Do not allow your teen to listen to music, or talk or text during family mealtimes or times designated for spending quality time together (e.g., family game night).

Once you have your teenager's attention, how do you have a conversation that does not degenerate into fighting or withdrawing? A very effective way to begin a conversation with your teen is to insert yourself into his or her space. If your son is watching television, sit down next to him. Don't talk, just sit. You might comment upon an actor, a situation, the commercial, but just sit. If your daughter is in her room doing homework, knock on the door and walk in with your own reading material, sit down on the floor and begin to read. Sitting in their space is like parallel play, in which you join them in a similar activity without interacting. Stay as long as you want unless it becomes uncomfortable. If that seems the case, make light of the situation and exit. You may be surprised when your adolescent asks if you are dropping in the next night.

For all adolescents, indirect communications can provide the gateway. Initiating a conversation about a movie, TV program, or friend offers a way to engage your teenager in conversation, particularly if you talk about something he or she is interested in. Sometimes, recounting a story about your own history or one of your friends or relatives can also work effectively. If the story suggests some weakness, mistake, or poor judgment on someone else's part it may become particularly compelling to your teen and can result in conversation. These stories are not about bravado or hard luck, but include an element of humiliation or poor decision making. By using a personal story to illustrate to your child that you understand feelings of vulnerability, your child may choose to share his or her concerns with you. Remember, the goal is to elicit conversation, not shut it down.

If you can't beat them, join them. Even though competition is not the goal, maintaining communication and ensuring that your voice is heard is the aspiration. When talking results in tension, conflict, or unresponsiveness, parents must find other ways to communicate with their teens. Try texting, emailing, or instant messaging your adolescent.

These modes of communication are preferred by teens and, because they do not require face time, it may be easier for your child to open up to you. Conversations may last longer online than they would in person, allowing both you and your child time to think about responses. In addition, communicating electronically may reduce conflict and tension.

Your job as the parent of an adolescent is to slowly and safely allow your teen to take control of his or her own life. This is a long and arduous process, because teenage brains (and even some adult brains) are often not developed enough to consistently make good decisions. Part of your job is to help your child with decision making by alerting him or her to risks and helping him or her consider alternatives. You should do your best to avoid threatening your teen or passing judgment. Warm, supportive, positive communications that focus on effective problem solving will help the locus of control shift. Effective parenting of an adolescent requires an authoritative style. This means that you set the rules, explain them, and then follow through with consequences. Permissive or overly lenient parenting, in which the limits remain unenforced, or authoritarian parenting, which is overly controlling, strict, and requires unexplained obedience, is not effective with adolescents and will not result in successful communication between you and your teenager.

When it comes to the last word, you can always give it up, particularly if you identify the need. If you are in an actual verbal exchange with your teen, and a struggle develops, the most important thing to do is identify any negative consequences that may result from a bad decision on your child's part. Once you have "said your piece," your child may have the last word. If you and your teen continue to go back and forth, you may simply step away from the struggle and give up the last word. As stated earlier, all teenagers want to do is take control of their own lives. It is your responsibility to help them think through and make good decisions. If having the last word gives your teenager a sense of control, and you have already stated the risks and consequences, let it go. Your teen will be more likely to listen to you the next time around.

WHEN TO SEEK PROFESSIONAL HELP

How do we know when an uncommunicative child needs professional help? When children's behavior suggests an emergency—that is, they cannot be calmed down, or they threaten to hurt themselves or someone else—they need outside help and possibly consultation in an emergency room. If they exhibit dangerous behaviors such as running away, destroying property, harming animals, harming peers or parents, or fire setting, they need professional help. These kinds of situations and behaviors require consultation with a mental health professional.

You should seek professional help when the situation requires more help than you feel confident giving on your own. You may wish to consult your child's pediatrician, who can help you find a professional who has expertise in your area of concern. If it is not an emergency, you may wish to seek a consultation on your own (without your child present). The professional may suggest that you bring your child in for an assessment and/or psychological treatment. Often, child psychologists want to see the parents first, in order to understand the challenges and concerns observed by the parents.

SUMMARY

Maintaining a dialog with your children provides the means to keep them safe and affords you the opportunity to develop and maintain a positive parent–child relationship. Staying in touch with your children can prove challenging because of their age, temperament, or self-esteem. Communication can also be difficult because, as parents, we do not have the tools to listen or respond in ways that our children can hear. Although it can be difficult, finding ways to be available to your children, listening carefully to their verbal and non-verbal cues, and responding in such a way that they know you care about them and value their point of view are hallmarks of effective parenting. If these strategies fail to yield results, seeking professional consultation can prove quite helpful.

WHERE TO FIND OUT MORE

Books

Barkley, R.A. and Robin, A.L. (2008). *Your defiant teen: 10 steps to resolve conflict and rebuild your relationship.* New York: Guilford.

Greenspan, S.I. and Salmon, J. (1995). *The challenging child: Understanding, raising and enjoying the five "difficult" types of children.* Cambridge, MA: Perseus.

Lippincott, J. & Deutsch, R. (2005). *Seven things your teenager won't tell you and how to talk about them anyway.* New York: Ballantine.

Riera, M. (2003). *Staying connected to your teenager : How to keep them talking to you and how to hear what they are really saying.* Cambridge, MA: Perseus.

Taffel, R. (2001). *Getting through to difficult kids and parents.* New York: Guilford.

Websites

American Psychological Association
Communication Tips for Parents
   http://www.apa.org/helpcenter/communication-parents.aspx
Free Parenting Basics
   http://www.freeparentingbasics.com/

CHAPTER 12

Coping with the Birth of a New Sibling

Amanda Gordon

Tammy and Adam are such great kids. Tammy has loved Adam since the day he was born, and now, at 4 and 2, they get along terrifically together. But Mummy's tummy has begun growing, much discussion about a new baby has taken place—and suddenly the bickering has started. Has Adam become a "terrible two" at the worst possible moment? And what about this nastiness Tammy seems to have picked up at preschool? Now they won't share, they cry easily, push and shove, tease each other . . . and that's before the baby has even arrived. What is happening to their family?

Seven-year-old Wendy had slept in her own room since she was 2. Suddenly, she has been waking in the night and crawling into Mummy's bed, which surely can't be good for her—and isn't great for her parents' sleep either. The new baby wakes her, and she wakes them.

The imminent birth of a new baby can evoke all sorts of emotions in the other children. Older children are often excited, and younger kids may experience some anxiety or confusion. It is important to understand that young children often express emotions through changes in their behavior. We can understand both Tammy and Adam's behaviors as expressions of their own excitement and anxiety about the birth of the new baby. You need to keep this in mind as you respond to your own children's behaviors. Of course, you will want them to feel excitement and anticipate with pleasure the changes to come. Your task is to reduce your children's anxiety and hopefully assist them to express any uncomfortable emotions in a less disruptive way. Obviously, you do need to talk about the fact that you are having a baby and that the baby's arrival will change the composition of the family, so the real questions involve how and when to have those conversations.

HOW DO I TALK TO MY CHILD ABOUT THE NEW BABY?

The ages and the curiosity of your children will provide your best guide as to how and when to speak to them. Although very young children may initially show little curiosity about your growing belly, you need to be the one to let them know that a new sibling is coming. Your children should not hear about the new baby from relatives or family friends. Keep the discussion brief and the focus on your children. Do not force your children to talk about their feelings. Young children do not yet have the capacity to contemplate future events or even imagine what the future may be like. When they seem ready, you should start talking about what the future holds, with an emphasis on the idea that the new baby will become a part of the life that your family has been building together.

Follow your children's lead in determining the amount of detail you give them about how a baby is made or the birth process. When children ask technical questions, take care not to make the answers too scientific. However, don't insult them by making up stories about the stork delivering babies when clearly they want to understand better why Mom started growing a baby at this time. There are many good books available that can help you talk to your children about the new baby (see Where to Find Out More).

Story time can be used as a tool to help your young children adjust to the idea of a new baby brother or sister. Allow your children to sit on your lap as you read to them, so that they can get used to your changing body. With daily cuddly contact, the changes won't seem so dramatic, and your children will feel more accepting of them. So, although the baby will not necessarily become the subject of every discussion, the fact of its growing will become evident and helpful for your children in their ultimate acceptance of the new baby in their lives.

In a family such as that of Adam and Tammy, storytime for Tammy might include stories about new babies, and Adam could be included but not necessarily expected to join in the discussion about what life will be like at home when the new baby arrives. For Adam, these stories will seem no different than any other bedtime stories or fairy tales. For Tammy though, such stories will provide an opportunity to talk through what life at home with a new baby will be like.

Older children will have a rather different reaction to the news that Mom is having another baby. They will more likely have preconceived ideas about how a new baby may change their lives, and they may not like what they envision. They may worry that you won't have time for them once the baby arrives, that they will get stuck doing all the household chores while you care for the new baby, or that the new baby will use up all the family's money. It is important to talk honestly with your older children about the changes the new baby will bring. Don't pretend it will bring only joy and celebration—even though it is important to stress the positives that you believe will come with the new child.

Girls may look forward to a new baby with great delight and see it as a chance to play with a real live dolly. Share your daughter's joy and invite reasonable participation, but make it clear that the baby is a real person, fragile in some ways, and not a toy. Older girls may feel challenged by the idea of their mother having a baby, as it provides evidence of their mother's sexuality. They may not recognize that this is the cause of their discomfort, but may need to talk to you more intensively about relationships at this time, so recognize this and make yourself available. Female siblings of different ages will have different needs in anticipation of the birth of the baby—try to tune in to what makes your daughters anxious.

HOW DO I PREPARE MY CHILD FOR THE BIRTH OF A STEP- OR HALF-SIBLING?

The complexities of an impending birth increase in blended families, where the new baby may only have one parent in common with older siblings. In this situation, where the child already has to cope with sharing their own mother or father with a person who does not truly belong to them, the likelihood for jealousy and/or resentment increases greatly. These children may already have had to learn new rules when a stepparent has joined the family and may resent having to modify things again in anticipation of the new baby.

In this situation, the ideal response involves ensuring that all of the parents take a part in discussing the way family life will change, before the baby arrives. The more open the discussion, the better for all the children involved. Following are some tips you can use to help your children and stepchildren deal with the arrival of a new sibling.

- When a pregnancy occurs in one of the child's households (i.e., either the child's mother or stepmother), discuss it with the parent in the other household as early as you can, so that the child doesn't feel they must keep the new baby a secret. Be aware that your ex-partner, who is also your child's parent, may not feel as happy as you about the new child in your new relationship, and if that proves true, allow for open discussion with your child.
- Develop a shared language between households to make life easier for the older child who moves between them. For example, when your child asks whether the new baby is her sister, make sure you have an answer that makes sense in both households. Even if you don't like your child's new stepparent, her life will be easier if you encourage her to feel part of each of her parent's families. Avoid feelings of having to compete with the new stepsibling for your child's attention.
- Ensure that the stepparent, who is the parent of the new baby, engages with the older child as well, and reflects in their actions the value placed on the older siblings.
- Have age-appropriate play and stories with the older children, and continue that even after the birth of the new baby.
- When a child has a stepparent, they do better when they can establish a relationship with that parent independently of their biological parent, who brought them into this relationship. So, encourage special time between your child's pregnant stepmother or expectant stepfather and the older children. Then, when the baby arrives, the older siblings will have a place in the life of the stepparent and be able to fit in as a sibling for the new baby.

HOW DO I PREPARE MY CHILD TO HELP?

Take the opportunity to share with your older children the delight you have had in watching them grow and take increased responsibility for their own things. In that way, when you point out the sorts of things that you'll need them to help with once the baby arrives, it won't seem solely a matter of the new baby meaning that they have more work to do. Instead, help your children to feel pride in their own ability to do more tasks around the home (such as setting the table or clearing the dishes after meals), and see the value of tidying up their own possessions. You can begin by asking them to take on more responsibility during the pregnancy. The goal is to ensure that the new baby does not get "blamed" for extra tasks. Your children should come to see that helping around the house is a valuable way for them to contribute to the family, regardless of whether or not there is a new baby on the way.

You may wish to practice with your older children some of the tasks they will be expected to perform once the baby arrives. Be sure to praise your children for their help, as this will enhance their sense of pride and make it more likely that they will enjoy helping you after the birth of the baby. As they help out, you may want to take the opportunity to point out the "benefits" of the new baby's arrival, including their new status as "big brother" or "big sister." Don't wait until the baby arrives and then throw chores at your children—give them a chance to feel competent in an age-related way before the baby's birth, and give them loads of attention and praise as they increase their contribution to the household.

The best course of action is to gradually increase the contribution your children make to the family, so that they begin to feel as though they have become part of making the household tick. Young children can put their toys and books away, and older children can help prepare dinner or separate the laundry. The following are some suggestions for getting your children to help with household responsibilities:

- Frame increases in responsibilities for chores as part of the process of growing up and helping out, rather than the result of a new baby taking up too much of your time.
- Take care to define appropriate jobs for your children based on their ages. This will allow your children to be successful in completing tasks and will help instill a sense of pride.
- Help your children learn new skills and take pleasure in their newfound competence—they have more to do because they are "big girls" and "big boys."
- Work together with your children to accomplish tasks. Helping out around the house can turn into shared fun—doing things together helps people feel connected and supportive.

HOW SHOULD I MODIFY MY ROUTINE BEFORE THE BABY ARRIVES?

After the baby's birth, your daily schedule runs the risk of interruption, as the baby will place demands on you and your spouse or partner at inconvenient and unpredictable times. One way to make sure this interruption does not become too problematic is to make some changes prior to the birth of the baby. For example, if it has always been Mom's job to read bedtime stories and get the kids ready for bed, perhaps this responsibility should shift over to the other parent before the children blame the new baby for Mom's unavailability. Begin early in the pregnancy, bringing your spouse or partner or even the babysitter in to learn and become part of the revised routine. The real trick involves minimizing surprises for children who are accustomed to reassuring routines.

Here are some suggestions for modifying your household routine before the baby arrives:

- Have your children teach your spouse or partner or other caregivers (e.g., baby-sitter, nanny) about their daily routines, including how to pack their book bags and prepare their lunches and snacks. This will help your children feel that they have access to fully competent support, not merely shallow substitutes for unavailable Mommy.
- If grandparents plan on coming from out of town once the baby is born, help your children prepare for their visit by having them create welcome signs and decorate the house. In this way, your children will become excited about their grandparents coming to visit, as well as about the baby's arrival, and feel engaged in the preparations.

WHAT DO I DO WHEN I BRING THE BABY HOME?

In most cases, the actual birth will occur in the hospital with both parents present, so it is important to make arrangements for someone else to watch your children while you are away. Plan ahead of time, and share your plans with your children so they know what to expect. Do your best to minimize your children's anxiety about your absence. Try to make this a calm time and engage familiar people who can support your children. Consider having a special treat prepared for your kids, as they wait at home for news of the birth of their brother or sister.

Don't forget to let your children know as soon as you can of the baby's birth and when you expect to return home. Some people find it useful to bring a gift home for the siblings from the new baby, but children will have more interest in knowing that their parents still care about them than that the baby sent a gift. If you plan on bringing gifts to your children, do it yourself when you bring the baby home. Give your children their gifts, and spend some time playing with them, rather than just handing the presents over and continuing to coo over the new baby.

No matter how old your children are, they will want and need to get to know the baby. It is hard not to feel protective of the new baby, but you will be amazed at how even the wildest 2-year-old will sit in awe as a new baby is placed carefully in his lap. However, do not leave the baby in the care of your young children in your absence. The responsibility is too great. Make sure you let your older children know the "rules" of handling their new sibling. For example, touching the baby's face is not okay, but holding the baby's hand (once your own hands are clean!) can be fun. Older children can be encouraged to talk and sing to the baby as well.

Remind your children that a baby cries when he or she wants to communicate, and that even baby may not know what he or she wants to say. It is okay to speak soothingly to the baby as it cries, rather than having to do anything, and the older children who understand this will thus become less anxious about a baby's cries and more likely to respond gently.

Older children often fight for the chance to hold the baby and then may want to take on full responsibility for their new brother or sister. Allow your children a chance to play with their new sibling, but don't be persuaded to allow them to immediately take over. Remind them that the baby is a new little person and needs to spend a lot of time with Mom in the beginning. Although older children can be very big helpers to you and the new baby, they should first form a sibling relationship and establish a bond. As time goes on and your children adjust to the baby's presence, they can assume more responsibility for caring for the baby, such as preparing bottles and changing diapers.

HOW DO I MANAGE CHANGES IN MY CHILD'S BEHAVIOR?

As noted earlier, children's emotions often find expression through changes in their behavior. Tammy and Adam, from the first example at the beginning of the chapter, started acting mean to each other and expressing defiance toward their parents. On the other hand, Wendy, from the second example, expressed her concerns about the changes to her family by regressing to a younger stage of development, wanting to sleep with her mother and refusing to go to bed by herself. In each case, the children's behaviors are responses to the changes in the family structure, and in particular to having to share their mother with another demanding creature. Once you understand that your children's behaviors are an expression of their emotions, it becomes much easier to respond to them. Try the following suggestions:

- Always make sure to notice when your children are behaving appropriately. Reward them with praise and attention. This will help maintain their good behavior.
- Remind your children that they won't get what they want be behaving naughty— and respond really positively when they change their behavior.
- If you need to, respond to naughty behavior by withdrawing your attention from your children. When your children resume appropriate behavior, find time to respond promptly and warmly to them.
- When your children come into your bed at night, give them a cuddle and then put them right back in their own rooms. Promise them a special story or quality time together if they manage to stay in bed until the morning.
- Reduce the anxiety underlying your children's behavior by reassuring them that they occupy a most important place in the family.
- Praise your children for age-appropriate behavior and reward them with an extra story before bed or a special treat for just the two of you.

SUMMARY

Following the birth of a first child, we advise the new mother to rest when the baby rests, and to do only the most vital of chores, leaving things that don't matter until her strength returns and she finds herself able to do more. However, with other children to attend to in the house, it proves much harder for mother to put her feet up at any time, let alone sleep during the day. But if your 2-year old still naps, try to put the baby down for a nap at the same time, and go straight to bed yourself. Go for gentle walks with both children. Try to go to bed early—even if the toys are not all put away.

When parents put energy into looking after themselves, including getting as much rest as possible as well as putting time into their own loving relationship, they will manage all the challenges that bringing a new baby into the household can create. Take good care of yourself and reduce your expectations for a while, and your children will put aside their own anxieties more quickly and adjust to their new little brother and sister. Before long, you'll all wonder how life was possible before the baby was part of it!

WHERE TO FIND OUT MORE

Books

Ferguson, Alane. (1999). *That new pet!* Illustrated by Catherine Stock. Unpaged. New York: Lothrop, Lee & Shepard Books. (Ages 3 to 8.)

Manushkin, Fran. (1986). *Little rabbit's baby brother.* Illustrated by Diane de Groat. Unpaged. New York: Crown Publishers. (Ages 2 to 5.)

Harper, Anita. (2007). *It's not fair!* Illustrated by Susan Hellard. Unpaged. New York: G. P. Putnam's Sons. (Ages 1 to 5.)

Sheldon, A. (2008). *Big brother now: A story about me and our new baby* (Illustrated by Karen Maizel). Washington, DC: Magination Press.

Sheldon, A. (2005). *Big sister now: A story about me and our new baby.* Illustrated by Karen Maizel. Washington, DC: Magination Press.

Brooks, Robert. (1983). *So that's how I was born!* Illustrated by Susan Perl. New York: Simon & Schuster.

Websites

Health 24.com
    http://www.health24.com/child/Parenting/833-852,27049.asp
Dr. Lawrence Kutner
    http://www.drkutner.com/parenting/articles/sib_rivalry.html
Baby Center
    http://www.babycenter.com/0_helping-your-preschooler-adjust-to-a-new-sibling_3636582.bc
suite101.com
    http://parentingresources.suite101.com/article.cfm/preparing_older_children_for_a_new_sibling

CHAPTER 13

Sibling Rivalry

Rebecca A. Jones and Casey J. Moser

Raphael is 11 years old and says his younger sister Elizabeth started annoying him the day after she was born. They often fight and take each other's possessions without permission. Sometimes their arguments get physical. Their mother is worried that they will never get along.

Sibling relationships can sometimes provide tremendous safe havens of friendship, understanding, and mutual fun. As adults, many of us value our siblings over almost everyone else in our lives. One study of college women found that most felt as close to or even closer to a sibling than to a parent. Many times, however, sibling relationships can become war zones of jealousy, competition, and rivalry. Children learn roles such as "caretaker," "controller," "competitor," "always in last place," or even "bully" through repetitive play with their brothers and sisters. Many times, those roles carry over into later relationships with friends, partners, and co-workers. Interactions with siblings help form the blueprints for the relationships we build later in life, and we often find ourselves in the same roles in adult relationships that we played with our brothers and sisters.

There is not a lot of research available on sibling rivalry, but several wonderful books and websites can help parents struggling with their children's rivalry (see *Where to Find Out More*, at the end of this chapter). These materials will prove particularly helpful for understanding complex issues such as gender differences, adopted siblings, attention deficit disorder and learning differences in siblings, chronic illness in a sibling, etc. In this chapter, we provide a general overview of sibling rivalry and offer some guidelines for parents regarding when and how to intervene.

THE FIGHT FOR PARENTS' LOVE AND ATTENTION

Many times, siblings fight or compete in order to feel competent. When an older child accomplishes a new task, for example, a younger sibling might try to sabotage the achievement out of pure frustration at her inability to demonstrate the same level of skill. However, the primary source of sibling rivalry flows from competition for the attention and affection of parents and other caregivers. Thus, when siblings compete, they are essentially struggling to maintain a sense of security in the family. When they feel there is not enough love or attention to go around, they sometimes express their frustration by picking fights with one another.

BIRTH OF A SIBLING

Sibling rivalry may become most dramatic when a younger sibling arrives. When Mom gives birth to a new baby, she isn't able to give her other children the same amount of attention as she did before the baby arrived. This experience may serve as a tremendous opportunity for emotional growth for the older child, but as 11-year-old Raphael expressed in the example at the beginning of the chapter, the birth of a younger sibling can also trigger sibling rivalry. The older child may come to resent the younger child for taking up all of his parents' time, energy, love, and affection. In contrast, a younger child may come to resent an older child for her status as the older, more competent child. The following are some suggestions for minimizing sibling rivalry upon the arrival of a younger child:

- On the birth of a new child, provide older children with extra support, attention, and affection to keep them from feeling deprived. Extra hugs, more quality time with you, and verbal expressions of affection and pride can help make up for having to share your time and attention.
- Encourage older children to play an active role in caring for the new baby, but also provide them chances to act as young and innocent as they were before their sibling's birth. Don't alter expectations too rapidly or dramatically.

SIBLING ENVY AND JEALOUSY

As young children mature, they become more conscious of their mixed feelings for their siblings and often express feelings of envy or jealousy. Envy is sometimes described as a wish to possess attributes that a sibling has, including physical attributes such as hair or eye color. Envy can also extend to other characteristics such as talents, intelligence, or athleticism. Children also may feel jealous of the time and attention that their siblings receive for those attributes and talents. A wish to possess a sibling's attributes may actually help in establishing a positive identity, in that siblings may serve as important role models for younger brothers or sisters. However, intense, unresolved sibling envy can lead to lasting interpersonal difficulties. A child who perceives himself as "less than" his siblings may internalize an enduring sense of inadequacy or inferiority.

FAMILY ROLES AND IDENTITY DEVELOPMENT

As a parent, it is likely that you are looking for a clear vision of your children's identities or personalities. Even during pregnancy, mothers often label their children based on their behavior. Parents sometimes describe very young children as "active," "calm," "easy," or "a troublemaker," and it often seems as though only one child can fill any given role in a family. Therefore, one child may often find herself referred to as the "serious" or "smart one," and the other as the "rebellious" or "funny one." If one role appears already taken, future siblings may try to find a different path or be assigned one by their parents, even without realizing it. For example, an older child sometimes fills the role of the "competent one" because he has spent an extended period of time in the company of adults. In this case, the younger child may seek his parents' attention by acting silly, clingy, or demanding. Rigid roles make rivalry more likely, especially when one role seems more socially desirable and/or more valued by parents. Ideally, you should allow your children's roles and identities to be flexible. It is okay for more than one of your children to be recognized for the same traits. The "funny" child needs her competencies recognized, and a child labeled "serious" or "smart" needs permission to act silly and playful as well.

Another common dynamic that may lead to increased jealousy involves messages from parents that one child seems more similar to a particular family member. For example, we often hear parents exclaim, "Sam is just like his mother, and Matthew is just like his father." This type of forced identification can also breed rivalry, because children want to feel valued and cherished by both parents equally. In addition, some parents or extended family members may criticize an adult in front of the children, leading to problems for the child perceived as like that parent.

LONG-TERM CONSEQUENCES OF FAVORITISM

Many experts describe the long-term struggles of children who believe they received less care or attention than their favored siblings. Children who feel less favored may develop grief, anger, and resentment toward their siblings, poor self-esteem, or feelings that they are inadequate or "damaged" in some way. Favoring one child over the other can make the unfavored child believe that she does not deserve equal love and care, and she may take this expectation into later relationships. A favored child, on the other hand, may develop an inflated sense of self and expect others to value him or her more highly than others.

RECOGNIZING UNIQUENESS IN EACH CHILD

Research has shown that the best thing you can do to minimize sibling rivalry in your family is to accept and cherish the uniqueness of each of your children. In the life of every family, episodes will occur when a parent prefers one child over others. But overall, in order for children to feel motivated to negotiate and make peace with their siblings, they must believe that the family has enough love for everyone. Or, as one creative mother put it, "I just remind them that there is plenty of time for everyone to be the favorite sometimes." Children who earn recognition for their unique abilities can more easily tolerate and appreciate the talents and skills of their brothers and sisters. To avoid favoritism and rigid roles among siblings, we offer these suggestions:

- Make an effort to reflect and value each child's unique characteristics, even those that may differ from your own or other siblings.
  - For example, say "Mary, you really seem to love playing the guitar, and you have really gotten good at it;" or "Henry, that Lego castle you built looks fantastic."
- Express to your children that you value their different talents and traits equally, and always avoid comparing one child to another.
- When one child's interests and talents differ from the typical family culture (e.g., an artistic child in an athletic family), make an effort to spend special time with that child, sharing his or her unique pursuit, and to value that child's productions as much as any athletic accomplishment.
  - For example, accompany your child to her first concert or art show. For the young girl interested in horses, order an equestrian magazine, read it together, and spend time discussing the articles.
- Make an effort to balance the distribution of time and resources for your children.
  - For example, make every other Friday "dinner out with Mommy," and allow each child one night out each month.
- Attend children's events and activities equally. If both parents attend a son's baseball games and practices weekly, both can watch a daughter's swimming lessons as well. In this way, children whose activities are less "public" still receive equal attention.
- Ask questions about your children's behavior and interests, rather than labeling.
  - For example, say "How did it feel to serve so often in volleyball today?" Or "I noticed you were the first to tell a joke today. How'd you like getting all those laughs?"

REALISTIC EXPECTATIONS FOR SHARING AND COOPERATION

Sibling fighting can stress everyone in the family. With very young children, fights often revolve around "sharing." As a parent, you likely expect your children, even if they are very young, to *want* to share and to have the skills to cooperate with each other peacefully. However, it is unrealistic to expect children to share their toys and other belongings, particularly given that adults do not share in this way with other adults. It is rare to find an adult who will loan his or her car to a friend without hesitation, for example. Rather than insisting that your child give up her possession just because her sibling wants it, you might instead validate each child's feelings in the struggle, in order to build empathy for other's positions. It is important that you maintain realistic expectations for cooperation and sharing, especially with young children.

WHEN SIBLING RIVALRY INCREASES

There are bound to be times in your family's life when your children's influence on one another will be stronger than usual. Children increase their focus on one another during times of family stress (divorce, parental job loss), during times when parents are away from the home or generally inaccessible (while traveling on business or busy caring for a sick relative), and when they feel stressed on account of having difficulties in another area, such as academics or friendships. Sometimes children fight and compete with one another to distract from losses or greater problems in the family, or to gain parental attention that feels lacking. A dramatic increase in sibling rivalry also could signal that parental arguing has reached a toxic level and warrants professional attention. Sometimes children's expressions of anger toward their brothers and sisters represent displaced anger toward their parents. The following are some suggestions for dealing with increased sibling rivalry in your family:

- If sibling rivalry increases dramatically, evaluate the level of stress in the whole family. If parental discord may have provided the cause, seek couples or family counseling.
- Listen closely to your children's worries and complaints about school and friend-ships. A child may act out his frustration about an academic difficulty or friendship trouble by fighting at home. Patiently and persistently, ask your children to share their concerns with you, so that you can help them solve real problems outside the family.
  - For example, "The fighting between you and Jasmine has really become rough this week. I keep wondering if something at school or with your friends might be upsetting you." Follow up with concrete advice and consultation with teachers and other professionals as needed.
- Reassure your children during times of stress that you love and care for them. When children experience loss, such as the death of a pet or grandparent, they tend to harbor fears of other losses as well (e.g., loss of a parent or sibling). They may act out these fears with aggression toward siblings. Take time to talk with each of your children about the meaning of the family-level stressor in language they can understand.

MODELING AND REINFORCING COOPERATION

Sibling aggression serves an important function in that it gives children the opportunity to practice their interpersonal skills, such as tolerating anger from other people, being assertive, negotiating, and taking turns. In this way, it becomes a part of normal interpersonal development and an important learning opportunity.

However, sometimes children lack the skills to constructively resolve their conflicts and therefore resort to violence or manipulation. Children learn new skills by observing someone like them using those skills (modeling) or through instruction and rewards. In other words, they may learn to negotiate or take turns by watching an older sister use these skills. Or, they may learn because a parent makes suggestions and then congratu-lates them for listening and following through. Children need practice in pro-social con-flict skills such as deal-making (negotiation), taking turns, working together, and changing course in an argument. Family therapists recommend that families intentionally build rituals of cooperation and collaboration into their daily and weekly routines, so that they have a chance to model and teach these skills, and so that collaboration and peaceful time together become the norm. The following are some ways you can accomplish this in your family:

- Spend family time in cooperative pursuits (rather than competitive games) such as hiking, biking, household projects, jigsaw puzzles, or making music together. Model simple skills such as turn-taking and deal-making during these peaceful times.
- Establish rituals of cooperation with "equal time" for everyone to receive attention.
  - For example, establish conversations at dinner time that allow each child to report an interesting or funny experience from the day. As the parent, gently interrupt your children when they talk over each other. You may say something like, "Give Robbie a chance to talk; he was telling a funny story too. We want to hear about science lab. You'll get your turn."

Finally, children may need incentives to practice cooperation. When children express their rivalry in the most annoying ways—picking on each other, annoying each other, or hurting each other—we cannot avoid paying attention. You may be tempted to punish your children during these times either by separating them or taking away their privileges. Sometimes this approach works temporarily. However, it may be more effective to set up a reward system in which your children are awarded small gifts for cooperating. When they feel motivated, children can often find ways to cooperate that would otherwise not emerge. For young children, setting small easily attainable goals (3–5 minutes of "gentle hands and words") and immediate and tangible rewards (treats or fun activities) will work best. Refer to the following tips for setting up a reward system:

- Promise your children a valued reward if they behave cooperatively for a specified period of time or until completion of a task.
  - For example, say "If you guys can use gentle hands and voices during this car ride, we'll get those cookies out when we get home."
  - For older children, "If the two of you can clean the kitchen without an argument, you can watch the movie we rented today." If the task becomes a battle, you might suggest a skill, such as "I would suggest you discuss and agree on each person's job ahead of time."

As a busy parent with lots of responsibilities, it will prove a challenge not to give in and grant rewards to children even when they have not cooperated with each other. This becomes particularly hard when the reward or activity is something *you* would really enjoy. If you really do not want the family to miss some special activity or event, we suggest planning it without strings attached. When you have provided adequate opportunities for children to cooperate and negotiate with one another, and they still fail to do so, they may need more direct help from an adult. In cases like this, when children consistently fail in their attempts to negotiate with each other, help them each to express themselves assertively. For example, say "Lisa, tell Sharon exactly what you want in a big girl voice and look her in the eyes. Great. Now listen to Sharon. Okay, now we know Lisa wants to swing and Sharon wants to jump rope. Do you need to drop both ideas and find a game you both enjoy, or can you think of another solution?"

LISTEN TO FEELINGS AND USE "TIME OUT" FOR AGGRESSION

A moderate amount of aggressive sibling interaction (a noninjurious wrestling match on the living room floor or spirited verbal criticism about fashion sense) may be necessary, and may even prove to be a positive part of some siblings' relationships. Therefore, parents need to tolerate a certain amount of sibling conflict.

Sometimes children need to talk to parents privately about their frustrations. Allow your children to express anger, jealousy, resentment, and hurt feelings about their siblings. Validate these feelings, while at the same time clearly prohibit inappropriate behaviors such as hurtful physical aggression. In other words, we expect everyone to feel and talk about a range of different emotions, but we can't accept hurtfully acting them out against someone.

- Find an appropriate response to aggression, such as time away or "time out" from parental and siblings' attention, and use it as consistently as possible.
- If a child's aggression intensifies, or you find yourself unable to manage conflicts consistently, find a local parent training course. These small group classes offer an array of skills for parents in similar situations.

SUMMARY

At times, it might prove best to let your children work out their conflicts without your help, especially when the conflicts are not aggressive or hurtful. However, keep in mind that research has shown that parents who avoid getting involved in their children's more serious conflicts do a great disservice to each child and to the sibling relationship. When parents don't pay attention, siblings often act out to regain that attention. And, if rivalry escalates to aggression, failing to respond appropriately may result in the development of a destructive pattern for a child. Children must learn that they can't get their way in the world by harassing or hurting others. Overall, we recommend an approach to sibling rivalry and conflict that includes maintaining realistic expectations for children's social skills, acknowledging other stressors that can affect the sibling relationship, setting up rituals that encourage turn-taking and collaboration, rewarding children's pro-social behavior, and openly treasuring each child's unique identity and contributions to the family.

WHERE TO FIND OUT MORE

Books

Alley, W. (2007). *Bratty brothers and selfish sisters: All about sibling rivalry* (Elf-Help Books for Kids) St. Meinrad, IN: Abbey Press.

Bank, S., & Kahn, M. (1997). *The sibling bond.* New York: Basic Press.

Brazelton, T.B., & Sparrow, J.D. (2004). *Understanding sibling rivalry – The Brazelton Way.* Cambridge, MA: Decapo Press.

Cicirelli, Victor G. (1995). *Sibling relationships across the lifespan.* New York: Plenum Press.

Faber, A & Mazlish, E. (2004). *Siblings without rivalry.* New York: Harper Collins.

Goldenthal, P. (1999). *Beyond sibling rivalry: How to help your children become cooperative, caring, and compassionate.* New York: Henry Holt and Company.

Kennedy-Moore, E. and Katayama, M. (2005). *What about me: Twelve ways to get your parents' attention without hitting your sister.* Seattle: Parenting Press.

Sheldon, A. (2008). *Big brother now: A story about me and our new baby.* Illustrated by Karen Maizel. Washington, DC: Magination Press.

Websites

Kids Health
    http://kidshealth.org/parent/emotions/feelings/sibling_rivalry.html
University of Michigan Health System
    http://www.med.umich.edu/1libr/yourchild/sibriv.htm
Child Development Institute
    http://www.childdevelopmentinfo.com/parenting/sibling_rivalry.shtml

CHAPTER 14

Temper Tantrums and Noncompliance

Alison R. Zisser and Sheila M. Eyberg

Georgey is a highly noncompliant 5-year-old. His parents describe him as a stubborn and willful little boy who has meltdowns whenever he doesn't get his way. His public behavior is particularly embarrassing to his parents, and all of their discipline attempts have failed. In grocery stores, when Georgey's parents deny his demands, his extreme tantrums draw disapproving looks from shoppers. In the past, these reactions led his mother to give in to his demands. His father simply refused to take him along on errands. At this point, neither parent takes him out in public, but instead trade off watching him at home while the other parent completes errands.

Sarah is a 13-year-old described by her mother as rebellious and argumentative. Sarah has always had a strong personality, but with the exception of occasional tantrums as a young child, she seemed mostly compliant and well behaved. Over the past year, however, Sarah has become increasingly defiant, refusing to complete homework or chores at home, and often staying out later than allowed. Her mother attributes Sarah's behavior to a new group of girls she began spending time with when she entered middle school. She describes outbursts in which Sarah yells and cries and storms to her room whenever her parents attempt to enforce limits. Sarah's mother expresses helplessness in managing Sarah's behavior and distress about losing the warm relationship that she and her daughter used to share.

If either Georgey or Sarah sound like your child, you have likely experienced frustrations and feelings similar to their parents. Frequent tantrums and noncompliance become disruptive to the family system and not only affect parent–child relationships, but also affect the child's relationships with siblings. Frequent noncompliance often affects the relationship between parents as well.

NONCOMPLIANCE ACROSS CHILDHOOD

Some struggles with parents occur normally in childhood. Sometimes, though, noncompliance begins a vicious cycle of interaction between parent and child in which both parent and child trigger increasingly negative behavior in each other. To illustrate, when a child refuses a parent's request (e.g., Georgey's mother tells him to put back the candy he grabbed from the grocery shelf and he refuses), the parent might unintentionally reward escalating negative behavior with attention (e.g., Georgey's mother angrily repeats her demand and Georgey screams "no" and falls to the floor in a full-blown tantrum). The parent might continue to increase her negative behavior until she gains control (e.g., Georgey's mother yanks him up by the arm, yelling her demand more fiercely, and Georgey puts back the candy). The child's compliance then rewards the parent for using harsher methods to obtain control, and the coercive cycle continues. Changing your child's disruptive behavior often requires changing your relationship with your child to include more healthy interactions that promote positive behavior.

Whether parents interpret their child's behavior as problematic partly depends on their tolerance for their child's behavior. For example, most preschoolers are very messy eaters. Parents who know and accept the fact that their preschooler is still developing the fine motor skills needed for eating independently can teach their child about keeping food on the plate and provide positive attention for small gains during meal time. In contrast, parents who have little tolerance for a mess may provide negative attention for their child's eating behaviors and may begin a negative cycle of interaction that increases the child's risk of developing disruptive behavior at the dinner table. In the same way, if parents fail to recognize their child's difficulty with self-control when frustrated, they miss opportunities to teach more effective self-control methods. They also miss opportunities to reward their child's developing self-control, leading to increased tantrums and other disruptive behavior.

Children throw temper tantrums for a multitude of reasons. Maybe their parents didn't give them something they wanted or took away something they wanted to keep. Children's tantrums are largely goal directed—they seek to get their way in a conflict by crying and yelling. Georgey's tantrum in the grocery store demonstrated a fervent attempt to keep the candy bar he took from the shelf.

DEVELOPMENTAL CONSIDERATIONS

The ways children express noncompliance differ as they mature. Between 18 months and 4 years, children commonly resort to saying "no" and tantruming. In fact, up to 3 or 4 years of age, many children average one tantrum per day. Within limits, tantrums and noncompliance at this stage qualify as developmentally normal, as children learn to assert their independence. Your resonse to your child's misbehavior during this period often determines whether the tantrums escalate into serious behavior problems or decline over time.

By the time children reach school age, noncompliance and tantrums may still occur on occasion. But if you have successfully navigated the preschool years, the elementary school years typically prove the calmest, when children seem most cooperative, and parent–child conflict remains low. Still, whenever your school-age children test the limits by ignoring requests, back-talking, or making up excuses, you must stand ready to deal with such behavior immediately to prevent it from escalating. Good communication and relatively straightforward limit-setting and follow-through tend to resolve issues more easily than at the earlier or later stages of child development.

As children approach their teenage years, new challenges emerge for parents. Although this generally becomes a time of increased parent–child conflict, most teen-agers make it through this period without major emotional, behavioral, or social difficul-ties. The increase in bickering that families experience during early adolescence occurs when teens (much like toddlers) attempt to exert their independence in the family and assert themselves in decision making. Teens also spend more time with their friends and become more influenced by peers than at earlier stages.

Many parents believe their teen's moodiness stems from hormonal changes and see their noncompliance as a stage that will pass with time. However, scientific evidence shows that hormones have little to do with noncompliance—social influences play a much more important role. Recall 13-year-old Sarah from the example at the beginning of this chapter. Her mother's belief that Sarah's new friends influenced her behavior was likely correct. Sarah and her friends may all be testing out their developing sense of freedom from family as they enter the new environment of middle school. Their interactions may reinforce one another's desires for greater independence from family rules about friends, chores, and after-school activities. Sarah and her parents have had little success in negotiating these changes. Parents' tolerance of the changes that take place in early adolescence, and the way they react to them, largely determine whether serious conflicts emerge.

HOW DO I DEAL WITH MY CHILD'S TANTRUMS AND NONCOMPLIANCE?

People learn acceptable and unacceptable behaviors (children are not born with specific genes to say "please" or to back talk), and they can unlearn almost any learned behavior. Parent training programs teach strategies for reacting to children's behaviors in ways that cause the positive behaviors to happen more often and the negative behaviors to decline. Parents can also learn how to teach children new positive behaviors, especially behaviors that can take the place of negative ones.

With practice, you can learn to pay attention to your child's positive behaviors and to ignore most negative ones (unless those behaviors pose a danger). In this chapter, we describe several ways to apply these principles on your own to reduce child noncompliance and tantrums. Some techniques, such as positive attention, prove useful for children at any age. Others work best at specific stages of development. However, all techniques require new twists at each stage because of the rapidly changing cognitive, physical, emotional, and social development that takes place between toddlerhood and the teenage years.

Praise Your Child's Positive Behaviors

Although they may not admit it, children and adolescents all seek attention from their parents. Giving positive attention can take many forms (e.g., giving smiles, joining in your child's activity). One of the easiest ways to give positive attention involves praising your child's positive behavior (e.g., "I'm proud of you for being so good in the store"). Making your praise specific (e.g., "Thanks for bringing the car home on time"), instead of non-specific (e.g., "Thanks"), makes it more likely that the specified behavior will continue.

When you praise your child for positive behavior, be sure to add reasons for why the behavior is important to you (e.g., "A storm is coming, and I'm so glad to know you're safe"). Even preschoolers benefit from hearing reasons why their good behavior is important. Stating the reason serves to amplify the praise to emphasize how important the child's behavior is to you and how it may benefit the child as well (e.g., "When you mind me so quickly, it gives us more time for bedtime stories").

Ignore Your Child's Negative Behaviors

Ignoring means actively taking away your attention. You say nothing, look away from your child, and pretend nothing has happened. Ignoring only works with some behaviors—the negative behaviors that children do to get your attention, such as tantrums. When you first ignore a negative behavior, it may get worse before it gets better. This happens because, at first, your child will likely try harder to get your attention by making the tantrum louder and longer until you give in. If you give in then, your child has learned to begin using worse behavior to get the reward of your attention. But if you don't give in—if you consistently ignore the behavior, even when it worsens—the behavior will fade away.

If you decide to use ignoring to get rid of a negative attention-seeking behavior, you must stay alert while ignoring so that you can immediately give your positive attention to whatever non-negative behavior you can find, once the negative behavior stops (e.g., "Thank you for standing up" or "Thank you for asking quietly"). One of the fastest ways to change negative attention-seeking behavior involves ignoring it and then praising a positive behavior.

Ignoring will not work for noncompliance. Children generally do not disobey to get parental attention. Instead, they disobey to avoid doing something they do not want to do. A child told to clean up toys who does not want to clean up is more likely to refuse the task in order to get out of doing it than to gain parental attention. Noncompliance is rarely an attention-seeking behavior. Other examples of disruptive behavior typically not performed for parental attention include hitting a sibling (rewarded most by the reaction of the sibling) and sneaking cookies from the pantry. To change these kinds of disruptive behaviors, other discipline methods are needed.

Give Your Child a Time Out

A time out provides a powerful method for changing noncompliant behavior in young children when correctly applied. Many parents say that time out doesn't work. This often happens because they did not follow all the steps needed to make it work. Time out works most effectively with children ages 2 through 6. In this age group, five components are critical to reducing noncompliance with time out:

- You must be prepared to use the time out procedure every single time your child disobeys a direct instruction.

- The time out place should be boring, out of reach of toys or parental attention.
- Do not give attention to your child while in time out.
- The time out should last the same amount of time every time (we recommend 3 minutes for children ages 2 through 6).

To make the process of learning to comply as fair as possible for a child, we recommend that, after you give a direct instruction ("Please bring me the brush"), you allow your child 5 seconds to begin obeying your directive. If your child has not started to obey within 5 seconds, you should give *one* brief statement of the consequence for not minding ("If you don't bring me the brush, you will have to go to the time out chair"). After this statement, again give your child 5 seconds to obey. Five seconds is a good length of time to wait, because it allows your child enough time to begin complying, but it prevents dawdling. If your child chooses not to obey after hearing the consequence, you need to take your child to time out promptly and calmly, without giving additional attention (words). When your child is in time out, you must ignore any negative behavior, such as complaining or whining. Successful time out requires time away from your attention.

After your child has completed the designated time (e.g., 3 minutes on a time out chair), you should wait for 5 seconds of quiet before letting you child know that time out has ended. The 5 seconds of quiet plays an important role. If the 3 minutes ended as your child yelled, and you ended the time out right then, your child might believe that yelling is the secret to ending the time out. Waiting for 5 seconds of quiet makes it clear that you have control over the time out. When the time out ends, give the original instruction again, and if your child still does not obey, return your child to time out for 3 minutes more. When your child does obey the instruction, remember to give specific praise (e.g., "Thank you for doing what I told you to do").

Keep Behavior Charts

Behavior charts work well for decreasing noncompliance in school-aged children. Completing chores typically becomes the major source of noncompliance at this age. Behavior charts provide a concrete method for rewarding successful completion of daily responsibilities. Using material rewards (e.g., a small toy) or activity rewards (e.g., going to the park) helps to motivate children.

To create an effective behavior chart, the best strategy involves working together with your child to decide on the behaviors that cause conflict and seem helpful to change. Behavior charts typically start out with two to five behaviors, depending on the child's age, and gradually increase as the child experiences success. Your child might feel overwhelmed and discouraged if the chart includes too many behaviors at once. Behavior charts should not include more than seven behaviors at any one time.

It works best to involve your child in deciding the reward for completing tasks on the chart. The more your child feels involved, the more likely your child will understand the chart and work hard to earn the rewards. Behaviors on the chart require very specific description. For example, if your child resists completing household chores, the chart might list behaviors such as "take out garbage" and "feed the cat" instead of "complete chores."

After selecting the target behaviors, decide how to keep track of your child's progress on the behavior chart. School-aged children often like stickers or smiley faces. You then need to determine how many stickers your child needs to earn in one day (or across the week) to get a reward. For example, if a 9 year-old boy has four behaviors on his chart, he may need to earn two stickers to get a small reward for the day (e.g., watching a favorite TV show). The number of stickers needed to earn a reward should start at a level your child can likely achieve easily. Along with daily rewards, you may also establish a weekly reward for the total number of stickers earned in a week. For example, if the chart has four target behaviors for completion each day (28 possible points in a week), you might begin with a weekly reward, such as going to a movie on Sunday if your child earns 15 points or more in the past seven days. Assuring your child's success and ability to earn rewards for good behavior is your first goal.

Withdraw Your Child's Privileges

For most school-age children and adolescents, withdrawal of privileges proves effective for reducing noncompliance. For example, if you have made a rule that your child must return home with the car by 10:00 P.M., and your child repeatedly disobeys, you might tell your teen that every time this happens again, the car keys will stay in your pocket for 5 days. For this technique to work effectively, it is important to (a) select a consequence that you have control over, such as car keys; (b) remain totally consistent in following through with the rule you set; and (c) limit the time of the consequence. With teens, loss of privileges should typically not exceed one week. With school-age children, we recommend one day.

Create If-then Plans

"If-then" plans can work effectively with children from toddlers to teens, if you state the plan in words the child understands. Parents can apply this technique on-the-spot for a single behavior. An if-then plan involves an activity that your child enjoys (e.g., snack after school) and a condition you require for the activity to take place (e.g., eating the snack in the kitchen to prevent crumbs from falling on your carpet). If children have become accustomed to having these treats without having to "earn" them, they may feel angry about these new rules. But if the rule is important, then stick with it! Do *not* let your child have the "then" before completing the "if." In other words, the child who does not sit at the table does not get the snack, now or later.

When applied consistently and when children understand the rule, an if-then plan can help make future tantrums unlikely. Because the consequence has a positive focus, this technique will prove less likely to evoke tantrums than withdrawal of privileges. For example, if Sarah whines about not wanting to do her homework but knows that she may not use the computer before completing homework, Sarah's mother might say, "If you do your homework right now, then you may use my computer."

SUMMARY

Child and adolescent noncompliance frustrates parents and disrupts the family system. Although occasional tantrums are normal for young children, these behaviors can escalate to problematic levels if left unchecked. Your reactions to your children's noncompliance and tantrums greatly affect their development of emotion-regulation skills. Through consistent discipline, attention to desirable behavior, and maintenance of positive relationships, children learn to express their autonomy appropriately, negotiate disagreement, and communicate their thoughts and feelings with others.

WHERE TO FIND OUT MORE

Books

Clark, L. (2005). *SOS! Help for parents* (3rd ed.). Bowling Green, KY: Parents Press.

Faber, A. & Mazlish, E. (2004). *How to talk so kids will listen and listen so kids will talk.* New York: HarperCollins.

Faber, A. & Mazlish, E. (2005). *How to talk so teens will listen and listen so teens will talk.* New York: HarperCollins.

Websites

Nemours Foundation: KidsHealth for Parents (2005). *Temper tantrums.* http://kidshealth.org/parent/emotions/behavior/tantrums.html.

Nemours Foundation: KidsHealth for Parents (2005). Teaching your child self-control. http://kidshealth.org/parent/emotions/behavior/self_control.html.

CHAPTER 15

Traveling with Children

Sanford M. Portnoy and Joan F. Portnoy

Tom and Cathy stand on a Metro platform in our nation's capital at the end of a day of sightseeing with their two children, aged 2 and 4. The mid-July temperature has reached the high 80s, as they wait for the train to take them back to their hotel. The long day full of sightseeing has included the Air and Space Museum, the Museum of Natural History, the Washington Monument and Lincoln Memorial, lunch at McDonald's, and ice cream in the afternoon: a day of wondrous discovery. As they await their train, Tom turns to Cathy and irritably growls, "I'm not having a very good time, you know!" Cathy responds angrily, "Neither am I, and you're not doing much to help!

As evening falls, Fred and Frieda have finished a full day of touring the sights of San Francisco with their two children who are, purely by coincidence, aged 2 and 4. They have driven out to Sausalito for lunch, toured Muir Woods across the Golden Gate Bridge from the city, and taken in the sights and sounds of Fisherman's Wharf. Having finished dinner, they head back to the hotel in a rather unusual way. Fred and Frieda are each pushing a child in a stroller (although Bruno, the 4-year-old, has been mostly out of a stroller for years). Even more unusual, Fred and Frieda are running! Fred suddenly makes a sharp right into a side street as Frieda continues straight ahead. The kids are screaming with delight, urging their respective pushers to go faster. It's a stroller race to see who can get back to the hotel first: a fun end to a fun day.

To put our cards on the table, we are Tom and Cathy. But we are also Fred and Frieda. Both of the scenarios just presented are quite real. We have had wonderfully successful trips with our children across all ages. And we have had a few pretty awful ones. Following our disaster in D.C., we began to research successful versus unsuccessful travel with children and eventually wrote the first family travel book. We want to share what we have learned and experienced since, with you.

Traveling well with children of any age involves observing and putting into practice a few basic principles.

KNOW WHAT YOU WANT TO GET OUT OF YOUR TRIP

A trip to the beach is great if you want rest and relaxation, but it's the wrong trip to take if you crave excitement or a physical adventure. Touring cities can provide an exotic experience (depending on the city), culture, educational enrichment, or some of each. Making the decision about what your goals are becomes a bit more complicated when you tote the tots because you need to consider everyone's needs. How to do that?

Think about what has gone on in your family's life of late. If you have just moved or changed jobs, you will likely feel a bit more stressed than usual and find yourself in the process of making adjustments. You may need a vacation that simply allows you to chill out. The same holds true for the kids. Have any significant changes in their lives occurred that necessitate some time to kick back? If so, this would seem the wrong time for the hectic pace of visits to foreign cities, and the perfect time for a beach cottage or an all-inclusive resort (i.e., the kind where nice attentive people keep asking you if you would like anything to eat while you lounge by the pool?).

On the other hand, if you have felt closed in near the end of a snowy winter or if your life has felt a bit tedious for any reason, then something a bit more challenging or adventurous might provide just what the doctor ordered. Go ahead and try your hand at foreign languages and customs, hike the Grand Canyon, or spend a week at a dude ranch.

Remember that any trip can bring family togetherness that potentially leads to a sense of unity or to family growth. But this happens in different ways. Just spending time relaxing with each other is different from learning together, and different from the exhilaration of conquering new physical challenges. All can be good. Just know what you want for your clan.

ACCOUNT FOR YOUR CHILDREN'S AGES AND WHAT THEY CAN DO

Toddlers have short attention spans and little legs. Activities that require sustained concentration or patience, such as museums or fine-dining restaurants, will present a challenge. This does not mean that you have to rule them out, but it does require thoughtfulness and creativity about how you engage them. We will discuss this in more detail a bit later.

As children come of school age, their sense of the world broadens and their awareness of others expands. Visiting places that strike them as different or unique will have more meaning and increase their tolerance for new experiences, leading to fewer frustrations with customs and behaviors they don't understand. Children at this age also begin to take pride in newfound abilities. They are more likely to enjoy visiting foreign capitals and physically demanding trips, although you will still need to make adjustments based on your children's abilities.

By middle childhood, physical capabilities have expanded, so that trips demanding stamina become more feasible, whether they involve hiking, camping, or strenuous city touring. Children of this developmental era also begin to experience a sense of self and a desire to establish relationships outside the family. Travel becomes an opportunity to broaden that sense of self, so that newly experienced routines and cultural differences become incorporated more easily. Children at this age can also contribute more to family vacations, both in the planning stages and during the trip.

Adolescence brings individuality and the establishment of primary connections outside the family. Your teenager may decline to go on a family trip at all. On the other hand, teens can become wonderful companions, able to fully engage the travel experience in every way. The key to travel success with this age group is to be flexible and allow your teens some time to pursue their own interests. Some Caribbean resorts, for instance, offer separate teen programs. When it feels safe, allow some time for your adolescent to go off on a separate exploration excursion. Accounting for developmental needs, abilities, and flexibility often provides the keys to successful family trips.

PLAN YOUR TRIP SMARTLY

Some trips require more planning than others. Renting a beach cottage for the week and relaxing on the sand seems a simple matter. But even here, anticipating your children's needs becomes important. Find out what activities are available nearby for those times when your children feel bored with the beach, or when weather turns cold and rainy. Know your kids' tolerance for quiet and restful times and when they will likely need a chance to move around and be entertained. Miniature golf courses, climbable sand dunes, or bike trails might prove just the thing; so know what opportunities exist near your planned destination.

A touring trip involves even more challenges. You will want to make sure that you don't overestimate how much distance you can cover by car in a day, how many ruins the little ones can tolerate without turning your trip into one, or for how long you can successfully negotiate the Louvre during one visit.

Once you have decided the type of trip you want to take, have chosen your location, and have researched the sights and activities available and desired, sit down with the kids and discuss it. This makes them feel a part of the process and helps them to develop some anticipation for the coming experience. Then plan your itinerary so that it allows for Timmy's unexpected car sickness on the way to the Grand Canyon, takes into account your family's eating schedule and preferences, and anticipates that the first thing your toddler will want after a 7-hour plane ride is a dip in the swimming pool at the hotel.

On the Road

Car travel can provide the most relaxed form of family travel, and it can also be the most disastrous. Nothing will turn a potentially wonderful vacation into a nightmare quicker than *too much driving at one time!* Make sure you carefully research driving times and distances before you leave home. Then plan to drive just a little bit less in a given day than you think you and your kids can handle.

Give the children little jobs to do to help you get ready. It gives them a sense of involvement and anticipation. Even toddlers can take on simple tasks, like choosing their favorite stuffed animal to take in the car, and putting it with the luggage.

As the day of departure approaches, try to create as little tension as possible for both yourselves and the kids. Pack early—preferably a day or two early—so that the bags can sit by the door ready to go, or, even better, go in the car the night before. Make a list of those items you cannot pack until the last minute (e.g., the stuffed animal your child sleeps with every night) and consult the list last thing before you leave the house.

Part of your research about the trip should include what sights and attractions along the way can provide for a needed break from the tedium of the car and inject a little energy into flagging spirits. Something as simple as stopping at a playground or a planned picnic along a river bank can prove sufficient to keep your spirits on course. Even those attractions that sound silly like "the world's biggest . . . (fill in the blank)" do help. We once happened across a pretzel factory while driving through Pennsylvania Dutch Country when our kids were quite young. Not only did it give them a much needed break; we actually found it fascinating. You never know what you may discover!

A few other rules of the road:

- Try not to put two long driving days back to back. You really want to avoid the killer, "drive, eat, sleep" syndrome.
- Instead of using your breaks to sit at a fast-food restaurant, do something physical. Find a playground. Use the Frisbee you have brought just for this occasion. Buy food at a deli or supermarket and have a picnic.
- Don't arrive at night. You will feel hurried to bring in the luggage, grab dinner, and then quickly get to bed. This is not a recipe for the kids to wind down so that they *can* sleep. If, on the other hand, you stop in mid-late afternoon and the kids have some time to take a dip in the motel pool, or flop in the room and watch TV before dinner, your evening routine may go more smoothly.
- Adapt if things are not going well. If, on the third day of your driving tour of the West Coast, you realize that you are not having fun, change something! First, look at your itinerary. Trying to pack too much in is the most common mistake in family travel, especially when going by car. Decide whether you ought to stop at that amusement park you read about, or at a book or toy store to add something new to the armamentarium. If some minor change won't do it, you may have to swallow hard and make the *big decision!*
- Cut something out of the itinerary. As hard as that may feel at the time, it can slow your pace and save both your trip and your blood pressure.

In the Air

If your trip involves air travel, you will want to know which airlines fly to your destination, whether some flight times will accommodate your family's needs better than others, and of course, which fares will suit you best. But a couple of other questions can prove at least as important, if not more so.

First, will you have to change planes en route? There are pros and cons here. On a very long flight of, say, 6 hours or more, it may prove beneficial to break it up and have some time to exercise those large muscles in an airport terminal. On the other hand, most people prefer to get to their destination more quickly and thus prefer nonstop flights. Just remember that if you do not want to stop, then what you indeed want is a *nonstop* flight. A *direct* flight, on the other hand, simply means that the plane you leave on will take you to your destination. But it may stop along the way to discharge and pick up passengers. One absolutely critical point: if you do change planes, schedule your flights *farther apart than you might if you were traveling without the kids.* While we mentioned the benefit of exercising those large muscles in the terminal, some of those large muscles are in small legs. The last thing you want is to race through a terminal to catch your connecting flight, with the kids struggling to keep up and the tension mounting.

You should also plan to arrive at the airport earlier than you would when traveling without the kids. Early arrival allows for a slower, less frenzied pace; and as we all know, airports seem the center of the frenzy universe amid potential weather and security complications. It will also help for parents to split up the chores. One of you can check baggage while the other supervises getting drinks or handles restroom stops. Alternate responsibility for child management during the flight as well. Give each other some breaks to read or look out the window. Or, decide which of you will have responsibility for which children during the flight.

If you will need to have your infant's formula or food warmed up, let the flight attendant know as soon as you board. This would also be a good time to ask for blankets and pillows. These are particularly useful on flights long enough to show in-flight movies. These serve a double purpose. Movies can provide an entertaining diversion for older kids (or alternatively, your own movies brought from home to view on a portable player or laptop computer), but they also help with the younger ones in a different way. When the movie comes on, passengers usually pull down the window shades and the flight becomes quieter. This creates a great chance for the tiny tots to catch 40 winks. Hence, have the pillows and blankets at the ready.

Try to have a variety of activities on board, and space them out so that the kids don't become bored or restless quickly. Reading stories, watching movies, playing games, and even working on simple art projects offer different sorts of diversion. When junior gets tired of one type of activity, switch to something that calls on a different skill set or a different interest. On flights of several hours or more, get the kids up to stroll the aisles every once in a while. There are also stretching exercises that you can do together while seated. Some airlines have brochures that describe them. Finally, pack some snacks or simple meals. Snacking both satisfies hunger and provides another in-flight activity.

TAKE THE RIGHT STUFF

Assembling the right assortment of clothing, food, toys, and activities is the final step to preparing a successful family trip.

If you are traveling with infants or younger children, it is smart to bring a change of clothes in case of spills or other accidents. Make sure to keep these readily accessible. Have them in your carry-on bag when flying. For car trips, pack them at the top of a suitcase that should be on top of the other bags in the trunk or back of the minivan.

Chewing gum, raisins, or hard candy, and baby bottles often help during takeoffs and landings when you are flying. Air pressure changes can block up the ears. Sucking, chewing, and swallowing can help. Check with your pediatrician about medicines to carry along if your child tends toward nasal congestion, blocked ears, or upset stomachs.

Take along those special objects that give your children a feeling of home, like their favorite stuffed animals, baby blankets, and some favorite bedtime books. These will all help your children to get to sleep in new surroundings or can be pulled out when your child feels fragile or overtired.

Have an assortment of toys, books, and activities at the ready to keep children entertained, not only in the plane or car but in restaurants, while standing in long lines, and other slow-moving situations. Keep these items relatively small for easy packing, and keep them in a bag or backpack for easy portability. Portable electronic devices that can play movies or cartoons can prove a godsend. Music and story CDs for the car can make the trip move by smoothly. Children's music can provide "sing-a-longs" for the whole family. As the children get older, you may share the same taste in some CDs, but when parents don't appreciate their children's music, headphones save the day.

Have that backpack or bag of activities with you for static times, but also bring along your imagination for spontaneous games that don't require props. Find ways to incorporate children into adult activities. For example, when our children were young, we would pick them up and bring them very close to an impressionist painting so that everything looked like blobs or dots of paint. Then we would slowly move backwards until, like magic, those blobs would turn into a person, a boat, or something else recognizable. The kids loved this game, even when they were very young! Make a family tradition out of eating snacks in museum restaurants and comparing them as a way to recharge your children's interest in the museum. Standing in a long line to get into an amusement park ride can prove brutal if your only strategy involves standing still quietly. Play old classic games such as "20 Questions," "I Spy," or "Going on a Picnic." Adjust the difficulty of these games depending on your children's ages. For example, pick big and easy to see objects when playing I Spy with your young children. With our teenage children, we played more sophisticated word games that made car trips whiz by when the scenery became dull and they tired of other activities.

In a restaurant or a long line, break up the monotony for children by taking them out of the situation briefly for a quick stroll or to go look at the fish tank at the front of the seafood restaurant. Sometimes your teenage child (who also gets restless) will jump at the chance to take a younger sibling out of that long line to sit on the grass and play with small toy cars or read a book.

Always have some staples to get you by, such as granola bars, dried fruit, trail mix, and juice boxes. Children often get the munchies in a car or on the plane apart from meal time. At times, your children simply won't eat restaurant food, and peanut butter crackers and a juice box will save the day. Have adhesive bandages and antiseptic lotion available for taking care of the little cuts and scrapes that are bound to occur at the most inconvenient times.

Most importantly, bring along your sense of humor, your most flexible frame of mind, and sense of adventure.

SUMMARY

Things will not always go as planned on family vacations but those things sometimes make the best memories, like the pigeon on Lincoln's head that delights your child at the Lincoln Memorial while she pays no attention to the monument itself. Enjoy the trip, and the whole family will grow together as a result, reliving the adventures over and over again into adulthood.

WHERE TO FIND OUT MORE

Books

Jeffrey, N. (1996). *Adventuring with children: An inspirational guide to world travel and the outdoors.* Avalon House Travel Series.

Kaufman, E. (2007). *The travel mom's ultimate book of family travel: Planning, surviving, and enjoying your vacation together.* (Compact Disc). New York: Random House.

Lanigan, C. (2002). *Travel with children.* Oakland, CA; Lonely Planet Publishing.

Meyers, C.T. (1995). *The family travel guide: An inspiring collection of family-friendly vacations.* Berkeley: Carousel Press.

Meyers, C.T. (1992). *Miles of smiles.* Berkeley: Carousel Press.

Portnoy, S. & Portnoy, J. (1995). *How to take great trips with your kids.* Boston: The Harvard Common Press.

Rivoli, S. (2007). *Travels with baby: The ultimate guide for planning trips with babies, toddlers, and preschool-age children.* Berkeley: Travels with Baby Books.

CHAPTER 16

Helping Your Child Cope with Divorce

Robin M. Deutsch

Eleven-year-old Evan's parents, Sarah and John, separated, and Evan was residing primarily with his mother. His father had taken a new job in another part of the state, and Evan saw his father on alternate weekends. Evan's mother worried about Evan's adjustment, and she tried to compensate for his loss by letting up on the usual routine, structure, and rules in the house. In addition, she felt very sad and found it difficult at times to enforce rules. John, on the other hand, felt very angry about the divorce and blamed Sarah. When John and Sarah spoke, they tended to argue and Evan often heard them yelling at each other. When Evan spent time with his father, John often asked Evan about his mother's activities, and also criticized her for letting Evan get away with so much. When the school called to let Sarah know that Evan seemed more distracted and seemed to have difficulty following the rules, Sarah sought help from a psychologist. The psychologist suggested that John may also want to meet to discuss how they might best parent Evan, given their different parenting styles. Sarah and John decided to meet separately with the psychologist. After meeting with Sarah for a few sessions, she then met with John and was able to help each of them understand the impact of divorce on Evan and how they might best meet his needs.

Divorce is very painful for most parents. They often experience feelings of sadness, anger, betrayal, and disappointment, and they worry about the future. The children also often experience these difficult feelings. The extent to which parents can focus on their children's needs directly influences a child's adjustment to the divorce. While most parents put their children in the forefront in those moments, it will often prove hard to keep them front and center as parents try to figure out how their lives will change, begin to rethink themselves as divorced parents, and assess what their futures will hold. This chapter will help you focus on the things you want to think about and do to help your children cope with your divorce.

WHAT MATTERS TO CHILDREN

Sarah and John provide an example of what we want to avoid for our children. We know that all children, regardless of age, need certain things from their parents—whether the family remains intact or the parents have divorced. What matters to children is avoiding exposure to conflict between their parents, as it undermines their sense of security and stability. Conflict can mean a silent, tense, disengaged standoff, or it can mean yelling, swearing, and screaming. The research on the effects of divorce on children indicates that two main factors predict children's adjustment to divorce. One of them is conflict between parents. The research concludes that, to the extent that children experience conflict between their parents, the children's adjustment fares worse. For all children, conflict threatens their sense of security and safety. It also results in confusion as children try to figure out what is true and what is false. When the conflict seems to focus on them, they will feel prone to blame themselves. Their perceptions and interpretations become challenged and confused as the two people whom they love and trust most in the world see the world so differently and, as children, they lack the skills to negotiate or resolve those differences. Finding ways to shift your parenting relationship to a business-style relationship focused on rearing your children poses a major challenge for parents as they navigate a post-divorce relationship.

The second major thing that children need from their parents involves good enough parenting after the separation. Not uncommonly, parents become so consumed with their own issues, the stress they feel, and the need to recreate their identities and lives moving forward, that their usual parenting practices shift and may not work as effectively as before. They may not act as attentively, and they may not parent as well as they previously did. Sometimes, parents become more permissive because they feel guilty, or believe that doing so compensates for the losses their children experience, or simply because they do not have the energy or focus to discipline their children as consistently as needed. Other parents believe that they must counteract permissive parenting and they become too authoritarian with their children, not allowing the child to have a voice in decision making. Neither of these parenting styles teaches children how to make choices or decisions, nor do they encourage an understanding of responsibility or consequences.

What does make a difference for children after their parents divorce? Parental warmth, involvement, appropriate expectations, and confident authoritative parenting all exert positive influence. That kind of parenting involves loving, but firm and consistent limit-setting, taking the child's views into account and being willing to explain the rules and limits. Using the *Three Little Bears* as an analogy, authoritarian parenting involves too much control, permissive parenting involves too little control, and authoritative parenting is just right. No matter the age of our children, we want to teach them to function independently. Explaining the necessity for a rule or limit teaches children how to assess situations and make choices and decisions.

It matters to all children that they have continued love and support from both of their parents regardless of how much they see them. Ideally, they will feel that both of their parents remain available for them and that he or she, the child, is most important. That means children feel that their parents tune in to them emotionally, understand their needs, and are willing try to meet those needs.

Consistency and parental involvement also matters to children. Remaining responsive to your children's activities and schedules helps your children to feel important. And, unless one parent behaves in an abusive or dangerous manner, maintaining contact with both parents is very important for children's short- and long-term adjustment. Having a good relationship with both parents matters to all children. To have a good relationship with a parent, the child needs to feel known and understood by both parents, and to have their parent involved in their activities, needs, and life.

Another thing that matters to all children of separation or divorce is being able to make a smooth transition between their parents, with their parents' help. When parents cannot adequately communicate about their children, or the children feel that they must cross the great divide between the two homes by themselves, they miss the sense of feeling "held" by both of their parents and expend energy to keep the details of life with each parent in separate compartments. To the extent that parents can communicate about their children's needs, schedules, and activities, and the children are not put in the position of managing that communication or of being stuck the middle by transmitting important information, they adjust better.

HOW DO I TELL MY CHILD ABOUT THE SEPARATION/DIVORCE?

When parents decide to separate and/or divorce, one of the most sobering thoughts focuses on how they will tell their children. They worry about how their children will react in the moment and what will happen to them in the long term. All children need to know about the separation/divorce, and ideally that communication should come from both parents. If it seems impossible to avoid conflict and to stay focused on the children's needs without blaming the other parent, then parents should not attempt to tell their children together. No matter the age of the children, they need to know what arrangements have been made (i.e., where each parent will live and when the children will see each of their parents). They also need to know that both of their parents will always love them and that, although as parents you will not live together, you will always be there as their mom and dad because parents do not get divorced from their children. This explanation should be simple, and should not include the personal detail and circumstances of the decision to separate.

What parents tell their children will change, depending on the children's ages and developmental level. The older the children, the more detail they need and the more questions they will ask. Timing of telling your child also relates to age. Younger children should hear about the divorce close to the time that one parent moves out. All children need to know the details of who will go where and when, and when they will see each parent. They will want to know what it means for their daily life. Will they stay in the same home, go to the same school, live in the same neighborhood? If a move to a new home looms, it can prove helpful to bring your children to visit the new home and allow them to choose some of the things in the rooms where they will sleep (e.g., picking out new bed sheets, choosing toys to bring to the new home, choosing posters or pictures for the walls). Ideally, the non-relocating parent will also visit the new home, so that the children know that their other parent knows where they will relocate. Most children will have more questions over time, and they need to know that you and your former spouse or partner will each remain available to answer those questions. No matter their ages, most children have fantasies that their parents will get back together. Some children may even construct events or situations to try to get their parents together. Parents need to be very clear with their children that, even if the family does some things together, you will not get back together as a couple.

PLANNING PARENTING TIME

Parenting plans will vary depending on the age and developmental level of the children. Infants and toddlers need frequent contact with each parent. Depending on how involved each parent was before the separation, they may each see the children every day or on alternate days. In order for the relationship to develop closely, where children can continue to regard each parent as a trusted caretaker, each parent should try to stay involved in the children's care-taking routines. For infants and toddlers, communication between parents about children's sleep, eating, and toileting schedule, as well as any developmental changes and health issues remains critically important. Whether this happens via email, a parenting notebook that goes back and forth with the child, by telephone, or in person, information exchanged on these topics should occur at each transition.

Preschoolers need more social contact with peers, whether in play group, preschool, play dates, or at a neighborhood park. They do not need as frequent contact with each parent but, depending on the level of involvement each parent has previously had in child care, children generally do best if they do not spend more than 4 or 5 days apart from a parent. They also need their parents to communicate regularly about eating, sleeping, health, developmental changes, activities, and strategies for managing behavioral issues. School-aged children need the ability to maintain their chosen activities with both practical and emotional support from both of their parents. Whether sports, music lessons, art, theater, dance, or social play activities, they need both parents to support, share, and value attendance and practice. Many types of schedules work for school-aged children, and they can tolerate longer regular absences from the other parent. However, they do need their parents to communicate regularly about school, homework, activities, and health issues.

Adolescents need different considerations and a voice in planning the parenting schedule. It is critical for parents of adolescents to communicate about schedule changes, rules, and potential risks. Adolescents can easily fall through the cracks and engage in risky behaviors when the parents do not communicate closely about these issues.

For all children, a very clear and specific parenting plan works best. It should include all elements of who, what, where, and when: who picks up and drops off the children, where, when, and under what circumstances. Parenting plans generally need to evolve over time, based on the age, developmental level, and needs of the children. To avoid future conflict and to create assurance that parents will continue to see things through the eyes of their children, it is often helpful for parents to build in a protocol for making future changes to the parenting schedule.

HOW CAN I MAKE THINGS EASIER FOR MY CHILD?

There are certain things within your control that you should pay attention to and manage as you are going through your divorce, in order to make the transition easier for your children. The following are some suggestions:

- Communicate with your former spouse or partner, specifically when it comes to discussing your children. There are several benefits of effectively communicating about your children. First, when both parents have information about their children's activities, health status, sleeping and eating routines, developmental changes, behavioral issues, and school and friend issues, the level of trust between parents rises and keeps the children's interests in the forefront. Second, when their parents communicate well about them, children feel important and the focus of their parent's attention. Even if the parents do not get along, they can put other issues aside because of their love and devotion to their children. Third, children do not get caught in the middle, expected to manage the communication between their parents. When children must serve as the link between their parents, the information may not flow with complete accuracy, and the burden can result in anxiety for the children. When parents effectively communicate, important issues, experiences, risks, and behaviors do not go unattended, unheeded, or lost between homes.

- Separate your own disappointments about your marriage or relationship from your role as a parent and be sure to respect your former spouse or partner for his or her parenting role. This can prove difficult for parents who have very different parenting styles or for the parent who feels that his or her ex-spouse was not a good husband or wife. However, if your children see you behaving cordially and respectfully, hard as that might be to accomplish, they will gain comfort and confidence. Children who must worry about how their parents will behave when they encounter each other, or how to transition from one home to another, must expend their energy on those worries instead of on their own developmental tasks.

- Tolerate differences in parenting practices and values. Unless the other parent truly causes harm to your child because of abusive or neglectful parenting practices, know that you will do things differently and your child will not suffer damage. Children can adapt to different practices and values much better than they can adapt to conflict about those differences.

- Value what the other parent offers your children. When you married, you valued things about your spouse. That parent brings some of those things to your children. Your children will become fuller and have more experiences and exposures because you each offer different things. Your child should know that mommy or daddy can do different things with them or see things differently from each other, and can feel fortunate about that. When children believe that a parent does not value the other parent, they worry about the parts of themselves that may seem like their other parent. This can lead to confusion, compartmentalizing different parts of themselves, and poor self-esteem.

- Focus on your children's needs, and don't share your problems with your children. Your children cannot give you the support that you need, nor can they solve your problems. Find outside parenting groups or individual psychotherapy to help you become the best parent you can be and to find the assistance you may need to help you move into this new stage of your life.

WHEN TO SEEK PROFESSIONAL HELP

Divorce initially stresses the children. They need loving, firm, and consistent parenting, and enough contact with both of their parents. To the extent that some things in their life remain the same, they do better. Most children move through the first early years of divorce quite well. However, if your child's behavior changes for a few weeks and becomes more aggressive, more withdrawn, or excessively clingy, you may want to seek help from a mental health professional. And, if you notice that your child has become increasingly worried or sad, or if she has difficulty concentrating or sleeping, those also may signal a need for professional help. Some children fear expressing their feelings to their parents, not wanting to hurt or burden them. However, they may talk to other important people in their lives, such as extended family, teachers, coaches, neighbors, or clergy. Sometimes, school- or community-based groups which include other children whose parents have separated or divorced prove quite helpful. Psychotherapy for parents can also be helpful so that you, as the parent, can get help for your own issues in order to provide better emotional availability for your children. The key: your children need your support and attention and, with the appropriate help, have a very good chance of a good adjustment.

SUMMARY

Making life perfect or even normal for your children following a divorce or separation may prove impossible. However, you can help your children by keeping a focus on effective parenting. This means creating as secure and stable an environment as possible for your children, and keeping any negative comments about your ex-spouse or partner to a minimum. Remember, children cope best following divorce when each parent tries to help the child retain a good relationship with the other parent. Take your children's age-related needs into account and focus on helping them to feel loved without fear of divided loyalties.

WHERE TO FIND OUT MORE

Books

Emery, R.E. (2004). *The truth about children and divorce.* New York: Plume.
Lippincott, J.M. & Deutsch, R.M. (2005). *7 Things your teenager won't tell you.* New York: Ballantine.

Long, N. & Forehand, R.L. (2002). *Making divorce easier on your child: 50 Effective ways to help children adjust.* New York: Contemporary Books.

Ricci, I. (1997). *Mom's house, dad's house.* New York: Fireside.

Thayer, E. & Zimmerman, J. (2001). *The co-parenting survival guide: Letting go of conflict after a difficult divorce.* Oakland, CA: New Harbinger Publications.

Websites

HelpGuide.org

Children and Divorce: Helping your kids cope with the effects of separation and divorce
http://www.helpguide.org/mental/children_divorce.htm.

CHAPTER 17

Siblings in Stepfamilies

James H. Bray

Christy has been remarried for 7 months. Her husband Rick has two children from his previous marriage, and Christy has three kids of her own. Prior to their marriage, Christy and Rick lived together for 1 year. During that time, their children visited every once in a while and had few problems getting along. Since their marriage, however, Christy and Rick's children are on a more formal visiting schedule and spend more time with each other than they had previously. This has led to frequent disagreements and fighting. Rick's oldest son Ricky has been getting into trouble and exerting a negative influence on Christy's children. She and Rick have been arguing a lot lately about how to discipline their kids. Family conflict and stress is at an all-time high.

This scenario is not uncommon in newly formed stepfamilies. The process of integrating two different families with different histories, rules, and expectations for both the parents and children frequently triggers stress and conflict.

Stepfamilies have become increasingly commonplace due to the high rates of divorce, remarriage, and children born outside of marriage. Other names for stepfamilies include remarried families, blended families, or reconstituted families. Also, in many situations, couples live together without formal marriage. In all of these cases, stepfamilies are born out of loss, either due to the death of a parent or the loss of a marriage or prior relationship. Connections to the prior marriage and family vary, but have both direct and indirect effects on the resulting stepfamilies.

WHAT ARE THE EFFECTS OF STEPFAMILIES ON CHILDREN?

Children in stepfamilies have a higher risk of developing psychological problems, and they make use of mental health services more often than do children from first-marriage families. Given the added stress, changes, and complicated family makeup of remarried families, it is not surprising that children in stepfamilies may experience more psychological difficulties than do children from other types of families. The link between stepfamily relationships and the problems that trigger help-seeking may not be readily apparent in the beginning. However, in most cases, the interactions of members within the stepfamily can create or contribute to the child's problems. Solutions to these problems lie in understanding and changing stepfamily relationships.

Parenting and integrating children into a stepfamily is the most stressful aspect of life in a new family unit, both early after remarriage and even a decade into stepfamily life. This chapter discusses common issues that siblings in stepfamilies encounter and describes some potential solutions for dealing with these issues. Keep in mind that stepfamilies deal with different issues over time, and these challenges intersect with the developmental changes that children undergo through their lifespans. In addition, different issues come into play for families with young children compared with families including adolescents because of their varying developmental needs.

HOW DOES A STEPFAMILY INFLUENCE THE PARENT–CHILD RELATIONSHIP?

Parent–child relationships often change after a remarriage. An initial disruption often occurs during the early months after remarriage in the custodial parent–child relationship (i.e., when divorced parents split custody and one or both remarry), but this typically improves over time, and fewer differences occur between parent–child relationships in stepfamilies and first-marriage families. The remarriage of the custodial mother often proves more disruptive for preadolescent girls and may contribute to an increase in girls' behavior problems. Following divorce, school-aged girls often develop close relationships with their mothers, whereas boys typically develop more distant and conflicted maternal relationships. The remarriage of the mother interferes and disrupts this close bond between mother and daughter. For boys, the remarriage of the mother usually seems a neutral or positive event, because the boy has a male adult to relate to in the family. Fewer gender differences seem typical in parent–child relationships for adolescents in stepfamilies.

The stepparent–child relationship often seems characterized by more distance and negativity than do biological parent–child relationships, and these differences can persist for many years following the remarriage. This type of relationship seems the norm for stepparents and children. Stepparent–child relationships may also change after the remarriage, as both adults and children begin to view family members differently and new overt and covert expectations come into play. The Boyd family's experience of more conflict provides examples of such changes.

Many stepparents desire a close relationship with their stepchildren and expect that this closeness will develop quickly. However, if you are a stepparent, you must allow sufficient time for the relationship to develop and understand that this may take several years, rather than months. The expectation for instant love (or even liking) between siblings is unrealistic and may create undue strain and conflict in the relationship, especially among adolescents. It also appears that, even if the stepparent has lived with or known the children prior to the marriage, as in the case of the family at the start of the chapter, it still takes time to develop this relationship because the children view the new stepparent differently after the marriage. The stepfather is no longer mom's boyfriend—he now holds parental status, with a different set of expectations.

Assessing these relationships is necessary for understanding the child's problems because behavioral issues often develop in response to changes in these relationships, as happened with Ricky in the example at the start of the chapter. Children frequently want to know if the stepparent will replace their nonresidential parent, what might happen to them if their custodial parent died or left, or what the stepparent can do with and for them. Normalizing conflicts, providing reassurance, and exploring unrealistic expectations of family members can facilitate the children's adjustment and promote better sibling relationships.

TYPES OF SIBLINGS IN STEPFAMILIES

Three different types of sibling relationships exist in stepfamilies. These include full biological siblings, half-siblings, and stepsiblings. In the first case, children have the same biological parents. They usually enter a stepfamily because of divorce or the death of a parent. Half-siblings share one biological parent in common, whereas stepsiblings have no biological relationships to each other. A variety of sibling relationships can be present in a blended family, and matters may become even more complex if a stepfamily breaks up and the partners remarry yet again. In addition, siblings of all types may live primarily with one family and/or visit on a part-time basis. The complexity of these relationships means that stepfamilies vary considerably and that each family needs to consider its unique situation when dealing with sibling relationships. It can take longer for visiting siblings in stepfamilies to develop good relationships because they do not live together full time.

COMMON ISSUES IN INTEGRATING SIBLINGS IN STEPFAMILIES

Respect among Siblings

Respect involves a *feeling or attitude* of admiration and deference toward someone. One must earn respect, rather than demand it. Demanding that your and your new partner's children respect one another won't work, but setting reasonable expectations for certain behaviors in your family can help the children adjust to the new family makeup. As an alternative, requiring that siblings treat each other with *courtesy* affords a sensible way to behave toward others with politeness and consideration. Our research and clinical work has shown that having a family rule requiring everyone to treat each other with courtesy creates a positive atmosphere, setting the stage for good relationships.

Rule Setting

In most stepfamilies, different expectations for parenting and rules for the household exist from the start. Such expectations flow from the adults' families of origin, life experiences, prior relationships, and marriages. Most people regard their views as "normal" and "right," and they consciously and unconsciously develop expectations based on these views. It is critical that the adults in the stepfamily discuss their expectations for the children and come to a common set of explicit rules and expectations between themselves. *Compromise is the key to success,* as no *one* right way exists for all stepfamilies to function. Making a set of three to five basic rules and specifying the consequences for violating the rules is an important first step in developing common ground in parenting. Once you and your spouse or partner have agreed upon the house rules, explain them carefully to the children and enforce them in a consistent manner. In the case of adolescents, you may need to negotiate the rules in consideration of your teenagers' developing independence.

For example, in some families, children and adults eat their meals in front of the TV and in other informal settings. Other families take their meals together at a dining room table. Neither pattern is "right"—they just differ. Compromise and allow some flexibility, especially when stepsiblings visit.

Generally speaking, visiting siblings should also expect to follow the rules of the house. Most children can show flexibility and can adapt to changing expectations. However, it is essential that you explain the rules carefully to the visiting children. In addition, during the first day of visitation, the children may need some gentle reminders (in an age-appropriate manner) about the rules of the house. Posting the list in an obvious place, such as a refrigerator door or bulletin board can serve as a reminder about the rules and consequences.

Loyalty Conflicts

A client came for a consultation because of conflicts with her new husband over their children. She said, "When he criticizes my daughter, I just see RED and go on the attack—it even happens when his daughter argues with my daughter." She explained that her previous husband had behaved abusively to her and their daughter, and any hint of that caused a strong emotional reaction in her. Two issues contribute to her reaction: loyalty conflicts and unresolved emotional events, which we call "ghosts at the table."

Common issues for siblings in stepfamilies center on loyalty conflicts. A sense of loyalty to one's family probably has its roots in our biological connections and need for survival. Children usually feel a loyalty to each biological parent, because they are half that parent. Criticism of their biological parent will trigger a natural defensive response because, in a sense, they are defending themselves. Biological parents feel a sense of protectiveness and will typically quickly defend their biological children from criticism or threats from others—that includes stepsiblings and stepparents. While this qualifies as a "normal" response, it also represents an issue that parents should address openly to help siblings integrate into a stepfamily. Avoiding criticism of a biological parent in front of the children will also avoid triggering threatened loyalty feelings and defensiveness. Over time, as a good relationship develops between siblings, stepsiblings, and stepparents, fewer loyalty conflicts occur because a sense of loyalty to the stepfamily usually develops.

Unresolved Issues: Ghosts at the Table

Strong emotional reactions to situations that don't seem to warrant that level of emotionality usually signal an unresolved anger, hurt, or wound from a previous family experience.

For example, Mark's mother and stepfather brought him to a psychologist for evaluation after he suddenly lashed out and hit his younger stepbrother, Bobby. After talking with the family, it became apparent that Mark felt that Bobby had made fun of him because his father did not come to get him for a scheduled visitation. Bobbie said that he simply asked Mark a question—"Mark, why are you here? I thought you were going to visit your dad this weekend?" Bobby said that Mark yelled at him and then punched him. Mark initially denied this, but then admitted that he "over-reacted" because he felt so upset that his dad "ditched him again." Mark felt that his father had frequently made promises to spend time with him and do things for him, even before the divorce, but did not keep his promises. Mark had especially looked forward to an event this weekend. Mark looked at his mother and stepfather and said, "and I hate it when you make your snide comments about my dad when he does not show up—it just makes things worse." Mark's sense of abandonment and hurt had led him to act out and negatively affected his relationship with his stepbrother. Mark later apologized to Bobbie for punching him. Bobbie said he understood because his dad had done that to him a few times, and it really made him feel sad and hurt. This revelation seemed to bring all of the family members together and created greater empathy for Mark and his situation.

Age Differences

Many families have broad age ranges of children, and this becomes an issue when stepfamilies come together, because an oldest child may become a middle child or the "baby" of the family after he or she is used to being leader of the pack. Older children and adolescents may model problem behaviors to younger children who want to emulate their older brother or sister. Creating positive sibling relationships can pose a challenge in stepfamilies in which children are far apart in age, with varying interests and histories.

Remember that each child has his or her own unique strengths and interests. It is particularly important in stepfamilies to avoid comparing one child to another. Comparisons invoke strong loyalty conflicts and arguments. Use your children's differences in interests and strengths as a way to expose them to new opportunities and experiences. For example, in Josh's family, he and his kids had often engaged in sports and outdoor activities, while Alicia's family had no exposure to camping and tended more toward quiet activities such as reading and "surfing the net." Forcing Alicia and her kids into a wilderness camping adventure created significant conflict, particularly when Josh's kids started making fun of Alicia's kid's for being city nerds. After the parents stepped in, they used this as an opportunity for Josh's kids to show Alicia's kids about camping, while Alicia's kids showed Josh's children how to use the Internet to improve their schoolwork.

Space for Each Sibling

Remarriage of parents often brings changes in the physical households for both adults and children. When a household originally shared by two or three people is now shared by five or six, thoughtful change becomes a necessity. Moving to a larger home is often a good idea, if the family can afford it. A new house creates a fresh start for the family, eliminating feelings of invasion or loss. However, relocation may not be financially possible, and the family may have to move in together in one party's home. The key to integrating siblings is to make your home a home for all of the children, even if they just visit on the weekends. If siblings have to share rooms, then it becomes important that each person has some personal area in which to keep his or her things and have that space remain off-limits to the other siblings. This is essential, even when siblings visit only on the weekends and holidays.

Appropriate Boundaries

Appropriate boundaries around dress and romantic relationships need careful consideration. The passion of a new marriage and open displays of affection often feel upsetting to adolescents who do not like to think of their parents as sexual. In addition, in households where all males or females reside, family members may feel very comfortable wearing few clothes or being nude in the home. However, this may not feel as appropriate once different genders begin living in the same house. It is important to discuss this issue openly. Develop household rules about clothing, and move some expressions of affection behind closed doors if necessary.

Nonbiological siblings may have prior feelings or develop feelings for one of their stepsiblings. At one level, this may not seem a challenging issue, since the adolescents only relationship comes via their parents' marriage. However, these types of feelings and relationships warrant open discussion and discouragement because of living arrangements. For example, erotic feelings between adolescent stepsiblings in such families can add considerable tension to the household.

SUMMARY

While it may prove challenging to integrate siblings in stepfamilies, these relationships have many potential benefits. For only children who have longed to have a sibling, stepsiblings can serve this purpose. Children close in age can develop close relationships, and they may become best of friends, helping each other adjust to the changes in creating a successful stepfamily. As previously mentioned, siblings may have different talents, skills, and interests, and these can help broaden the exposure of siblings to new and different possibilities. Finally, research indicates that stepsibling relationships often have less negativity, but similar amounts of positivity, when compared with full and half-sibling relationships. So, they may serve as a good role model for other sibling relationships in stepfamilies.

WHERE TO FIND OUT MORE

Books

Block, J.D. & Bartel, S. (2001). *Stepliving for teens: Getting along with stepparents, parents, and siblings (plugged in)*. New York: Price, Stern, and Sloan.

Bray, J.H., & Kelly, J. (1998). *StepFamilies: Love, marriage, and parenting in the first decade.* New York: Broadway Books.

Philips, S. (2005). *Stepchildren speak: 10 Grown-up stepchildren teach us how to build healthy stepfamilies.* Vancouver, WA: ANWY Publications.

Visher, E. B., & Visher, J. S. (1991). *How to win as a stepfamily.* New York: Brunner-Routledge.

Websites

Stepfamily Network
   http://www.stepfamily.net/
The National Stepfamily Resource Center
   http://www.stepfamilies.info/

CHAPTER 18

Nontraditional Families

Nathan D. Doty and Anne E. Kazak

Stacey is cared for by her grandmother. She doesn't know what to say when her classmates at school ask about her mom and dad.

Timothy has two dads. He loves his dads, but sometimes wonders about his birth-mother.

Families, like the people in them, are diverse. There is no right or wrong way to build a family. Nonetheless, children growing up in nontraditional family structures may encounter unique and sometimes difficult questions. This chapter provides tips for helping children cope with the challenges often faced by nontraditional families.

WHAT DEFINES A NONTRADITIONAL FAMILY?

According to the U.S. Census Bureau, in 2007, only 41% of all American families consisted of a married heterosexual couple raising their own children, thus making the so-called "traditional" American family not so typical. Children may grow up in a wide variety of family structures. Some of the most common types of nontraditional families include:

- *Single-parent families.* Single parents head up to 28% of all households with children under the age of 18. Although divorce triggers the majority of single-parent families, growing numbers of men and women have chosen to become single parents through adoption, uncommitted relationships, or reproductive technology.
- *Kinship caregiver families.* Extended family members sometimes take on child rearing duties when biological parents have died or can no longer provide care. In the United States, extended family members take full responsibility for rearing

approximately 3% of children, with grandparents heading up over half of these families.

- *Families with lesbian or gay parents.* Increasing numbers of children live in families with gay or lesbian parents. In the past, most of these children had been born into previous heterosexual marriages or relationships. Today, growing numbers of lesbians and gay men choose to have children, either as same-sex couples or single parents, through processes involving adoption, reproductive technology, or surrogacy. Broad estimates of the number of gay and lesbian parents in the United States range from 2 to 8 million, with nearly one-quarter of all same-gender couples rearing children.

Contemporary families take many forms, and research suggests that most Americans hold flexible definitions of family. Family can focus on immediate relations, but for many, family also means love, togetherness, and caring for those held dear. In 2005, a large-scale national survey found that only one-third of Americans defined family in the most traditional sense as "mother, father, and children," "wife, husband, and children," or "parents and children." With the growing diversity of family structures, it seems that most Americans agree, "love makes a family."

NONTRADITIONAL FAMILIES AND CHILD DEVELOPMENT

Do nontraditional family structures have any consistent or unique effects on children's development? What does the research tell us? In some cases, studies have found children from nontraditional family structures to have poorer mental and physical health than do children growing up with both biological parents. For example, children of single parents sometimes have lower self-esteem, poorer academic performance, and more behavior problems than do those in two-parent households. Similar studies have found increased rates of emotional, behavioral, and physical health problems among children reared by their grandparents. However, these problems may relate to social challenges, such as poverty and lack of support, that often affect nontraditional families. In recent studies taking into account these social challenges, family structure alone did not coincide with any differences in children's emotional, behavioral, academic, or social functioning. Recent studies have increasingly emphasized the strengths and resiliency of children in nontraditional families.

Public debate on the effects of gay and lesbian parenting on children remains somewhat contentious, with nearly half of all Americans opposing adoption by gays and lesbians. However, research comparing children of gay and lesbian parents with those of heterosexual parents consistently shows no differences in children's mental or physical health. Based on these findings, several major professional organizations, including the American Academy of Pediatrics and the American Psychological Association, have made public statements affirming that gay and lesbian parents can and do rear happy, healthy children.

Studies to date suggest that healthy child development occurs in a wide range of family structures. Strong evidence exists to show that communication and caring in a family are far more important than the family's structure or outward appearance.

NAVIGATING THE CHALLENGES OF
NONTRADITIONAL FAMILY LIFE

In addition to the normal stressors encountered by all families, children in nontraditional families may face additional challenges related to their unique family structures. Here, we discuss some of the most common concerns of nontraditional families, including those related to institutional barriers, lack of social support, experiences of discrimination, and children's perceptions of their families as "different."

Institutional Barriers

Policies in the United States generally apply to families made up of two married hetero-sexual parents and their biological or adoptive children. As a result, nontraditional families may confront a variety of legal or institutional barriers. For example, extended family members serving as primary caregivers may not be legally recognized for their cus-todial role, particularly since kinship caregiving arrangements often evolve informally. Gay or lesbian parents may also face particularly challenging legal obstacles. Although same-sex marriages and civil unions have gained recognition at the state level in some parts of the United States, many gay and lesbian parents simply cannot legally form a family. The lack of widespread legal recognition for same-sex couples creates ripple effects that undermine parental rights. Gay and lesbian parents, for instance, cannot obtain joint or second-parent adoptions in many states, meaning that only one caregiver may have legal authority to act as the parent. Caregivers in nontraditional families may lack parental rights, including the ability to make decisions on behalf of the child, receive access to school or medical records, obtain family and medical work leave, access social services, and exercise custody or visitation rights. These barriers affect children of all ages by impairing a caregiver's ability to provide typical forms of stability, support, and decision-making.

Lack of Support

Some nontraditional families may struggle with diminished levels of support from outside the family. In particular, lone parents, who lack the daily support of a co-parent, may have difficulties obtaining much-needed emotional or practical assistance during times of stress. Similarly, families with gay or lesbian parents may experience reduced support from extended family members or neighbors, particularly if they do not accept the parents' sexuality. Without adequate social support, nontraditional families may have greater difficulty coping with daily strains or responding to family crises when they arise.

Experiences of Discrimination

Unfortunately, some children experience discrimination or prejudice as a result of their nontraditional family structures. In particular, children in single-parent families or those with gay or lesbian parents may face societal stigma associated with these groups. In addi-tion to institutional forms of discrimination that may deny nontraditional families rights and privileges, children may encounter personal discrimination, ranging from overt victimization to more covert discrimination in the form of persistent assumptions or

misunderstandings by people outside the family. These experiences, whether discrete events or more chronic strains, may trigger emotional reactions in children, including shame, fear, sadness, confusion, and anger.

Feeling Different

Even children who do not experience stigma related to their nontraditional family structure may still recognize that their families are different from most other families. For example, children of single or non-heterosexual parents may wonder what it might be like to have both a mother and a father. Similarly, adoptive children may face issues surrounding their knowledge, or lack of knowledge, about birth parents. Youth in kinship-care families may also become aware of unique challenges, such as the physical limitations of an elderly caregiver. Children's awareness of their family as "different" may become keenly felt during later childhood and adolescence, as they compare themselves to peers and attempt to develop personal and group identities. Support and validation from friends becomes increasingly important with age, and youth may feel isolated if they sense that others outside the family cannot relate to their experiences. Throughout the normal course of development, feeling "different" may lead to a wide variety of emotions, including sadness, worry, and frustration, self-consciousness, and pride.

BUILDING AND MAINTAINING SUCCESSFUL NONTRADITIONAL FAMILIES

Although the challenges faced by nontraditional families may be stressful and even over-whelming at times, family members play an essential role in helping children and adolescents to cope. The following suggestions can help build and maintain strong, healthy families capable of navigating the obstacles of nontraditional family life.

Recognizing and Addressing Legal or Institutional Barriers

Nontraditional families often experience a lack of fit with the policies and procedures of institutions such as schools, healthcare providers, and legal systems. Caregivers can avoid potential life stressors by becoming aware of and addressing potential pitfalls before they occur. In some cases, local and federal laws may provide parental rights through processes of adoption or guardianship. However, some families, such as those with gay or lesbian parents, may require the services of a private attorney or advocacy group who can help the family to navigate complex legal loopholes in order to establish some degree of protection. Caregivers in nontraditional families must remain especially vigilant to potential barriers, as too often, caregivers assume they have certain parental rights, only to find themselves unable to navigate social and legal institutions when crises arise.

Providing a Strong Family Structure

Children fare best in consistent and predictable home environments. As in all families, daily routines (e.g., dinner together, age-appropriate bedtimes) and family rituals (e.g., holiday celebrations) are essential in developing a sense of control and security,

especially during times of stress or crisis. Similarly, children benefit from clear boundaries and consistent limit-setting by caregivers. Although nontraditional families may look different from families headed by married or heterosexual couples, establishing clear boundaries and consistent routines remains essential in promoting healthy child development.

Developing Dependable Support Networks

Because nontraditional families may lack support from outside the family, they must pay special attention to developing and maintaining relationships that provide both emotional and practical assistance in times of need. Families who lack traditional ties with extended kin may create "families of choice," made up of close friends who are considered part of the family. In addition, both children and caregivers may benefit from regular contact with other nontraditional families who share the same strengths and challenges. Beyond personal relationships, it is also important that nontraditional families foster supportive relationships with professionals (e.g., teachers, doctors, dentists, mental health professionals) who understand and affirm the family's nontraditional structure.

Encouraging Open Communication

Children in nontraditional families benefit from frequent, open discussions about the family and its unique challenges. These conversations provide opportunities to allay concerns, problem-solve tough situations, and talk about the many different ways of being a family. It is also important that caregivers remain aware of their own attitudes and emotional reactions. A child's concerns about the family's differences may trigger strong parental emotions of guilt, sadness, or frustration that, if not recognized, may undermine the parent's ability to offer support. Finally, children need some degree of control over the information they choose to share with others. Caregivers can help by assisting children in finding developmentally appropriate ways of explaining the family, but should also understand that children may not want to share this information in all situations.

Developing a Coherent Family Story

All families develop stories to give meaning to particular events and to help in understanding past and future development. Forming a coherent "family story" is especially important for nontraditional families because the notions of family presented in media and popular culture may not fully apply. Parents play a key role in helping children to understand the family's history and appreciate its differences. Nontraditional family stories may include unique elements, such as information about how the child came to live with the family or stories of how friends eventually came to be viewed as members of the family. Younger children in particular may benefit from opportunities to learn about their families in creative ways, such as drawing a picture or creating a family map. Older children may need support in grappling with complex issues of family and individual identity. What to tell children about the family depends on their developmental stage, but sharing accurate facts about the family's history usually provides a good start.

SUMMARY

Family members play a central role in the lives of all children and adolescents, providing emotional and practical support as well as a context for growth and learning about themselves and the world. Nontraditional families draw upon the unique experiences of their members to create their own definitions of family. Although children reared in these families may face unique and sometimes challenging situations, the vast majority grow up to lead fulfilling and productive lives. Caring and supportive family relationships, no matter how defined, remain among the most important factors in helping young people cope with both traditional and not-so-traditional life stressors.

WHERE TO FIND OUT MORE

Books

Card, E. and Kelly, C.W. (1998). *New families, new finances: Money skills for today's nontraditional families.* New York: John Wiley & Sons.

Erera, P. (2002). *Family diversity: Continuity and change in the contemporary family.* Thousand Oaks, CA: Sage Publications, Inc.

Fox-Lee, K. and Fox-Lee, S. (2004). *What are parents?* Los Angeles: StoryTyme Publishing.

Lamb, M.E. (Ed.). (1999). *Parenting and child development in "nontraditional" families.* Mahwah, NJ: Lawrence Erlbaum Associates.

Parr, T. (2003). *The family book.* New York: Megan Tingley Books.

CHAPTER 19

Discussing Family Secrets with Your Child

Karen J. Saywitz and Anna S. Romanoff

You find your 8-year-old son crying at the family reunion. When you ask him what's wrong, he tells you that he and his 16-year-old cousin had talked about why they don't look anything alike. His cousin told him, "It's because you don't really belong to the family." Another cousin jumped in, adding that your son's biological parents abused drugs. You have never told your son that you had adopted him from foster care as an infant. Of course, your parents, siblings, and their older children knew this at the time. A casual conversation at a family reunion changed your son's perception of his identity and how he came to live with his family.

Parents often feel at a loss when it comes to deciding whether or not to include children in discussions of sensitive family matters. These can involve emerging issues, such as impending divorce or diagnosis of parental cancer, or past issues, such as adoption or conception by sperm donor. Some secrets are difficult to hide, suspected by children, and best handled with honesty. Some secrets may be best saved for when children are older or not disclosed at all during childhood.

If you have a family secret, and you decide to share it with your child, how should you go about it? How much information is too much? How can you tell your child in a developmentally sensitive fashion? How can you help your child understand without becoming overwhelmed?

WHY PARENTS KEEP SECRETS

Most family secrets involve events perceived as potentially embarrassing, shameful, humiliating, or painful: an untimely pregnancy, financial mismanagement, mental illness,

criminal history, alcohol or drug abuse, gambling, divorce, adoption, abuse, undisclosed paternity, or cause of death. Most parents want to shield their children from hurt, fear, worry, and upset; do not feel equipped to cope with their child's reaction; or want to forget the issue themselves to avoid evoking emotions that might interfere with their ability to function at an optimal level. A parent may find that saying, "Your father died in a car crash when you were a baby" feels a lot easier on everyone than saying, "He died from a drug overdose or suicide." Parents fear telling children at the wrong time or before children have developed the understanding and coping skills to manage the thoughts and feelings that may emerge. Parents worry that knowing the secret will harm the child psychologically, disrupt school performance or friendships, and cause excessive worry. If the secret has to do with the child, parents may fear that disclosing the secret will damage the child's self-image and confidence. For example, adopted children might assume that they were "given up" because there was something wrong with them. This feeling of inadequacy can lead children to fear abandonment or rejection by adoptive parents as well. If the secret involves parents, a child's sense of safety and security may seem at risk (e.g., impending divorce, mother's breast cancer, or father's job loss could increase worry over instability and continuity of care). Some parents fear that knowing the secret could lead children to reject them or become ostracized from their friends (e.g., an HIV-infected mother). Often, secrecy offers a sense of control and protection, avoids shame, and protects the family's public image. The less others know, the less vulnerable family members are to hurt, criticism, blame, or judgment.

WHAT SHOULD I CONSIDER WHEN DECIDING WHETHER TO DISCLOSE FAMILY SECRETS TO MY CHILD?

Before making the decision to tell your child about a family secret, you should address the following questions:

- *How long can you keep the secret? Has the moment of disclosure become inevitable or unavoidable?* Often, relatives and friends also know the secret. People who know or suspect may confuse the child or ask for verification at the most inopportune times, without the presence of supportive parents to help children integrate and interpret the information, correct inaccuracies, or cope with emerging reactions and questions.
- *Does your child suspect something already?* Children are highly attuned to their parents' emotions—keen observers of our facial expressions, intonation patterns, and nonverbal interactions. As children's cognitive abilities mature between the ages of 7 and 9, they become better able to take another's perspective, recognize contradictions, and draw more sophisticated inferences from what we don't say, as well as what we do say. Does the secret create a source on ongoing tension for people the child interacts with daily? If so, will the child likely suspect something "bad" is going on?
- *Has the secret required you to tell smaller lies to cover up or maintain secrecy and to ask others to do so as well?* To keep a secret, parents may intentionally block further information or evidence from reaching their children. Family communications

can become a confusing maze of concealment, silence, and camouflage. Deception can create family mistrust, shame, and guilt. Secrecy can generate feelings of exclusivity, loneliness, or alienation, leaving the family member who does not know the secret feeling powerless or disconnected from everyone else without knowing why.

- *What assumptions has your child made?* Ignoring painful realities can allow the issue to become even larger in children's minds, to the point at which their fears can become worse than the reality warrants. Unanswered questions foster misperceptions and unrealistic expectations. Children feel forced to make sense of the family narrative without the facts—with gaps, guesses, and assumptions based on immature logic and limited experience that lead to a distorted sense of reality, confusion, and anxiety.

- *How will your child react?* Past coping patterns provide a good place to start in predicting future behavior. In addition, children's reactions flow as a function of how much the news will change their own lives and relationships. Some secrets will not impact the child's daily life at all (e.g., grandfather died in a bar fight, rather than on the battlefield); others may impact a parent much more than the child (e.g., father learns his birth resulted from an extramarital affair; however, the child's longstanding relationship with the loving grandfather he has always known will not likely change). You can help your child adjust to the news by teaching resilience in the face of adversity; how to bounce back and how to calm down when upset. As distressing as the information may feel, it can prove a relief to finally fill in the missing blanks.

- *Are your fears founded? How much of the decision comes as a function of your inability to cope with the ramifications of the secret rather than your child's?* Adults need to examine and anticipate their own reactions; put their own support systems in place so that they can focus on their children's reactions rather than their own. For example, in the case of adoption, parents may need to address feelings of shame associated with infertility or their fear of children's desire to reconnect with birth families. Many times, avoidance increases rather than prevents anxiety. In studies of parents with a terminal illness or breast cancer, children's levels of anxiety related more to whether someone told them about the illness and to the quality of communication with their parents, than to the fact of the illness itself. Higher anxiety was linked to an inability to discuss the illness with the parents.

- *What are the costs of keeping the secret?* Children learn through imitation and internalization of role models. You need to consider what style of coping and problem solving you want your children to learn. A family culture of secrecy teaches the less said, the better. If we don't talk about it, it can be forgotten, denied, as if it never happened. This style of communication runs the risk of undermining family trust and intimacy. Children may continue to wonder whether they can they trust what parents say, undermining their ability to feel confident and secure in their knowledge when they face the outside world. In return, children may learn that it is acceptable for family members to lie to each other if a good reason exists (to protect someone's feelings). This will include children lying to their parents about anything they perceive will upset their parents to know (sexual advances by older brother's friend, feeling bullied at school, offers of drugs by peers).

- *What are the benefits of telling the secret?* Discussing the secret with your children can afford an opportunity to teach them something profound about overcoming adversity, confronting realities, taking risks, being resilient, and coping with stress. It can enhance closeness and deepen family relationships when parents have the attitude that "we will all get through this together." Telling children expresses the parent's trust in the child's ability to cope, and that increases the child's sense of self-confidence. In one study, mothers infected with HIV who told their children of their diagnosis reported achieving a greater sense of emotional intimacy with their child.

- *How do I know when my child is ready? Should I wait until my child asks me?* If children have received the message to avoid the topic, they will feel reluctant to raise issues they believe will upset you. It is best to disclose family secrets earlier rather than later, before a crisis ensues, when the news can be delivered in a thoughtful, planned manner, and you can stay attentive to your children's reactions and provide the needed follow-up.

FOLLOW THE PRINCIPLES OF OPEN COMMUNICATION AND EMPATHIC ATTUNEMENT

While every family situation has unique aspects and demands consideration on its own merits, generally psychological studies suggest that open, honest, sensitive communication between parents and children creates a gateway to healthy psychological development. Studies suggest that family-process variables, such as communicative openness, parental warmth, emotional sensitivity, nurturance, and involvement play a greater role in children's psychological development and well-being than do structural factors, such as whether they live in single- or two-parent families or whether parents are divorced. For example, adopted teens who grow up in families in which their adoption is an open topic (rather than a forbidden one), also report more trust of their parents, less alienation, and better overall family functioning.

Communication openness involves not only the information exchanged but also support of the feelings associated with the information. Feelings of support often become less about the content of the secret and more about empathic attunement; the sharing and supporting of related emotions within the family. Healthy adjustment to the new information depends on:

- The ability of parents to create a safe way for children to express their thoughts, questions, and feelings about the information without fear of repercussions (e.g., angering/hurting a parent)
- The sensitivity of parents to the child's reaction, which often involves parents putting their own concerns (e.g., reactions of extended family members) in perspective to focus on supporting the child

In general, parents promote healthy psychological adjustment by open, honest, non-defensive, emotionally attuned family dialogues on important issues in the child's and family's life.

HOW DO I DISCUSS FAMILY SECRETS WITH MY CHILD?

Children require different kinds of explanations at different stages of development.

Preschoolers

Young children younger than 5 to 7 years of age tend to focus on the here and now and the environment's ability to meet their needs for safety and security. They do not need to know every detail. They need basic, concrete information. (For example, if parents plan on divorcing, preschoolers will want to know where they will sleep or go to school, where each parent will live, when they will be with each parent. If someone has cancer, the basics can include the name of the cancer, the part of the body affected, how treatment will occur, and how all of this will affect their own lives.) Young children's anxiety is about whether the news will disrupt their daily routine, who will take care of them, and what to expect.

Preschoolers have difficulty viewing the world from perspectives other than their own, and in combination with their limited understanding of cause and effect, such children assume they have more responsibility, control, and power in a situation than they actually do. If the secret involves a problem the family has kept hidden, young children need to know they did not cause it, cannot cure it, and cannot control it.

Elementary School-aged Children

Older children will need more information. Between 7 and 11 years of age, the child's knowledge base expands rapidly along with the ability to draw accurate inferences and take the perspectives of others. School-aged children begin to anticipate long-term consequences to others as well as to themselves. They may become worried about inheriting family problems. Feelings of self-consciousness begin to emerge. They need help planning how to explain the news to friends, if that becomes necessary. Children in this age range begin to develop the thinking skills necessary to treat their own ideas, behaviors, and feelings as objects of analysis and discussion. These skills enable them to engage with parents in more complex conversations about the past and future; to begin to anticipate how they might feel about different scenarios; and to plan anxiety-reducing coping strategies to prepare for anticipated problems.

Adolescents

Teens focus heavily on separating from their parents and exploring their own autonomy and identities. If you are the parent of a teen, you will need to walk a fine line and respect your adolescent's emerging sense of independence and need for privacy. You must recognize that your teen is more likely to rely on friends, rather than on you, to process and integrate new information. Show teens that you take their thoughts and feelings seriously by using reflective- and active-listening skills. Look for opportunities to praise teens for past efforts at handling challenges, and show confidence that your teen will cope with the new information equally well.

If teens become overly dramatic or self-involved in their reactions, do not escalate the emotion of the moment. Adolescents can seem rejecting or make extreme statements that feel hurtful to parents because they have kept the secret for so long. Wise parents will recognize that if they want their children to eventually become confident, competent, independent young adults, then their teens will need to practice separating in manageable doses. To provide guidance, share your own life experiences facing adversity (both successful and unsuccessful) rather than criticize, control, or correct your teen's reactions. Provide perspective, and share your view of the immediate difficulty as being a mere bump in the road that the family will overcome.

DO'S AND DON'TS OF DISCUSSING FAMILY SECRETS

The following are some do's and don'ts for disclosing a family secret to your child.

- *Approach the topic in a truthful, straightforward, positive, clear manner.* Use a calm, warm, matter-of-act tone of voice; do not approach the discussion in anger or crisis. When parents model honesty, they build trust. When you believe your children lack the maturity to understand some of the details, tell them you will explain further when they get older and can understand more. Remain clear about the implications of the secret, rather than leaving them to the child's imagination. For example, when explaining a family member's addiction, tell your children that the individual is not a bad person, but they have a disease and when they get high or drunk, they can do things that feel mean or things that do not make sense. When children ask why this happened, explain that the person didn't know what was best for him at the time and consequently made bad choices or mistakes.
- *Use language and concepts children can understand.* For children under 7 to 10 years of age, simplify your language. Use short sentences, one- to two-syllable words, and simple grammatical constructions. Draw a picture with your words; use concrete visual words rather than hierarchical or abstract terms. Don't say, "Your Aunt is going into treatment for her alcohol problem." Instead, say, "Your Aunt is going to a place like a hospital to learn how to stop drinking so much, so that she can be happy."
- *Help children express feelings.* Ask children what they think and feel about the news. Ask them to clarify ("What makes you think so?") or elaborate ("Tell me more about that?"). Explain that feelings are neither right nor wrong. Everyone has them. Remember that young children take their cues about how to interpret information from their parents. It is okay to admit to your child that what you are telling them may be upsetting, and it is okay to have strong feelings about it. However, just because the revelation is upsetting, it does not mean the family will not find a way to deal with the problem. At the same time, show your children your genuine feelings, even tearfully if the news warrants that emotion, as long as you provide the reassurance your children need and model positive coping strategies.
- *Help children cope with distressing information.* Suggest that children keep a journal to write down questions, thoughts, or feelings that come up. The discussion does

not have to end after the disclosure. Children process information at different rates and, over time, their curiosity about what you told them may grow. They may have more questions as time goes on. Let them know that the topic remains open for future questions and discussion.

- Another way to help children cope is to create a family tree, scrapbook, or time-line of their lives, showing important events. Listing important events on paper can put the secret event in perspective in comparison to all the good events in the child's life.

- Positive self-statements can help your children deal with the secret. Remind them that everyone talks to themselves—you can tell yourself things that will make you feel worse (e.g., "Everyone will think I am stupid; I will never get it right") or things that will make you feel better (e.g., "No one is perfect. No one expects me to get it right the first time. I'll keep practicing or I'll ask for help if I need it."). Help your child make a list of positive self-statements to cope with anticipated problems.

- Last, help identify individuals who children can talk to if they feel upset or unsafe. Prepare extended family members to answer your child's questions sensitively.

- *Respect children's feelings.* In an attempt to reassure, parents may inadvertently devalue or shut down children's feelings ("Don't worry. Don't be nervous. There is no reason to feel that way."). It is best to avoid this type of reassurance. Instead, validate and normalize your children's feelings. If they say they feel sad, mad, angry, jealous, or embarrassed, reassure them that there is nothing wrong with them; we all feel like this at times and usually for good reasons.

- *Dispel unrealistic fears.* Children often imagine things to be worse than they really are (e.g., If a family member has cancer, children may worry that cancer is conta-gious, that they or their parents will catch it, or that everyone dies of it.). Verify the accuracy of your children's understanding by asking them to explain what they have heard in their own words. Then, repeat back what your children said to make sure you understand their meaning. Also, be sure to correct any misperceptions your children may have. It is particularly important to let your children know that whatever the problem, it is not their fault. For example, "Grandma isn't acting that way because of anything you or I have said or done."

- *Encourage children to ask questions.* Avoid an authoritarian, one-sided approach that leads children to respond with silence ("Now that you know, just forget about it."). You don't need to have all the answers. If you do not know an answer, take an honest approach. Tell your children you don't know, but you will try to find out. If children are worried about the future, say something like, "There's no way to know what's going to happen. When things change and I know more, I will be sure to tell you. You can always ask me any questions, and I will do my best to answer."

- *Normalize the situation when possible.* Children may ask, "Why did this happen to our family?" Explain that every family has problems. Most problems can be solved or at least managed. Let older children know how common an occurrence the event may be and that many families feel too embarrassed or scared to talk about it. For example, "Doctors don't know why people get mental illness, but we are not alone. One out of four families has someone with a mental illness and many manage to cope and stay together."

- *Discuss confidentiality.* Discuss with your children who else, if anyone, needs to know the secret and whether the information must remain within the family. Confidentiality can strengthen family unity, teaching family members to trust each other and still maintain healthy boundaries in sharing information with others carefully and thoughtfully. With school-aged children, anticipate others' reactions: Explain that some people won't understand and it may scare them. They may make fun of it, have ideas that are not true, change the subject, or say nothing when you tell them. It may be helpful to role-play telling others (e.g., "My mom does that because she is sick. If you really understood what was wrong with my mom, you wouldn't say that. She has an illness that makes her do that. She's taking medicine, trying to get better.")

SUMMARY

If you are concerned that your child will develop psychological or behavioral problems as a result of learning the family secret, seek advice from a mental health professional, such as a child psychologist or family counselor. However, for many situations, parents need only create an ongoing, interactive communication process focused on the child's evolving needs and growing capacity for understanding—a family atmosphere characterized by open, honest, emotionally attuned communication.

WHERE TO FIND OUT MORE

Books

Keefer, B. & Schooler, J.E. (2000). *Telling the truth to your adopted or foster child.* Westport, CT: Bergin and Garvey.

Long, N. & Forehand, R. (2002). *Making divorce easier on your child: 50 Effective ways to help children adjust.* New York: McGraw-Hill.

Websites

Family and Corrections Network
  http://www.fcnetwork.org
Mental Health Association of Southeastern Pennsylvania
  Helping Children Understand Mental Illness: A Resource for Parents and Guardians
  http://www.mhasp.org/coping/guardians.html
About.com
  What to Tell Children About a Parent's Addiction: How to Talk to Children About Family
  Substance Abuse
  http://alcoholism.about.com/od/children/a/talk_kids.htm
The Daily Telegraph
  Lifeclass: Should Parents Tell a Donor Child About Their True Origins?
  http://www.telegraph.co.uk/health/healthadvice/3356323/Lifeclass-should-parents-tell-a-donor-child-about-their-true-origins.html

North Carolina Cooperative Extension Service, North Carolina State University
  Family Communication During Times of Stress
  http://www.ces.ncsu.edu/depts/fcs/pdfs/fcs424.pdf
University of Missouri Extension
  Helping Children Understand Divorce http://extension.missouri.edu/xplor/hesguide/
  humanrel/gh6600.htm
American Cancer Society
  Helping Children when a Family Member Has Cancer: Dealing with Diagnosis
  http://www.cancer.org/docroot/CRI/content/CRI_2_6X_Dealing_With_Diagnosis.asp

CHAPTER 20

Witnessing Parental Arguments or Domestic Violence

Neena M. Malik and Kristin M. Lindahl

You and your spouse just had a horrible argument. One of you lost your temper to the point that, when you swung your arm to make your point, you knocked over and broke a large lamp. You thought your kids were in their rooms, listening to music or doing homework, but they ran right into the room, a look of terror on their faces. All of a sudden, neither of you can remember what you had been fighting about; you both feel terrible that the kids look so scared.

If this has happened to you, you are not alone. All couples have arguments. When this happens, two of the most important questions for parents are, "What does it mean to my children?" and, "What effect does it have?" The answers differ based on the nature of the arguments, the ages of your children, how your children think about and experience the arguments, and how your family as a whole gets along. In this chapter, we address those issues and give you some ideas about how to help your children deal with parental arguments. We also address what you can do if you find yourself becoming afraid of being hurt or of hurting your spouse or partner during an argument.

Decades of research inform us about children's exposure to marital conflict. One of the primary findings is that children can suffer very negative effects as the result of parental conflict. Potential negative outcomes for children include problems with aggression, acting out, defiance, and other overt behavior problems that psychologists call "externalizing problems." Other children may not have obvious behavior problems, but may develop "internalizing problems." These problems are less obvious but just as painful and problematic for children, such as depression, sadness, anxiety, and low self-esteem. Both externalizing and internalizing problems can radiate to cause difficulties in school, friendships and peer relationships, and relationships with parents and siblings. Because marital conflict poses a risk for children's adjustment, it is important to understand what makes witnessing family conflict bad—and perhaps at times even good—for your children.

NOT ALL ARGUMENTS ARE CREATED EQUAL

All couples, all parents have arguments. Part of intimacy involves resolving conflicts that inevitably arise. Many different types of arguments occur, and parents have different ways of arguing with one another. Research has shown that disagreements that occur frequently, involve intense emotions or hostility, and remain unresolved will likely have the worst effects on children. Some parents never argue openly; they just withdraw to their "separate corners" and stop talking to each other. Other parents argue occasionally, perhaps with increasing frequency during stressful times, but they resolve conflicts and communicate with their children about the resolution. Still other parents have a hard time managing their anger, and conflicts become a regular part of communication in the family. For some couples, those conflicts may even escalate to a level called "domestic violence," a separate and more serious kind of arguing that is addressed later in the chapter.

It may surprise you to know that one of the most important predictors of how children adjust or behave in response to their parents' arguments is *how the argument is resolved*. We do not suggest that parents shouldn't argue; that isn't a realistic or even a good solution. In fact, since conflicts and disagreements are a part of close family relationships, it is important that children see that arguments can happen and come to closure without destroying the relationship. Thus, "not talking to each other" is not particularly healthy for children, because even though no yelling occurs, children easily sense the ongoing and lingering tension and perhaps even hostile feelings. Similarly, seeing or hearing an argument without a resolution can prove very difficult for children.

Whether the form of the dispute involves withdrawal and hostility or overt anger and yelling, unresolved conflict may leave a child with many unanswered questions and worries. Some of those questions and worries can include unspoken thoughts or worries such as, "It must be my fault."; "What did I do to make them so unhappy?"; "I wonder if they hate each other?"; "Are my parents going to get a divorce?"; "Do parents ever get along?"; "Why is everyone in my family so mad at each other all the time?"; and "I wonder if other families are happier than mine?" to name a few. All of those questions have answers that can relieve children's worries, if parents can effectively resolve whatever issues caused the argument, and if the ways they use communication skills to solve arguments become clearly evident to the children.

Children, particularly young ones, cannot help but feel scared, angry, or hurt when their parents fight with each other. But when parents compromise, and when the process of conflict becomes constructive rather than destructive, the outcomes reach well beyond avoiding discomfort for the children. In fact, the outcomes become positive for children, who may show more positive emotions toward their parents and feel better about their parents' relationship.

Perhaps the most important concept to remember is that not all conflict is created equal. The key factor in changing parental arguments from a negative to a positive is constructive conflict resolution, including compromise and open communication.

CHILDREN'S REACTIONS TO CONFLICT

A number of other important factors, in addition to the key element of conflict resolution, can impact how children respond to parental arguments. These factors include how children ascribe meaning to the conflict, as well as their age and gender.

First, how children understand and interpret their parents' arguments is an important predictor of how they will respond, and whether or not they will develop externalizing or internalizing problems, or school and/or social problems. Investigators have studied the process of children's understanding and interpreting (or "appraising") the conflict by asking children how they feel about their parents' arguments. Children are at greater risk for difficulties when they feel threatened by the conflict (e.g., they believe that their parents may divorce), or they worry that it means that their parents will feel angry with them. When children blame themselves for the conflict, such that they feel responsible for the argument and its outcome, children suffer more, particularly if such conflict happens often. Parents and children may differ in how frequent and intense they believe the conflict to be, but the important predictor of children's functioning involves *how children feel about it*, rather than the parents' perspective. Some parents may feel that their arguments occur only infrequently and that they are not severe overall. However, if children feel that arguments happen often and involve significant negative emotions, such as parental anger or sadness, children are at greater risk for both short- and longer-term negative consequences to their psychological health and development.

Second, age matters. Different children, even siblings within families, may appraise or understand parental conflict differently. Younger children are the most vulnerable to parents' fighting. Even babies detect shifts in parents' emotions, and even if they can't understand the words, they sense and become affected by hostility between the people they trust and love. Exposure to parental conflict causes stress for babies and toddlers. Parents will find that their negative feelings toward each other can easily lead to a fussy or tantruming child, which only makes the situation more challenging. Research also shows that younger children feel much more threatened by parental conflict. As children become older and approach adolescence, they feel somewhat less threatened when parents argue. As children get older, they have more coping skills and more support outside the family. Infants, preschoolers, and young elementary school-aged children have yet to develop a range of techniques to cope with difficult events or negative emotions, and they do not have as many activities or supports outside the family; as a result, they are at greater risk for feeling very threatened by parental arguments. An exception to these age-related differences in children's distress pertains to self-blame. Children who blame themselves for parental conflict are at risk for developing adjustment problems, regardless of their age. In addition, earlier child behavior problems predict continuing problems as children develop, particularly if rates of family conflict do not decline.

Third, children's gender may play a role in their reactions to parental conflict, although many questions about gender differences remain. Some researchers find boys report more self-blame than do girls, perhaps because they perceive their parents as arguing more about their behavior than do girls. Other research suggests that girls typically attend to the emotional quality of relationships more than do boys, and thus girls may feel more threatened by parental conflict than do boys. The findings on gender differences vary across studies, however, so it is difficult to know for certain whether boys and girls differ in their reactions to marital conflict.

THE QUALITY OF FAMILY RELATIONSHIPS MATTER

One of the most important factors in understanding how parental conflicts affect children is the quality of the parent–child relationship. So often, when ongoing hostility and conflict exist in a marriage, it becomes very easy for that stress and tension to spill over into the relationships that parents have with their children. For example, couple conflict is associated with increased negativity, frustration, and inconsistency in how parents respond to their children. Couples who argue frequently are often less patient and more conflictual with their children and have a harder time applying rules, consequences, and rewards in a consistent and predictable manner.

One of the worst ways that parental conflict spills over to the parent–child relationship is by involving a child in the conflict. Making the child the focus of the conflict may take some pressure off of the marriage, but it is potentially very damaging to the child, and leads to children feeling they are to blame for parental problems. Similarly, if children feel they must take sides, it compromises their feelings of safety and trust in their parents. Such "triangulating" of children into the parents' conflict has long-lasting consequences for children that include social and emotional problems. On the other hand, when security, trust, and open communication exist between parents and children, even when parents argue frequently, children may find themselves spared from feeling the social and emotional effects of marital conflict, since their high-quality relationship with their parents buffers them from the stress that their parents are feeling.

WHEN CONFLICTS ARE EXTREME: DOMESTIC VIOLENCE

The term "domestic violence" refers to aggression or violent behavior within an intimate relationship. That aggression can show itself verbally, psychologically, or physically. Most often, domestic violence occurs in the form of verbal aggression, during which spouses or partners say threatening, intensely insulting, hurtful, or controlling things to each other. Sometimes verbal aggression escalates to physical aggression. Throwing objects, pushing, shoving, grabbing someone by the arm, or blocking someone's exit or entry with your body can qualify as a physically aggressive, domestically violent act. It may not carry the same intensity or danger as hitting, slapping, kicking, or punching, but such behaviors may qualify as misdemeanor criminal acts in most states, and they can have very serious consequences for the couple's relationship and for children exposed to such aggression. In some cases, even if partners never physically touch each other, the verbal aggression can prove so intense and hostile that the effects on children are the same as if parents actually hit each other.

In most couples, domestic violence happens when people get so angry that they lose control. For various reasons, people who engage in intensely bitter, angry, hostile, out-of-control, and at times dangerous conflict behaviors do not have (or feel that they have) the skills to manage their own angry outbursts. They almost always deeply regret their behavior when the storm clouds have passed and the dust has settled. However, some people use aggressive tactics as a means of controlling their spouses, partners, or children. In those circumstances, domestic violence presents a very dangerous situation for both spouses and children.

Domestic violence has the same effects on children as does intense marital conflict. Many parents think that their children do not see or hear aggression that takes place during arguments, but it does in fact have an effect. Children are at risk for a host of internalizing and externalizing problems if domestic violence exists in their home.

An additional consequence of domestic violence for some children is symptoms of acute or post-traumatic stress. Especially with younger children and infants, an atmosphere of danger or intense anger in the home or in the parental relationship compromises the child's sense of safety and security that is so critical to their well-being and development. Ongoing exposure to episodes of domestic violence erodes a child's sense of safety and security. This applies to older, as well as younger, children. Children may experience such high levels of stress that physical changes occur in their bodies and their brains, potentially leading to long-term problems with attention, learning, concentration, and emotional regulation or control.

HOW CAN I HELP MY CHILD DEAL WITH CONFLICT?

Substantial evidence indicates that fighting between parents that is intense, frequent, aggressive, and unresolved creates a significant risk for children's difficulties, across areas such as emotional well-being, social development and relationships, and behavior and learning. Research also tells us, however, that there are many strategies you can use to help your children deal with conflict, and that nonviolent domestic conflict can create important and positive learning opportunities for children. Consider the following:

- All parents have disagreements; you don't have to feel bad that you sometimes argue with each other.
- Some arguing is better than no arguing, when it leads to resolving the conflict and children learn of the resolution.
- Positive developmental effects come from children understanding that conflict occurs and can be resolved without violence. Positive emotions emerge and relationships can improve when children see that parents can compromise with each other and constructively resolve disagreements.
- Even if you think your children don't know about parental disputes, they most likely do. They sense tension and hostility, and will try to find ways in their own minds to understand why. Sometimes their imaginations or immature reasoning can lead them to unfortunate conclusions. Many children, especially younger ones, will potentially blame themselves.

- Talk to your children when you have conflicts. Let them know it isn't about them. Even if the origin of a discussion between parents focused on something involving a child, the fact that the conflict exists is not about the child, but rather about how the parents communicate and deal with co-parenting that child.
- Resist involving your child in your conflicts, either by getting angry with them or by asking them to take sides. This will prove very harmful to your children and can compromise your relationship with them.
- Even when emotions become very difficult between parents, children are spared many, if not most, of the negative effects, by preserving positive relationships between parents and children. This can take a lot of energy, but it will prove very important for children's well-being.
- Much marital conflict comes from not having communication or problem-solving skills. Everyone needs to learn these skills—that is why constructive conflict can prove so important for children to see in action. If you don't have such skills, there are many ways to learn them. Many clergy, community-outreach centers, and marriage and family counselors have tools for couples to use to improve their communication, and there are many books and programs you can access without going to a counselor for help (see *Where to Find Out More*, at the end of this chapter).
- If there is aggression or danger in your relationship, pay attention to your own fear—either of hurting your spouse/partner or of your partner hurting you. If you feel such fear, your children have it ten-fold. Most communities have women's shelters or advocacy programs based in the city or county government, with 24-hour hotlines. A national domestic violence hotline operates 24 hours every day (1-800-799-SAFE; www.ndvh.org). Even when matters seem out of control, there are ways to find help for you and your children.

SUMMARY

Fighting with your spouse or partner in front of your children is not necessarily a bad thing. If parents are able to resolve conflict in a positive way, children can learn valuable lessons. When children see that their parents can compromise and resolve conflict in a healthy way, they learn that arguments can be resolved without damaging the relationship of the people involved. Use disagreements as opportunities to teach your children good communication and problem-solving skills. If there is danger or aggression in your relationship, you should seek help right away.

WHERE TO FIND OUT MORE

Books

Gottman, J.M., Gottman, J.S., & Declaire, J. (2007). *Ten lessons to transform your marriage: America's Love Lab experts share their strategies for strengthening your relationship.* New York: Three Rivers Press.

Emery, R.E. (2004). *The truth about children and divorce: Dealing with the emotions so you and your children can thrive.* New York: The Penguin Group.

Markman, H.J., Stanley, S.M., & Blumberg, S. (2001). *Fighting for your marriage: Positive steps for preventing divorce and preserving a lasting love.* San Francisco: Jossey-Bass.

Websites

MINCAVA (Minnesota Center Against Violence and Abuse) Electronic Clearinghouse. http://www.mincava.umn.edu.

National Domestic Violence Hotline (2009). http://www.ndvh.org.

PREP, INC. (1996–2009). State-of-the-art tools for an extraordinary marriage. http://www.prepinc.com.

CHAPTER 21

Raising Resilient Children

Robert B. Brooks and Sam Goldstein

Billy and Mike, 10-year-old teammates on a Little League team, both struck out each time they came to bat. They responded very differently to their failure to get on base. After his final strikeout, Billy screamed at the umpire, "You are blind, blind, blind! If you weren't so blind I wouldn't strike out!" As he ran off the field before the game was concluded, he continued to shout, "The umpire is blind! It's not fair!"

In contrast, Mike approached his coach after the game and said, "Coach, I've been striking out a lot. Maybe you can figure out what I'm doing wrong. I think I can hit much better than I have been doing."

Susan and Linda, age 11, recently moved to a new town. Both worried about making new friends. On the first day of school, Susan saw an empty space at a table in the cafeteria. She asked if she could sit there, but the kids said, "Our table's already full." Although she felt upset, she told herself that the kids at the table were not very nice, and she went to another table. When she asked if she could join, the group said, "Sure" and within a few minutes she was chatting with new friends.

A few minutes later, Linda also asked the kids at the first table if she could sit there, and heard the same negative response they gave Susan. Linda immediately told herself, "I just don't fit in, no one wants to sit with me" and sulked off to the bathroom where she sat in a stall during lunch. The next day she sat at a table in the corner by herself.

The capacity of a child to deal effectively with stress and pressure, to cope with everyday challenges, to rebound from disappointments, mistakes, trauma, and adversity, to solve problems, and to interact comfortably with others demonstrates *resilience*. In the examples at the start of the chapter, Mike and Susan showed resilience, while Billy and Linda did not.

It is essential for parents to identify practices that nurture the skills, positive outlook, and stress hardiness necessary for children to manage an increasingly complex and demanding world. We must search for consistent ways of raising children that increase the likelihood they will experience happiness, success in school, contentment in their lives, and satisfying relationships. To realize these goals, children must develop the inner strength to deal competently and successfully, day after day, with the challenges and pressures they encounter.

THE CHARACTERISTICS OF A RESILIENT MINDSET

The opening examples illustrate how resilient children possess certain qualities and/or ways of viewing themselves and the world that are not readily apparent in youngsters who do not successfully meet such challenges. The assumptions children have about themselves influence the behaviors and skills they develop. In turn, these behaviors and skills influence this set of assumptions in a dynamically changing process. We call this set of assumptions a *mindset.*

Understanding the features of a resilient mindset provides parents with guideposts for nurturing inner strength and optimism in their children. Parents who follow these principles when interacting with their children will reinforce a resilient mindset. While the outcome of any one situation may be important, the lessons learned in the process of dealing with each problem provide essential skills. The mindset of resilient children contains a number of noteworthy characteristics associated with specific skills. These include:

- Feeling loved and accepted
- Setting realistic goals and expectations
- Believing they have the ability to solve problems and make sound decisions
- Viewing mistakes, setbacks, and obstacles as challenges to confront rather than stressors to avoid
- Relying on effective coping strategies that promote growth and are not self-defeating
- Recognizing and accepting their weaknesses and vulnerabilities, seeing these as areas for improvement, rather than unchangeable flaws
- Recognizing and enjoying their strong points and talents
- Having a self-concept filled with images of strength and competence
- Feeling comfortable with and relating well to both peers and adults
- Having the ability to seek out assistance and nurturance in a comfortable, appropriate manner from adults who can provide such support
- Recognizing aspects of their lives they can control and focusing their energy and attention on those, rather than on factors over which they have little, or any, influence.

The process of nurturing this mindset and associated skills in children requires parents to examine their own mindset, beliefs, and actions.

HOW CAN I HELP MY CHILD TO BE RESILIENT?

The following strategies and practices can help you reinforce a resilient mindset and lifestyle in your child. These guideposts apply to all interactions parents and other caregivers have with children whether coaching them in a sport, helping them with homework, engaging them in an art project, asking them to assume responsibilities, assisting them when they make mistakes, teaching them to share, or disciplining them. While these apply differently from one child and one situation to the next, the guideposts remain constant.

Show Empathy

Empathy forms the basic foundation of any relationship. In parenting, empathy is the capacity to put yourself in your child's shoes and to see the world through your child's eyes. Empathy does not imply that you agree with what your child does, but rather you attempt to appreciate and validate your child's point of view. Children can more easily develop empathy when they interact with adults who model it daily.

Parents often believe they have empathy, but in reality empathy is more fragile or elusive than many realize. We can show empathy more easily when our children do what we ask them, meet our expectations, and give us warmth and love. They test our empathy when we feel upset, angry, or disappointed with them. When parents feel this way, many will say or do things that actually work against developing a resilient child.

To strengthen empathy, keep in mind several key questions:

- "How would I feel if someone said or did to me what I just said or did to my child?"
- "When I say or do things with my children, am I behaving in a way that will make them want to listen to me?"
- "What words do I hope my child would use to describe me?"
- "Do I behave in ways that would prompt my child to describe me that way?"
- "How would my child actually describe me, and how closely does it match my hopes?"

Communicate Effectively and Listen Actively

Empathy is closely associated with the ways in which you communicate with your child. Communication is not simply how we speak with another person. Effective communication requires actively listening to your child; understanding and validating what your child is attempting to say; and responding in ways that avoid power struggles by not interrupting your child, not telling your child how he or she should feel, not derogating your child, and not using absolute words such as *always* and *never* in an overly critical, demeaning fashion (e.g., "You never help out." "You always act disrespectful.").

Resilient children demonstrate a capacity to communicate feelings and thoughts effectively. Their parents serve as important models in the process. When 10-year-old Michael insisted on completing a radio kit on his own but was unable to do so, his father angrily retorted, "I told you it wouldn't work. You don't have enough patience to read the directions carefully." The father's message worked against the development of a resilient mindset in his son by taking an accusatory tone and focusing on Michael's shortcomings, rather than on his strengths. It did not offer assistance or hope.

Reflect upon how you would respond to the following questions pertaining to your communication style with your child:

- "Do my messages convey and teach respect?"
- "Am I fostering realistic expectations in my children?"
- "Am I helping my children learn how to solve problems?"
- "Am I nurturing empathy and compassion?"
- "Am I promoting self-discipline and self-control?"
- "Am I setting limits and consequences in ways that permit my children to learn from me rather than resent me?"
- "Am I truly listening to and validating what my children are saying?"
- "Do my children know that I value their opinion and input?"
- "Do my children know how special they are to me?"
- "Am I assisting my children to appreciate that mistakes and obstacles are part of the process of learning and growing?"
- "Am I comfortable in acknowledging my own mistakes and apologizing to my children when indicated?"

If you keep these questions in mind, you will be able to communicate with your child in ways that reinforce a resilient mindset.

Change Negative Scripts

Some well-meaning parents apply the same approach with their children for weeks, months, or years, even when it has proven ineffective. For instance, some parents remind (nag) their children for years to clean their rooms without success. When asked why they use the same unsuccessful message for years, they often respond, "We thought it would sink in if we told them often enough."

Many parents show similar reasoning, believing their children need to change, not them. Others believe changing their approach would equal "giving in" to their child and feel concerned their child will take advantage of them. Parents with a resilient mindset of their own recognize that if something they have tried for a reasonable amount of time does not work, they must change their "script" if they hope to see change in their children. This position does not mean "giving in" to the child or failing to hold the child accountable. It suggests the parents have the insight and courage to consider what they can do differently, lest they become entangled in useless, counterproductive power struggles. It also serves to teach children that alternative ways of solving problems exist and helps them learn greater flexibility and accountability in handling difficult situations.

Show Your Children Love and Appreciation

A well-established foundation of resilience involves the presence of at least one adult (hopefully several) who believes in the worth and goodness of the child. The late psychologist Julius Segal referred to that person as a "charismatic adult," an adult from whom a child "gathers strength." Parents, keeping in mind the notion of a charismatic adult, might ask each evening, "Are my children stronger or less strong because of the things I said or did today?"

When asked to recall a favorite occasion from their childhood when their own parents served as a charismatic adult for them, adults most commonly cite memories involving doing something pleasant and alone with the parent. These "special times" yield powerful memories. We recommend that you create such occasions in the lives of your children. Parents of young children might say, "When I read to you or play with you, it is so special that even if the phone rings I won't answer it." One young child said, "I know my parents love me. They let the answering machine take calls when they are playing with me."

Time alone with your children does not preclude family activities that also create a sense of belonging and love. Sharing evening meals and holidays, playing games, attending a community event as a family, or taking a walk together all provide opportunities to convey love and help your children feel special.

Accept Your Children for Who They Are and Help Them Establish Realistic Expectations and Goals

One of the most difficult but challenging parenting tasks involves accepting our children for who they are, not who we want them to be. Before children are born, parents have expectations for them that may prove unrealistic, given the unique qualities of each child.

Acceptance does not imply that we excuse inappropriate, unacceptable behavior but rather that we understand this behavior and help to modify it in a manner that does not assault a child's self-esteem and sense of dignity. It means developing realistic goals and expectations for our children.

Identify and Nurture Your Children's "Islands of Competence"

Resilient children do not deny their problems. Such denial runs counter to mastering challenges. However, in addition to acknowledging and confronting problems, resilient youngsters can identify and utilize their strengths. Unfortunately, many children who feel poorly about themselves and their abilities experience a diminished sense of hope. Parents sometimes report that the positive comments they offer their children fall on "deaf ears," and they become frustrated, giving less positive feedback.

Wise parents will recognize that when children lack self-worth, they are less open to accepting positive feedback. Parents should continue to offer such feedback, but must recognize that true self-esteem, hope, and resilience grow when children experience success in areas of their lives that they and significant others deem important. This requires parents to identify and reinforce a child's "islands of competence." Every child possesses such islands of competence or areas of strength, and we must nurture these rather then overemphasize the child's weakness. When children discover their strengths, they more willingly confront problem areas in their lives.

Help Your Children Realize That Mistakes Create Leaning Opportunities

Resilient children view their mistakes in ways that differ significantly from youngsters who are not resilient. Resilient children tend to perceive mistakes as opportunities for learning. In contrast, children with less hope often experience mistakes as an indication that they are failures. In response to this pessimistic view, they will likely flee from or avoid challenges, feeling inadequate and often blaming others for their problems. If you wish to raise resilient children, you must help them develop a healthy attitude about mistakes from an early age.

You can help your children develop a more constructive attitude about mistakes and setbacks by considering how your children would answer the following questions:

- "When your parents make a mistake, when something doesn't go right, what do they do?"
- "When you make a mistake, what do your parents say or do to you?"

The first question shows how you, as a parent, serve as a significant model to your children in terms of handling mistakes. It is easier for children to learn to deal more effectively with mistakes if they see their parents doing so. However, if they observe their parents blaming others or becoming very angry and frustrated when mistakes occur or offering excuses in order to avoid a task, they will more likely to develop a self-defeating attitude toward mistakes. In contrast, if they witness their parents use mistakes as opportunities for learning, they are more likely to do the same.

The second question also deserves your serious consideration. Many well-meaning parents become anxious and frustrated with their children's mistakes. Given these feelings, they may say or do things that contribute to their children fearing rather than learning from setbacks. For instance, parental frustration may lead to such comments as: "Were you using your brains?" or "You never think before you act!" or "I told you it wouldn't work!" These and similar remarks serve to corrode a child's sense of dignity and self-esteem.

No one likes to make mistakes or fail, but you can use your children's mistakes as teachable moments. When your child makes a mistake, engage him or her in a discussion of what can be done differently next time to maximize chances for success. Using empathy, refrain from saying things you would not want said to you (e.g., how many parents would find it helpful if their spouse asked, "Were you using your brains?").

Provide Your Children with Opportunities to Contribute

Parents often ask what they can do to foster an attitude of responsibility, caring, and compassion in their children. Offering children opportunities to help others is one of the most effective ways of nurturing responsibility. When we enlist children in helping others and engaging in responsible behaviors, we communicate trust in them and faith in their ability to handle a variety of tasks. In turn, involvement in these tasks reinforces several key characteristics of a resilient mindset including empathy, a sense of satisfaction in the positive impact of one's behaviors, and a more confident outlook as islands of competence and the use of problem-solving skills emerge.

We recommend that you frequently tell your children, "I need your help," rather than "Remember to do your chores." In addition, it is a good idea to involve your children in charitable endeavors, such as walks to raise money to combat hunger or AIDS, or food drives. These activities foster self-esteem and resilience. Children do not learn responsibility and compassion from parental "lectures," but rather by opportunities to assume a helping role and feel part of a "charitable family," a family engaged in acts of compassion and giving.

Teach Your Children to Solve Problems and Make Decisions

Children with high self-esteem and resilience believe they are masters of their fate and can define what they have control over. A vital source of feeling in control is children's beliefs that they have the ability to make decisions and solve problems. Resilient children can articulate problems, consider different solutions, attempt the solution they judge most appropriate, and learn from the outcome.

To reinforce this problem-solving attitude in your children, you must refrain from constantly telling your children what to do. Instead, encourage your children to consider different possible solutions. To facilitate this process, you may wish to establish a "family meeting time" every week or so during which your family can discuss problems and consider solutions.

Use Discipline to Promote Self-Control and Self-Worth

Acting as a disciplinarian is one of the most important roles that parents assume in nurturing their children's resilience. In this role, parents must remember that the word *discipline* relates to the word *disciple* and the teaching process. The ways in which we discipline children can either reinforce or erode self-esteem, self-control, and resilience.

Two major goals of effective discipline are (a) ensuring a safe and secure environment in which children understand and can define rules, limits, and consequences; and (b) reinforcing self-discipline and self-control, so that children incorporate these rules and apply them even in the absence of parents and other caregivers. A lack of consistent, clear rules and consequences often contributes to chaos and to children feeling that their parents do not care about them. On the other hand, if parents behave in a harsh and arbitrary manner, or resort to yelling and spanking, children will likely learn resentment rather than self-discipline.

There are certain key principles you can follow to employ positive and effective discipline techniques:

- *Practice prevention.* It is vital to be proactive rather than reactive in your interactions with your children, especially regarding discipline. For example, discipline problems were minimized in one household by allowing a young hyperactive boy to get up from the dinner table when he could no longer remain seated. This approach proved far more effective than the parents' prior approach of yelling and punishing him; by removing a punitive atmosphere the boy also learned greater self-control
- *Work as a parental team.* In homes with two parents, it is important that parents set aside time for themselves to examine the expectations they have for their children, as well as the discipline they use. This dialogue can also occur between divorced parents. While parents cannot and should not become clones of each other, they should strive to arrive at common goals and disciplinary practices, which often involve negotiation and compromise. Parental negotiation should take place in private and not in front of children.

- *Act consistently, not rigidly.* The behavior of children sometimes renders consistency a Herculean task. Some children, based on past experience, believe that they can outlast their parents who will eventually succumb to whining, crying, or tantrums. If you establish guidelines and consequences for acceptable behavior, it is important that you adhere to them. However, you must remember that consistency is not synonymous with rigidity or inflexibility. A consistent approach to discipline invites thoughtful modification of rules and consequences, such as when a child reaches adolescence and seeks permission to stay out later on the weekend. When modifications become necessary, discussing them with children helps them understand the reasons for changes and offer input.

- *Choose your battlegrounds carefully.* Parents can find themselves reminding and disciplining their children all day long. It is important to ask yourself what behaviors merit discipline and which are not really relevant in terms of nurturing responsibility and resilience. Obviously, behaviors concerning safety deserve immediate attention. Other behaviors will flow from the particular values and expectations in the home. Punishing children for countless behaviors in an arbitrary manner will destroy any positive effects of discipline.

- *Rely, when possible, on natural and logical consequences.* Children must learn the consequences of their behavior. Ideally, such consequences are not harsh or arbitrary, but based on discussions you have had with your children. Discipline rooted in natural and logical consequences can prove very effective. *Natural* consequences are those that result from your child's actions without you having to enforce them, such as a child having his bicycle stolen because it was left outside the garage. While *logical* consequences sometimes overlap with natural consequences, logical consequences involve some action on the part of parents in response to their child's behavior. Thus, if the child whose bicycle was stolen asked his parents for money to purchase a new bicycle, a logical consequence might involve the parents helping the child figure out how to earn the money to pay for a new bicycle.

Most questions people ask us about discipline focus on negative consequences or punishment, but the impact of positive feedback and encouragement provide important disciplinary approaches. Parents should "catch their children doing things right" and let them know when they do. Children crave the attention of their parents. It makes more sense to provide this attention for positive rather than negative behaviors. Well-timed positive feedback and expressions of encouragement and love are more valuable to children's self-esteem and resilience than stars or stickers. When children feel loved and appreciated, when they receive encouragement and support, they are less likely to engage in negative behaviors.

SUMMARY

The day-to-day interactions parents have with their children are influential in determining the quality of lives that their children will lead. Parents can serve as charismatic adults to their children. They can assume this role by understanding and fortifying in their children the different characteristics of a resilient mindset, by believing in them, by conveying unconditional love, and by providing them with opportunities that reinforce their islands of competence and feelings of self-worth and dignity. Nurturing resilience is an immeasurable, life-long gift parents can offer their children. It is part of a parent's legacy to the next generation.

WHERE TO FIND OUT MORE

Books

Brooks, R. (1991) *The self-esteem teacher.* Loveland, OH: Treehaus Communications.

Brooks, R., & Goldstein, S. (2001). *Raising resilient children: Fostering strength, hope, and optimism in your child.* New York: McGraw-Hill.

Brooks, R., & Goldstein, S. (2003). *Nurturing resilience in our children. Answers to the most important parenting questions.* New York: McGraw-Hill.

Brooks, R., & Goldstein, S. (2007). *Raising a self-disciplined child.* New York: McGraw-Hill.

Websites

Dr. Robert Brooks
http://www.drrobertbrooks.com
Sam Goldstein
http://www.samgoldstein.com
Raising Resilient Children Foundation
http://www.raisingresilientkids.com/

PART THREE

Social and Peer Issues

CHAPTER 22

Helping Your Child Develop and Maintain Friendships

Kevin M. David and Barry S. Anton

Your first child, Claire, just turned 2 years old and you notice that she has started to interact and play with other children, and you're wondering about when and how she will begin to develop friendships. You also wonder what you can do to help get her off to a good start.

Your 8-year-old, Xavier, came home from school and told you that some kids were making fun of him. You want to find out more about his interactions with peers and help him deal with teasing and make lasting friendships.

Victoria, your 14-year-old daughter, has started talking more about boys, but when you ask her about them, she acts as if she doesn't know how to talk to them. You wonder whether it is normal for girls her age to hang around with boys and about what you can do to help her navigate her increasingly complex social world.

The nature of children's friendships and the related stresses vary considerably from child to child and across age ranges. Even so, there is a lot you can do to help your children make and sustain friendships. Although various definitions of friendship exist, some elements seem common to most perspectives on friendship. Researchers generally agree that friendships are reciprocal relationships between two or more people involving mutual affection or liking, voluntary participation, and a desire to spend time together. Children's interactions with friends hold special significance because they provide opportunities for children to learn to take others' perspectives, practice social skills, and develop an understanding of relationships and people. Close friendships can also help buffer children from stressors such as rejection by the larger peer group, harsh parenting, and marital discord, even as early as kindergarten. Understanding how to help your children develop healthy friendships can help you benefit your children's social, emotional, and intellectual development.

FUNDAMENTALS

Although children's temperaments can contribute to how they interact with peers, environmental factors also influence the development of friendships during childhood and adolescence. Parents can play a unique role in helping their children think about and behave in social relationships. For instance, children and adolescents who are well-liked by their peers tend to have parents who recognize and discuss emotions, explain their reasoning for decisions, and generally have positive interactions with their children. Similarly, parents' relationships with other people can serve as models from which children learn about relationships, what to expect from them, and how to interact with people. Not surprisingly, parents with satisfying marriages and positive friendships of their own tend to raise socially competent children.

Two important ways you can foster your children's peer relations are *gatekeeping* and *coaching*. Gatekeeping, which proves especially influential during early childhood, involves determining where your children go, with whom they interact, and when they interact with peers. Socially competent children generally have parents who make an effort to arrange play dates for them and ensure that their children play with peers who seem a good match for them. Coaching involves giving advice about how to interact with other children, especially during times of uncertainty, such as when your child attends a new school or encounters difficulty. You can coach your children on a variety of skills, including joining a group, dealing with teasing, and handling peer conflicts.

Here, we discuss the nature of friendships across childhood and adolescence, including common problems or challenges that become evident at different developmental periods, starting with the first signs of friendships in toddlerhood and ending with the more adult-like and intimate friendships that take place during adolescence. Along the way, we will make suggestions about how you can foster your children's social competence with peers at different ages during the first two decades of life. We conclude this chapter by summarizing the main points and by providing a list of suggested readings for more in-depth reviews of children's and adolescents' friendships.

FIRST FRIENDSHIPS (2–6 YEARS)

Children's first interactions with peers generally occur during play dates arranged by their parents, at family gatherings, or in childcare and preschool settings. Interestingly, even infants show awareness of other infants and back-and-forth play between children seems evident as early as 12 to 18 months of age. Furthermore, research suggests that toddlers seek out certain peers when in groups of children, reflecting the first signs of friendship. Although these first friendships generally emerge as preferences for play partners, they do involve mutual affection and companionship, two hallmarks of friendship. As with older children, toddlers tend to select as friends children who seem similar to them in activity level, social skills, and interaction style. In addition, children may prefer to play with same-sex peers as early as 2½ years of age, which likely contributes to the development of more same-sex friendships than opposite-sex friendships during childhood.

Some of the most important skills that foster positive peer relations during early childhood include communication, self-regulation, and group entry. Toddlers and pre-schoolers who can effectively communicate their desires, while maintaining harmony with other children, seem especially well-liked by their peers. The ability to successfully resolve conflict is the primary challenge in children's first friendships. Peer conflict during this period generally focuses on desired toys, and friends actually experience more conflict than do nonfriends. You can foster positive social skills in your young children by helping them handle peer conflict successfully. Although conflict among friends occurs frequently at this age, disagreements are not necessarily a bad thing. In fact, quarrels among friends often resolve more constructively than conflicts with nonfriends. Young children who have difficulty resolving peer conflicts may have trouble making and maintaining friendships during this early stage of life.

Learning how to approach and join a group of children already engaged in playing presents another important learning opportunity. Socially competent children can effec-tively enter a group and join the play, while not disrupting or significantly altering the group dynamics. Children who have difficulty successfully joining groups may either feel too timid to approach their peers or act too controlling and overwhelming toward the other children. In either case, parents can play an important role in teaching and encour-aging their children with regard to group entry.

You will likely be most involved in your children's peer relationships and friendships during early childhood. Here are some suggestions for helping your young children develop and maintain friendships.

- *Become knowledgeable about your child's friendships and peer relations in general.* During early childhood, observe your child interacting with others, so that you can evaluate his or her abilities in attracting and interacting with peers and identify good potential playmates.
- *Set up play dates and arrange other opportunities for your child to interact with peers.* Provide your child with opportunities to develop social skills.
- *Intervene when necessary.* Young children often will resolve conflicts on their own, but intervention sometimes becomes necessary. When it seems like your child is having a hard time sharing or resolving an issue with a peer, make suggestions for how your child should act. Toddlers and even older preschoolers may not spon-taneously share or give up a desired toy, but many children will comply with their parents' requests to do so. In addition, some rough-and-tumble play (e.g., wrestling) occurs commonly among young children, especially boys, and may not require parental involvement. Developing an awareness of your child's typical behavioral patterns becomes important, so you can accurately judge when "play" turns mean or clearly no longer feels like fun for one or both of the children involved.

- *Help your child to appreciate other children's viewpoints.* Talking to your child about how to act with other people and explaining why certain behaviors work better to make friends can foster emotional understanding, empathy, and friendly or help-ful behavior. For instance, explaining to your child that helping others and sharing will likely make other children feel good and share their things can encourage such behavior.
- *Coach your children on how to behave with peers,* especially during early childhood, when they first try to get a grasp on how relationships and specific interactions unfold and develop. You can make suggestions to your child for specific things to say or do when presented with particular situations. For instance, to help with group entry, you can encourage your child to first observe what the group is doing and then move closer and actively, without being intrusive, ask if he or she can play or join them. Children often respond positively to children who actively communi-cate their desires and contribute to their play without trying to take over or domi-nate the situation.
- *Model positive behavior.* Children's behaviors often resemble those of their parents. Children who have socially competent parents tend to be well-liked by their peers and generally successful in their social relationships.

FRIENDSHIPS DURING MIDDLE CHILDHOOD (7–12 YEARS)

During middle childhood, friendships focus more on loyalty, trust, and psychological similarities among children. Although sharing similar activities and interests is still impor-tant during this period, school-aged children develop a more sophisticated understand-ing of friendship that contributes to their choices of friends. Children in this age period also spend more time in larger groups, compare themselves to their peers more often, and develop closer relationships with their friends. Additionally, peer acceptance and popularity become increasingly important to children across this period. Unlike in early childhood, you generally will be less involved with your children's peer relations during this period, and keeping track of their friendships may prove more challenging. You may need to make an extra effort to keep track of how your child's peer relations and friend-ships are going during middle childhood.

One of the greatest challenges for school-aged children is finding a network of friends that serves as a source of support and validation for them. During this period, children become especially sensitive about their popularity, and cliques (small groups of friends ranging from about 3 to 12 children) become prominent. Although children's popularity can vary for many reasons (including personal ones such as physical appear-ance) and popularity does not always mean having good social skills, you should recog-nize and respect that popularity is increasingly important to your children during middle childhood. Therefore, you should take your children's friendships and concerns about popularity seriously and provide appropriate advice and support when necessary. As in early childhood, children in middle childhood often need encouragement and some coaching regarding their friendships and peer relations. During this period, you can help your children learn how to deal with peer acceptance and cliques.

Another challenge for children during middle childhood involves developing their first close relationships with peers. School-aged children take their friendships very seriously, placing value on loyalty and trust in their friendships. Not surprisingly, conflicts among friends during middle childhood often center on perceived betrayal or mistrust. Jealousy also becomes more common in this age group and may require parental assistance. Encouraging your children to talk about their friendships and peer conflicts can show them that you care about their social life and provide opportunities for you to influence how they approach their peer relationships.

One other important skill that can determine a child's peer status during middle childhood involves learning how to handle teasing from peers. Most children get teased at some point, and teasing occurs across childhood and adolescence. In fact, teasing often becomes a way of communicating among friends, especially for boys. Nonetheless, children become particularly sensitive to teasing during this period. You can help your children handle teasing in an assertive yet competent manner by offering suggestions about how they should respond when others tease them.

During middle childhood, friendships become more important to children, and peer groups play a more prominent role in their social lives. Important skills for children to develop during this period include identifying friends who may serve as sources of support and encouragement, learning how to develop personal relationships with their peers, and learning how to handle teasing. Fortunately, you can help your children develop these skills in several ways:

- Although you will find yourself less involved in your child's peer relationships as he or she gets older, you can still have a profound impact on your child's social life. You should monitor who your child hangs around with and pay attention to how your child gets along with peers. If your child seems to have problems with peers, approach the subject in an open, comfortable, and nonthreatening way. This approach can encourage your child to talk about his or her feelings and perhaps generate ideas about how to improve peer relationships.
- School-aged children are quite concerned with how their peers view them. Even if you do not think popularity is important, your school-aged child likely does. Therefore, you should listen supportively to your children's concerns and questions about their friendship status. Because loyalty and trust become important issues in children's friendships during this period, jealousy also may become a bigger part of a child's life during middle childhood. For most school-aged children, close friendships become their first voluntary personal relationships, and they become quite attached to their friends, especially if they have a "best friend." To parents, children's jealousy about a friend hanging around some other kids may seem trivial. However, you can bet it feels anything but trivial to the child. A parent who takes these issues seriously and listens empathically, while providing helpful suggestions, can do a lot of good in helping a child deal with these issues.
- Even the most well-liked and socially competent children get teased. What separates them from less well-liked kids is their ability to handle the teasing in ways that appeal to their peers and reflect confidence. You can help by explaining to your child that all kids get teased and that children who tease them do not necessarily

dislike them. In fact, many times the biggest teasers are trying to make good impressions on other children because they too very much want attention and peer acceptance. You also can suggest trying to respond to teasing with humor. By "laughing it off" or making a joke about the comment, the child avoids giving the teasing child what he seeks and the teasing becomes less enjoyable and rewarding for the teaser. Other times, the best approach may involve looking the teaser directly in the eyes and assertively telling him to "knock it off." However, if the teasing becomes frequent and your child feels bullied (See Chapter 24 on Bullying for more information), you may need to get involved by talking to school officials (if it happens at school) and/or the bully's parents. Often, talking with the bully in the presence of his parents can prove helpful.

ADOLESCENT FRIENDSHIPS (13–19 YEARS)

Friendships become more important to children during middle childhood, but they take on a new level of significance during adolescence. Not only do teenagers spend a lot more time with their friends than they do with their parents, but adolescents also report that friends provide as important a source of support as parents by age 13 and a greater source of support than parents by age 16. Moreover, although trust, loyalty, and closeness in friendships first emerge in the later years of childhood, self-disclosure and emotional intimacy become key features of friendships during adolescence. When selecting friends, adolescents seek peers with whom they feel comfortable sharing their thoughts and emotions, and who have similar beliefs, interests, and psychological qualities as themselves.

Compared to children, adolescents spend more time in large groups of peers consisting of both boys and girls. The increase in mixed-sex peer groups in adolescence seems tied to dating, which first emerges around early to middle adolescence. Despite the increased interest in dating during adolescence, not until late adolescence do dating partners become significant sources of support and emotional intimacy for adolescents. Initial romantic relationships serve to teach adolescents about becoming a romantic partner, establish social status, and further one's own gender identity. Nevertheless, the increase in cross-sex friendships during adolescence requires boys and girls to adjust and adapt their styles of interacting to accommodate opposite-sex friends. Although adolescents often learn to adjust their interaction styles on their own, parents can help them think about and adapt their behaviors with opposite-sex peers. Researchers believe that opposite-sex friendships may provide adolescents with important experience in dealing with the opposite sex prior to dating.

A major challenge during adolescence is the tendency of teenagers to engage in more risk-taking when with their friends. This behavior is particularly worrisome because adolescents spend much more time with their peers unsupervised by adults than do younger children. However, maintaining a supportive relationship with your teens, as well as an open line of communication regarding risky behaviors, can keep you informed about how your children spend their time and with whom. Further, it can prove quite helpful to make suggestions for how your children can handle risky situations and peer pressure.

Adolescence is a time of exploration and experimentation, and wise parents will remain mindful of that when evaluating their adolescents' seemingly distant and "cold" behavior. Despite the greater reliance on peers during adolescence, most teenagers report that they have positive relationships with their parents and that they often turn to their parents for support when times get tough. Thus, although parents of teenagers may often feel like their children no longer listen to them and that they have lost their influence over them, research does not support that conclusion. Rather, the most socially competent adolescents tend to report that they have parents who act supportively and grant them an appropriate amount of independence while maintaining high expectations for them. Keep the following principles in mind:

- *Choose your battles.*   As adolescents seek independence, they want to feel that they are treated with more respect and allowed to make more decisions regarding their free time and peer relationships. You can help your teens achieve this goal while maintaining strong, close relationships with them. One way to do this is to choose your battles wisely. Let your adolescent children make some decisions on their own (e.g., what to wear, where they plan to go) so that they feel empowered, but make your voice known on important matters (e.g., curfews, knowing who they plan to go with). When you do make a decision that affects your adolescent, provide your teen with explanations for your decision, so that he or she knows that you did not make the decision arbitrarily. This will also show that you respect your teen enough to provide justification for decisions that affect him or her. Further, despite seeking more autonomy, adolescents generally want their parents' continued love and support. You should continue to show affection toward your adolescents and to let them know that their safety is important to you, because whether or not these overtures seem welcomed with gratitude, they do need and they do want your concern.
- *Learn who their friends are.*   Because parents have less involvement in their adolescents' peer relations than when they were younger, continue to talk to your adolescents about their peer relations. Try to get as much information as possible without coming across as overbearing. Welcoming your teen's friends over is a good way to find out what's going on in your adolescent's social life. Your teenager's friends generally will tell you more about what's going on than your child will. Even if your adolescent will not tell you much, keeping track of where he or she plans to go and with whom remains an important part of monitoring adolescents' behaviors and relationships. Although such inquiries may seem intrusive, most adolescents understand and appreciate that their parents want to be involved in their lives and are concerned about their welfare.
- *Actions speak louder than words.*   Remain mindful of your own behaviors, during interactions with your adolescent as well as with other people. Children and adolescents pay close attention to their parents' behavioral patterns and often interact with their friends in ways that resemble their parents' typical ways of behaving. Therefore, think about the behaviors and traits that you would like to see in your adolescent and try to model those characteristics.
- *Find time to talk to your adolescent about risk-taking and peer pressure.*   If you can anticipate certain situations that may arise with your teen's friends and that may

involve risk taking (e.g., drinking alcohol, driving), ask your child how he or she would handle those situations and discuss ways of dealing with peer pressure. A discussion about these serious matters might prove most effective if you approach these topics tactfully, in the context of a more casual conversation about your adolescent's friends and social life in general. Moreover, approaching such a discussion with an open mind and without prejudging will increase your chances of influencing your adolescent's thinking about risky behaviors.

SUMMARY

Different challenges emerge at different ages, but it is reassuring that parents *can* and *do* contribute to their children's ability to develop and deal with friendships. We have tried to highlight just a few key characteristics and challenges common to friendships across childhood and adolescence and suggest some specific ways in which you can foster your children's social skills and help them handle the predictable crises and problems that confront many children and adolescents in peer relations every day.

WHERE TO FIND OUT MORE

Books

Brokamp, E. (2008). *Circle of three: Enough friendship to go around.* Washington, DC: American Psychological Association.

Brown, L.K. (2001). *How to be a friend: A guide to making friends and keeping them.* New York: Little, Brown Young Readers.

Caporale, J.D. (2005). *They call me chicken: A story of courage.* Philadelphia: Xlibris Corporation.

Frankel, F. (1996). *Good friends are hard to find: Help your child find, make and keep friends.* Glendale, CA: Perspective Publishing.

Lonczak, H. (2006). *Mookey the monkey gets over being teased.* Washington, DC: Magination Press.

Madorsky Elman, N., & Kennedy-Moore, E. (2003). *The unwritten rules of friendship: Simple strategies to help your child make friends.* Boston: Little, Brown and Company.

Meiners, C.J. (2004). *Join in and play (learning to get along).* Minneapolis, MN: Free Spirit Publishing.

Nowicki, S., Duke, M., & Van Buren, A. (2008). *Starting kids off right: How to raise confident children who can make friends and build healthy relationships.* Atlanta, GA: Peachtree Publishers.

Riera, M. (2003). *Staying connected to your teenager: How to keep them talking to you and how to hear what they're really saying.* Cambridge, MA: Perseus Publishing.

Rubin, K.H. (2002). *The friendship factor: Helping our children navigate their social world—and why it matters for their success and happiness.* New York: Penguin Books.

Slavens, E. (2004). *Peer pressure: Deal with it without losing your cool.* Halifax, Nova Scotia, Canada: Lorimer Publishers.

Websites

American Psychological Association. (2004).
Communication tips for parents.
   http://www.apa.org/helpcenter/communication-parents.aspx
Copeland, M. E. (n.d.).
Making and keeping friends: A self-help guide.
   http://mentalhealth.samhsa.gov/publications/allpubs/sma-3716/making.asp
Substance Abuse and Mental Health Services Administration. (n.d.).
A family guide to keeping youth mentally healthy & drug free: Teach kids to choose friends wisely.
   http://family.samhsa.gov/teach/

CHAPTER 23

Sportsmanship

Jeffrey L. Brown

The umpire yelled "strike three" after Monica watched the pitch glide over home plate. The inning was over, but Monica's tantrum had just begun. Her parents felt stunned and embarrassed as they watched their fifth-grader kick dirt toward the umpire, then throw her bat and helmet against the chain-link backstop. The crowd focused on how Monica's parents would react to the situation.

Across town at a city pool, swimmers stroked at top speed for the final meters of the 100-meter freestyle in a close contest between first and second place. As Gregory pushed himself toward a city-record finish, he noticed a less capable swimmer flailing his arms and gulping water in the lane next to him. Without hesitation, Gregory acted on his lifeguard training from summer camp and forfeited his win to save the life of a peer he didn't even know. Gregory later told a local newspaper reporter he had simply forgotten about the race when he realized the other swimmer needed help. Gregory's parents felt very proud of him.

In the two contrasting stories of Monica and Gregory, sportsmanship stood on display for everyone to see. Did the two have choices about how to behave? Could their parents have said or done something to possibly shape these critical behaviors before they happened? Does sportsmanship really matter as much as people think it should? The answer: A resounding *yes* across the board.

WHAT IS GOOD SPORTSMANSHIP?

The cluster of behavior we call sportsmanship reflects an internal attitude of respect, fairness, and self-control. It requires skill development just as much as a perfect golf swing or a free throw shot that's all net. The Greek philosopher Plato made a slam dunk when he said, "You can tell more about a person in an hour of play than a year of conversation."

Undoubtedly, games and strategies may have changed over the centuries, but the strong desire to win certainly hasn't. A child's behavior can tell a powerful story without using any words and, it can create a reputation in an instant.

When young participants lack sportsmanship, spectators wonder about a flaw in character, or a weakness in parenting or coaching as well. One of the most revered attributes a competitor can possess, sportsmanship traditionally aligns with athletics. But, it also has a necessary place in other competitive arenas today including academics, music, drama, student government, and Internet gaming. In fact, the apparently growing emphases on respect for peers, rules, and mentors seem sure signs that sportsmanship carries more value than ever before.

HOW CAN I TEACH MY CHILD GOOD SPORTSMANSHIP BEHAVIORS?

Parents play a critical role in shaping a child's sportsmanship behaviors in competitive situations. There's plenty to do on the home front to engender good sportsmanship and rear a healthy, respected competitor. For parents interested in developing sportsmanship in their children, making a game plan for developing sportsmanship is a prerequisite in today's culture. The following are some key strategies that can help your son or daughter be an all-star on the inside *and* the outside.

Understand the Values Taught to Your Child by Others

Coaches, mentors, and after-school administrators probably spend more time engaged in extracurricular activities with your child than you do.

- Make sure you ally with other adults in your child's life about the important lessons taught to them about infusing positive values into your child's belief system.
- While the culture of some sports, like football and ice hockey allow for aggressive play, it can prove detrimental and confusing for your child if a coach encourages aggressive behavior beyond the limits of a game.
- A coach who allows intensely competitive behavior on the field, but who also expects respectful disciplined behavior toward teachers and peers in the classroom models the type of behavior you'd want on your team.
- Knowing the philosophies and strategies of your child's coach can help you collaborate when shaping your child's positive sport behaviors.
- Talking with a coach individually may prove a helpful way to share your values about sportsmanship and at the same time let you know more about an adult who has a strong influence on your child's development.

Clarify Your Own Values About Sportsmanship

Inconsistent or mixed messages about sportsmanship can undermine the sense of sportsmanship you are trying to instill in your child.

- Telling your children to play fairly and respect their teammates, but then later heckling or mocking their opponents from the stands will weaken the strength of your words.
- Research strongly demonstrates that children imitate behavior of people they see as successful or as role models, including unsportsmanlike behaviors.
- You should send a clearly defined, consistent message to your children about how much you value good sportsmanship, both on and off the field.
- Your actions must back up your words in everyday life.

Reinforce Sportsmanship Behaviors

Help your children develop an understanding of sportsmanship by identifying and reinforcing specific behaviors, attitudes, and interactions.

- If your child loans a piece of equipment to a peer or speaks words of encouragement to a teammate when the teammate has made an error, let your child know you observed the positive action and felt pleased and proud.
- If you happen to notice your child make a negative, off-handed comment or become impatient with a peer during a practice or performance, take time as soon as possible to talk with your child about what he was experiencing emotionally and encourage him to think about how the other child might have felt.
- Helping your child develop new options or solutions about how he could respond differently provides a great way of concluding the conversation and helps develop a plan of action for the future.

Predict Situations Where Sportsmanship Is the Best Response

As a result of athletics or other organized competition, children often have meaningful experiences that teach them about how to relate to others and how to problem-solve as a group. Together with your child, it can be helpful for you to predict dilemmas that may arise in future competition. Examples of challenging situations which can arise include:

- Playing against another competitive child
- Listening to jeering fans
- Staying cool in the heat of a critical moment
- Reacting to an official who makes an arguable decision

In addition to having a conversation with your child, you may find role-playing such situations with her as a helpful way of giving her experience and confidence. It can be a fun play-acting different personalities or experiencing mastery over particular situations that could pose a troublesome challenge at some point in the future.

Require Ownership of All Behaviors

Placing blame on an opponent or rival provides an easy way of justifying one's own unsportsmanlike behavior. Take the lead to ensure your children know their peers have different motives and behaviors from their own, and that kids have a choice when it comes to interacting with respect. Insist that your children react maturely and peacefully when someone treats them in an unsportsmanlike manner. Learning to minimize their negative reactions to others' negative behaviors allows your children to strengthen their sense of sportsmanship from within. When it comes to controlling behaviors in competition, teaching personal ownership provides the key.

Keep Games Fun, Fair, and Interesting

If you serve as both a parent and a coach or volunteer in a supervisory role, make sure to keep kids engaged in activities by having fun. Historically, the primary reason kids quit sports is because they no longer have fun when participating. By partaking in an activity they enjoy, younger kids especially can benefit from variations in practice routines, developing good organization, and predictable schedules. Of course, emphasizing sportsmanship in both practice and games should remain a priority. When good sportsmanship disappears, then participation is rarely fun for anyone.

Talk to Your Child About the Importance of Sportsmanship

Research strongly suggests that compliance with a request increases when the person understands the reason for the behavior. Kids may comply with sportsmanship behaviors in competition if they also learn about the benefits of such behaviors. For example, if they know others will respect them more, that younger children may look up to them, or that coaches may give them extra responsibilities, children will more likely act in a way that reflects sportsmanship. Saying something like, "Monica, when you show respect to the umpire, others will respect you, too," can help kids understand the reasons for positive behavior and the value of modeling it.

Teach Your Child How to Both Win and Lose

Many hours of practice go into developing expertise, but rarely will a team or individual practice losing or performing poorly for the sake of negotiating a bad performance recovery. Following the sage adage, "Practice like you're going to play," makes sense. However, when a child begins to perform poorly, subsequent frustration ensues and unsportsmanlike behaviors can begin to surface. Reminding your children that they will not always win, and that losing is normal and okay may substantially reduce their risk of making poor stress-related decisions during competition. Sometimes it's just okay to fail. Create opportunities to practice dealing successfully with good and bad performances. It may help to share with your children examples of winning and losing by telling stories from your own childhood, too.

Identify Positive Role Models

Most adults can identify positive role models who played influential roles at one point in their lives. Your child has more options than ever when it comes to choosing someone from popular culture to look up to. In recent history, news media has taken stories of drug-enhancement and other sports scandals to frenzied levels. Imitating unsportsman-like behaviors can prove tempting. The media routinely provides illustrative examples in advertising, news reports, and online. Help your child choose a good role model or two, based on the person's positive behaviors. Then, do what you can to share the enthusiasm for that role model with your child and use that role model as a reference point for your child's behavior. You may help your child develop sportsmanship behaviors by asking your child what his role model would do in a particular situation.

SUMMARY

For many kids, role models are found in their parents. Because of that important duty and privilege, parents should strive to develop in their child the art of playing fairly, as much as they would try to cultivate any physical skill. Since actions do speak louder than words, parents who are committed to instilling sportsmanship in their child can now be equipped with a game plan for raising a true champion. Remember to play hard, play fairly, and have fun.

WHERE TO FIND OUT MORE

Books

Bigelow, B., Moroney, T., & Hall, L. (2001). *Just let the kids play: How to stop other adults from ruining your child's fun and success in youth sports.* Deerfield Beach, FL: Health Communications, Inc.

Brown, J. (2007). *The competitive edge: How to win every time you compete.* Carol Stream, IL: Tyndale House Publishers.

De Lench, B. (2006). *Home team advantage: The critical role of mothers in youth sports.* New York: Collins Living.

Doyle, D., & Burch, D.D. (2008). *Encyclopedia of sports parenting.* Kingston, RI: Hall of Fame Press.

Ginsburg, R.D., Durant, S., & Baltzell, A. (2006). *Whose game is it, anyway?: A guide to helping your child get the most from sports, organized by age and stage.* New York: Houghton Mifflin.

Simon, R.L. (2003). *Fair play: The ethics of sport* (2nd edition). Boulder, CO: Westview Press.

Stricker, P.R. (2006). *Sports success Rx! Your child's prescription for the best experience: how to maximize potential and minimize pressure.* Elk Grove Village, IL: American Academy of Pediatrics.

Websites

EduGuide
Parent sportsmanship checklist
   http://www.eduguide.org/Parents-Articles/Parent-Sportsmanship
KidsHealth
Sportsmanship
   http://kidshealth.org/parent/fitness/general/sportsmanship.html
The Educated Sports Parent
   http://www.educatedsportsparent.com

CHAPTER 24

Bullying

William S. Pollack and Susan M. Swearer

School has always been hard for Ben. The teasing started in kindergarten, with other students making fun of his last name, Swan. Now that he is in high school, the teasing has escalated into physical violence. Kids sometimes kick and shove him in the hallways, in addition to calling him names. Ben says teachers see this happen, but don't stop to help. Even those kids that Ben thought were his friends join in on the bullying, or they just stand by and watch. His parents haven't done anything to stop the bullying either. He feels betrayed by his peers and the adults in his life.

Sarah is an athletic, intelligent, and attractive eighth-grade student with a stable group of friends whom she has known since elementary school. Sarah and her friends like to use Facebook to post pictures and leave each other comments. When a cute boy, Jack, arrived at their school, Sarah and some of her friends posted comments about him on their Facebook pages. Sarah's comment that Jack was a "hottie" upset one of her volleyball teammates who "defriended" Sarah on Facebook and told everyone in school that Sarah was obsessed with Jack. Soon Sarah realized that no one was talking to her and, when she logged on to her Facebook account, all of the volleyball players had "defriended" her. Sarah is devastated and doesn't know what to do.

Bullying pervades childhood and adolescence in America. Given the regular daily experiences of harmful bullying in the United States and many other Western industrialized nations, we can certainly feel the pain expressed by Ben and Sarah, although their stories don't surprise us. Many adults feel helpless to stop bullying. Often, teachers and parents are not aware of the extent of the bullying. Perhaps children downplay the bullying because they are ashamed.

In this chapter, we hope to illuminate how common and hurtful, how psychologically toxic, as well as potentially physically harmful bullying is—to the "victim," the "bystander," and, yes, even, in some ways, to the bullies themselves. We want to help parents recognize the insidious signs of bullying and then to help them coordinate their efforts along with their children and with other adults responsible for the care of youth. Only with a coordinated effort among youth, parents, and caring adults (including teachers and other "mentors") can we help diminish and eradicate bullying.

WHAT IS BULLYING?

To solve the problem of bullying, you must accurately identify and differentiate bullying behavior. Bullying presents both an obvious and a subversive problem. Bullying, according to the classic definition levied by the pioneer in bullying research, Dan Olweus, has three components: (1) intent to harm; (2) repetition; and (3) power imbalance (sometimes referred to as gaining "power over" another). Thus, bullying involves negative physical or verbal behavior that occurs repeatedly and in a relationship in which the bullied person has a difficult time defending himself or herself.

Bullying differs from other forms of aggression in important ways. Aggressive behavior between youth of equal power or status does not qualify as bullying. If two students, both about the same size and equally as powerful, engage in teasing or even fighting, this does not qualify as positive behavior, but does not constitute bullying. If, however, the fighting or teasing occurs repeatedly, and the person who is under attack is weaker or less powerful, then the behavior qualifies as bullying. In the example of Ben and Sarah, the repetitive nature of the bullying and their inability to defend themselves made the bullying particularly detrimental.

Bullying behaviors span the gamut from verbal (i.e., name-calling) to physical (i.e., hitting, kicking, and serious beating) to electronic (i.e., using cell phones and computers/the internet). Bullying can also occur in *relational* contexts (for both males and females) in that individuals can manipulate relationships and damage the reputation of others in order to inflict harm (i.e., bully them). Involvement in bullying also spans a continuum of roles, from students who bully others to those uninvolved in bullying. Typically, involvement can occur in and in combination across five roles: (1) bully, (2) bully-victim, (3) victim, (4) bystander, and (5) "upstander." (These roles are discussed in more detail in the section that follows.) Parents and educators must recognize that these roles are not fixed in individuals, especially in the younger years; and that typically, children and youth engage in more than one role, depending upon the *context*, which may or may not protect them, or, support these behaviors.

HOW DOES BULLYING AFFECT MENTAL HEALTH?

Both the obvious and insidious nature of bullying connects involvement in bullying to mental health or daily emotional difficulties. Youth who bully others repeatedly will more likely express antisocial behavior, including conduct disorder and oppositional defiant disorder, disorders characterized by chronic behavior problems. Yet, these youth may also experience intense depression. Youth who experience bullying (victims) will more likely experience anxiety and depression. Youth who both bully others and who feel bullied themselves (bully-victims) fall somewhere in between on the spectrum of emotional pain. Bystanders, those who observe bullying but feel confused or frozen and unable to act, will also more likely experience anxiety and hopelessness/helplessness. "Upstanders," or those youth who feel connected enough to a supportive adult to either report the bullying behavior, or if it seems safe enough, stand up for the victims in a healthy school, after-school, or home environment, feel a sense of personal well-being. However, data suggest a likely longstanding connection between ongoing involvement in bullying and later mental health difficulties. Thus, it is imperative that parents, educators, and other adults responsible for providing a protective and safe environment for youth work together with youth themselves ("healthy empowerment") to effectively reduce this detrimental behavior. Bullying robs students like Ben and Sarah of successful and positive school and life experiences, and interferes with the experience of a growing sense of healthy emotional resilience.

IN WHAT CONTEXT DOES BULLYING USUALLY OCCUR?

In addition to the connection between bullying and mental health issues, it seems clear that bullying does not occur in a vacuum. Bullying happens when social relationships become unhealthy and when we permit a breakdown of human decency and kindness to occur and/or persist. If everyone acted in ways that were kind, nice, and *mutually respectful*, then bullying, by definition, could not occur. Bullying occurs when the conditions in the environment or context allow this negative behavior to exist and persist. Youth interact with their peer group, the school climate, their families, other significant adults, and their neighborhoods, and within societal norms and expectations. At any one of these levels (i.e., individual, peer, school, family, "caring" adults, neighborhood, society) conditions could occur that would support or, conversely, eradicate the involvement in bullying behavior.

What conditions in Ben and Sarah's lives supported the bullying behavior? Ben seemed a shy, anxious child who felt badly about teasing regarding his last name (individual level). He did not fit in as part of the popular peer group (peer), and he went to a school where the school culture supported or tolerated (actively or just passively) bullying behaviors. Ben's parents had busy lives and did not notice the results of his chronic victimization: lowered self-esteem, diminished mood, shifts of interest in attending school, and sometimes complaining about bodily pains that "appeared" to have no physical basis. Thus, all these conditions worked together to maintain the bullying behaviors perpetrated against Ben.

In Sarah's case, she had her own laptop and the family home had a wireless router. So, Sarah could have access to her Facebook pages at all times. In fact, she admitted that she spent about 3 hours a day on Facebook and text messaging. Many of these posts would happen late at night, after her parents had gone to bed. Her unsupervised access to technology contributed to the relational bullying that Sarah endured.

WHAT CAN I DO TO HELP MY CHILD?

For many youth who feel bullied, the scourge of bullying becomes so embarrassing and damaging that they typically do not tell their parents or other adults. For boys in particular, the embarrassment (shame) and devastation caused by the bullying can feel overwhelming.

These feelings may lead bullied youth to engage in a "code of silence" and decide to not talk about their experiences.

Parents or authority figures stand as the front-line adults in the war against bullying. Of course, to solve a problem, one first has to notice it! Bullying is both an *obvious* and a *hidden* epidemic. Sometimes, bullying can hide in plain sight. In other words, it goes on around other children too frightened to talk about it or intervene and around adults who are unaware of the serious nature of the problem and who either feel helpless to stop it or too afraid to try.

Parents and other responsible adults can take several actions to genuinely make a difference in their children's lives so as to diminish their hurtful experiences with bullying.

First, you must regularly talk with and /or remain "available" to your children. Your presence, as long as you are nonshaming, can help your children break their code of silence and open up to you. To help you in these tasks, educate yourself about bullying (see Where to Find Out More).

Second, establish a healthy ongoing relationship with your child's school and teachers/administration. Parents who stay involved in their child's education and who can observe their child's peer-group interactions have more information about the school and peer-group conditions (the "school/after school *climate*") that contribute to their child's experiences—for better or worse. Armed with this information, you can act more successfully in helping your child deal with or eradicate bullying.

Third, model healthy social relationships in your own life. Too often, students who become involved in bullying witness bullying interactions in their home and/or neighborhood. To protect your children from involvement in bullying (either as bully or victim), you must demonstrate healthy relationships. And, equally important, you need to connect with other like-minded parents with zero tolerance for bullying behavior and other helpful adults who can support you in your attempts to help your children. Remember that, although parents and school officials should maintain a "zero tolerance" for bullying behavior, they should not uniformly impose uniform severe penalties to *every* offender, or your credibility as a "go-to" person in times of trouble will be diminished in your children's' eyes.

Fourth, make sure you understand how text messaging, instant messaging, email, and social network sites operate. *NEVER* let your children have access to technology without some negotiated form of adult supervision. Computers should be kept in public, rather than private spaces around the house.

SUMMARY

The following steps will give you the chance to help your children avoid involvement in bullying and perhaps even eradicate it, or at least come close to stopping this devastating social problem:

- Recognize the warning signs of bullying.
- Find research-supported yet practical information about bullying.
- Create and maintain connected relationships and "shame free-zones" with your children that "bust" the code of silence.

- Establish connections with school personnel and peer groups.
- Model healthy social relationships.
- Find connections and support among other like-minded parents and caring adults to diminish a sense of isolation in your quest to end bullying.

Not only will our children and young adults gain protection from the present crisis of hurtful bullying, as well as its longstanding after-effects of trauma, but parents and caring adult mentors will experience a sense of healthy empowerment and joy in being able to provide a genuinely meaningful legacy from one generation to another in which we can all take pleasure.

WHERE TO FIND OUT MORE

Books

Brown, L.M. (2005). *Girlfighting: Betrayal and rejection among girls.* New York: NYU Press.

Devine, J., & Cohen, J. (2007). *Making your school safe.* New York: Teachers College Press.

Olweus, D. (1993). *Bullying at school: What we know and what we can do.* Malden, MA: Blackwell Publishing.

Pollack, W.S. (2001). *Real boys.* New York: Penguin Books (paperback edition).

Pollack, W.S., Modzelski, W., & Rooney, G. (2008): *Prior knowledge of potential school-based violence* (Article and helpful recommendations posted on www.williampollack.com). Washington, DC. US Secret Service and US Department of Education.

Rigby, K. (2008). *Children and bullying: How parents and educators can reduce bullying at school.* Malden, MA: Blackwell Publishing.

Rivers, I., Duncan, N., & Besag, V.E., (2007). *Bullying: A handbook for educators and parents.* Westport, CT: Praeger Publishers.

Simmons, R. (2002). *Odd girl out: The hidden culture of aggression in girls.* New York: Harcourt, Inc.

Swearer, S.M., Espelage, D.L., & Napolitano, S.A. (2009). *Bullying prevention and intervention: Realistic strategies for schools.* New York: The Guilford Press.

Underwood, M.K. (2003). *Social aggression among girls.* NY: The Guilford Press.

Websites

Education.com
    http://www.education.com/definition/bullying/
Stop Bullying Now
    http://stopbullyingnow.hrsa.gov
Take a stand, lend a hand, stop bullying now!
    http://stopbullyingnow.hrsa.gov
Dr. William Pollock
    http://www.williampollack.com
Bullying Research Network
    http://brnet.unl.edu

CHAPTER 25

Homesickness

Brandon G. Briery

Your child is getting ready to go away to camp for the first time. You insist that she call you any time she wants, no matter what—and maybe even slip a cell phone into her luggage, even though you know it violates the camp's policies. Clearly something must be amiss if the camp wants to limit your contact with your own child, right? Well, not necessarily. Those policies are likely in place for good reasons— that benefit both you and your child. To better understand homesickness, how it happens, how to prevent it, and how to deal with it when it can't be prevented, read on.

Homesickness occurs much more commonly than many might guess. In fact, researchers have found that homesickness may occur for as many as 83%–95% of children and teens, and that it affects boys and girls at similar rates. In simple terms, homesickness occurs when someone misses, or is afraid of missing, being at home or with loved ones to the point at which it causes that person significant difficulty in performing daily activities.

Homesickness is not a new, modern-day phenomenon, but opinions regarding its causes—and cures—have changed over the ages.

WHY DOES MY CHILD GET HOMESICK?

Today, most experts agree that homesickness results from a variety of factors that occur together. These factors typically include characteristics of the child, the environment that child finds himself or herself in, and the circumstances that led the child to be there to begin with.

Some characteristics of children that may make them more susceptible to homesickness include:

- *Developmental age.* Younger children (or those who may function on a younger level as a result of disability, illness, or environmental factors) are at greater risk of experiencing homesickness than older (or more cognitively developed) children.

- *Experience being away from home and parents.* Children who have never spent time away from home or away from their primary caregiver(s) are at greater risk of experiencing homesickness.
- *Anxiety/depression.* Children who have a history of experiencing symptoms of anxiety and/or depression are at greater risk of experiencing homesickness as well.
- *Health.* Children who experience some sort of health or disability issue (e.g., asthma or diabetes), particularly issues that may be new to them, are at greater risk of experiencing homesickness.

Some characteristics of the environment that may intensify experiences of homesickness include:

- *New/novel environments.* A child who finds himself or herself in a brand new environment (e.g., sleep-away camp, the hospital), especially one very different from anywhere else he or she has ever been, stands at greater risk of experiencing homesickness.
- *No or few familiar peers.* A child who goes off to camp (or some other new environment) without friends he or she already knows is more likely to experience homesickness.
- *Unexpected weather/environmental challenges.* A child who cannot fully participate in activities he or she anticipated getting involved in before going away may be more likely to develop homesickness.
- *Unexpected living arrangements.* A child who is surprised to learn that he or she will be sleeping in a large group setting, without certain amenities (e.g., plumbing or electricity), or in a more rustic setting than anticipated (e.g., a tent rather than a cabin), may be more likely to experience homesickness.
- *Less than desirable food.* A child who expects bad food may create a self-fulfilling prophecy, and if he or she experiences what is perceived as bad food, it may increase his or her likelihood of homesickness.

Circumstances that led to children going away from home may influence their experience of homesickness; these include:

- *Surprises.* Children and adolescents typically value structure and routine (even though it may often seem otherwise when living with them on a daily basis!). If you sign your children up for camp without telling them, they may feel resentful. This resentment can lead your children to feel homesick once they actually attend camp.
- *Forced attendance.* Children whose parents have decided to send them to camp (without surprising them), even though the children made it very clear that they do not want to go, are more likely to experience homesickness.
- *Bargaining.* Parents who have made deals with their children—promising they will come pick them up if they call and say they are not having a good time—are more likely to experience homesickness.

HOW DO I PREVENT HOMESICKNESS IN MY CHILD?

After reading the preceding list of potential risk factors for homesickness, you may begin to feel a bit ill yourself! Don't worry—there's good news! Experts widely agree that most instances of homesickness can be avoided with the proper investment in prevention strategies. The following are adapted from Thurber and colleagues (2007) recommendations for setting kids up for success:

- *Involve your children (to the extent possible) in the decision to spend time away from home.* This may prove easier for a stay at summer camp than for a hospitalization, but even the latter can include children in the planning stages. Allow your children to take part in even the smallest decisions (e.g., what bag or suitcase they will pack their clothes in). This will help them feel like they have at least a little bit of control. By contrast, if your children feel forced into leaving home, they are likely to experience intense homesickness.
- *Educate your children.* Let your children know that it is normal to miss home when they are away. You may say something like, "Almost everyone misses something about home when they are away. Homesickness is normal. It means there are lots of things about home you love. And the good news is that there are lots of things you can think and do to help make things better if homesickness bothers you."
- *Teach your children how to cope.* Practice with your children some of the following strategies that they can use during their time away from home. These exercises can help boost your child's confidence about the separation:
  - Arrange for *practice time away from home,* such as a weekend at a friend's or relative's house. Ideally, these 2 or 3 days do not include telephone calls but do include opportunities for writing a letter or sending a postcard home. After the practice time away, parents can discuss how things went and which coping strategies worked best.
  - *Practice basic correspondence.* Ensuring that children know how to write letters increases the likelihood that they will maintain some contact with home. Better yet, provide your children with prestamped, preaddressed envelopes and notebook paper.
  - Work together with your children to *learn about the new environment,* be it a hospital, school, new neighborhood, or summer camp. Websites, orientation booklets, and current students, alumni, or staff members are excellent resources. They increase familiarity and, thereby, reduce anxiety.
  - *Get to know people* in the new environment. Having at least one familiar face—be it an adult or a peer—in a new place can diminish feelings of homesickness by augmenting social support and connections.
  - Encourage your children to *make new friends and seek support* from trusted adults. Both kinds of connections ease the adjustment to a new environment. College students who feel socially anxious prove less likely to seek social support and more likely to feel homesick.
- *Avoid expressing anxious or ambivalent feelings about your children being away from home.* Well-intentioned parents have often exacerbated homesickness with comments such as, "I sure hope the food there is decent," "I hope you'll be okay," or

"Have a wonderful time. I hope I remember to feed your dog." Giving children something to worry about will increase the likelihood of their being preoccupied with thoughts of home. Ideally, you should express enthusiasm and optimism about your child's time away from home. If you feel anxious, talk to other parents who have experienced the same thing. Do not share your anxiety with your children.

• *Maintain predictability and perspective about the time away.* Use a wall calendar to show children the time between today and the day of the separation. Highlight the days or weeks your children will be away, so they can see that it is a discrete period, not an eternity. During the separation, calendars are also useful tools for helping your children keep a perspective on duration.

In addition to these strategies, you may wish to try some of the following if your child is going away to camp:

• *Openly discuss any concerns you have that your child may experience homesickness with your child's counselor, the camp director, or camp nurse.* You don't have to have the discussion in front of your child, but many times parents are reluctant to share such information because they are afraid the camp will not allow their child to stay. As noted earlier, an overwhelming percentage of people experience some sort of homesickness while away from home; this is normal, and camp settings deal with it every day. Still, it is helpful when camp personnel are able to anticipate it and work with you to develop some prevention strategies that they can help implement.

• *Please respect camp policies on limiting telephone contact—especially if they have policies regarding no cell phones* (and most do these days). Experience has taught us that telephone contact exacerbates, rather than relieves, homesickness. Cell phones also serve as a distraction, as campers may feel more inclined to spend time texting or talking with friends or family from home than meeting new people and trying the new challenges the camp environment has to offer. Furthermore, most camps cannot guarantee the security of items like cell phones, so if they are lost or stolen, the burden is on you.

• *Call to check on your camper.* Although counselors are usually "out in the field" with campers most of the time, your child's counselor, a unit leader, or someone else familiar with your child and his or her experience at camp, can usually call you back and provide you with an update. This will vary from camp to camp, but if you feel worried about your camper, ask about the camp's policies and who you can contact for updates. Many camps also now use technology to provide photos or video clips through a password-protected website that parents can access. Many parents I've spoken with have told me this has reassured them, and that seeing their child laughing, smiling, and engaged in activities has sometimes offered a pleasant contrast to content in letters or emails sent home. A picture can indeed be worth a thousand words!

• *Pack things that will likely comfort your child.* These could include a favorite stuffed animal, pillow, blanket, or photos of family, pets, or favorite things.

• *Send care packages to your child at camp* (if the camp allows this). You may want to send something before you even drop your campers off, so there is something waiting for them when they arrive or on the next day. In the package, include things that you know your children love—possibly some of the comforting objects listed above, or their favorite cookies or snacks (if the camp allows). Simply sending letters to your child may also feel reassuring to them—reminding them you have not forgotten them. Always try to focus on the positive, such as that you are looking forward to hearing about their adventures and accomplishments at camp. Being specific about activities you know they are likely to enjoy may also be helpful (e.g., "I can't wait to hear how you liked canoeing," or "I look forward to seeing the projects you are making in arts and crafts!").

HOW DO I DEAL WITH MY CHILD'S HOMESICKNESS WHILE IT IS HAPPENING?

By now you know that many different factors can affect homesickness, and even though there are many strategies you can use to help prevent it from occurring, you may not always be 100% successful in preventing it. The following are some strategies that may be helpful if, despite your best efforts, your child still becomes homesick while away from home:

- *Talk to your child's counselor, camp director, or other staff.* Give them ideas about your child's hobbies and interests. Camp staff (and hospital staff) typically prove very good at finding a connection with children in their care (e.g., an interest in theatre, or computers, or pets), but a suggestion from you may provide just the breakthrough they had not previously achieved.
- *If time is of the essence, try sending your child an email if that is possible.* If your child is not able to access a computer to check email (or doesn't have an account or know how), find out if one of the staff members can receive an email from you and then share it with your child.
- If a telephone conversation directly with your child becomes necessary for some reason, *have a conference call with your child that includes the child's counselor, camp director, or other personnel.* Children will less likely exaggerate conditions if they know someone right there with them knows better!
- In any communication with your child, *avoid the temptation to make "pick-up deals" with them* (e.g., "If you aren't enjoying things better by tomorrow, I'll come pick you up."). Instead, try making deals with them such as, "There are a lot of fun things to do at camp that I know you have been looking forward to. I want you to try horseback riding and archery tomorrow. If you are still feeling bad, let your counselors know and they can contact me to talk about other things we can try."

SUMMARY

Going away to camp—or to other programs or similar situations—can be challenging. It is likely difficult to find anyone who would dispute that. Still, trying new challenges, experiencing different things, meeting new people, acquiring new skills, and learning independence are all very positive outcomes associated with participation in camps and other programs that make the challenges worthwhile.

One other thing of note is that parents often find themselves "campersick" as well, missing their child greatly while the child is away. Resist the temptation to attempt contacting your child in order to solve your own "campersickness." Ultimately, the growth and learning that occur through these experiences are important aspects of the developmental process, helping to foster success and independence in children and adolescents that will continue to benefit them into adulthood.

I encourage you to do your homework in preventing homesickness in your children, but also encourage you to strongly consider offering them the opportunities that can be found through participation in camps and similar programs. I believe you'll find your kids thanking you, and you thanking yourself for making the experiences possible for them!

WHERE TO FIND OUT MORE

Books

Sileo, F.J., & Fisher, E.S. (2009). *Bug bites and campfires: A story for kids about homesickness.* Albuquerque, NM: National Health Press.

Thurber, C.A., & Malinowski, J.C. (2000). *The summer camp handbook: Everything you need to find, choose and get ready for overnight camp-and skip the homesickness.* Glendale, CA: Perspective Publishing.

Websites

American Camp Association. (2008).
How to choose a camp: Homesickness.
  http://www.acacamps.org/media_center/how_to_choose/homesickness.php
Camp Spirit. (2008).
For parents.
  http://www.campspirit.com/parents/
Nemours Foundation. (2008).
KidsHealth for parents: Homesickness.
  http://kidshealth.org/parent/emotions/feelings/homesickness.html
Nemours Foundation. (2008).
TeensHealth answers & advice: Homesickness.
  http://kidshealth.org/teen/your_mind/emotions/homesickness.html

CHAPTER 26

Coping with a Change in Caregiver

Barbara Siegel

Carrie and Trevor's moms decide to share a part-time nanny. This is the first nanny for 11-month-old Carrie; Trevor, age 17 months, has recently said goodbye to his nanny, who cared for him for 1 year. Carrie is a feisty little girl, constantly grabbing toys out of Trevor's hands, fussing when she eats and has her diaper changed, and crying when the time comes to go home from play dates. Trevor is rather mild mannered, and when Carrie grabs something from him, he easily finds another toy. When the new nanny arrives, Trevor acts impassively and a little curious. His mom warmly greets her and introduces her to Trevor. They sit together for a while as Trevor becomes engaged in the nanny's game of "hide the toy cars." But when Carrie and her mom arrive—late—they have less time to spend on introductions. Carrie's mom feels anxious about leaving Carrie with a stranger, takes out her multipage list of emergency numbers and instructions, and hastily goes over it with the nanny. When Carrie's mom gets ready to go, she places Carrie in the arms of the nanny. Carrie sobs and wiggles to get out of the sitter's arms. The moms leave, Carrie's with a heavy heart and feeling terribly guilty.

Many different dynamics account for the different reactions that Carrie and Trevor had to the new caregiver. First, is the age difference. Carrie most likely finds herself in a stage of development called *separation anxiety*, the term given to babies as young as 6 months and as old as 18 months who cry when separated from their primary caregivers—usually their mothers.

Second, is the children's temperaments. Some adapt quickly, like Trevor, while children with a temperament like Carrie's get very anxious whenever they experience a change or transition. Third, Carrie and Trevor's moms responded very differently to the upcoming change. Trevor's mom had time to help him see the new adult as someone *she* trusted and liked, while Carrie's mom felt frantic and expressed her anxiety by going over page after page of instructions.

IS SEPARATION ANXIETY NORMAL?

Separation anxiety is a normal and healthy stage of growth and development, but it can be unsettling. Most babies younger than 6 months adapt pretty well to other caregivers as long as they have their needs met. But sometime between 4 to 7 months of age, babies develop a sense of "object permanence" and learn that things and people exist even when they're out of sight. Your once easy, social baby may now become anxious and teary every time you leave the room, even when grandma or close friends are nearby.

When your baby can't see you, that means you've gone away. And since babies don't understand the concept of time, they do not know if or when you'll come back. Whether you're in the kitchen, in the next bedroom, or at the office, it's all the same to your baby—you've disappeared. As your child grows into a more mobile toddler, he or she becomes even more uncertain about separations from you.

As children get a little older, their memory of past experiences with you will comfort them when you're gone, and they'll have the ability to anticipate a reunion. But during the period of separation anxiety, your child is only aware of the present. When you leave your child with another caregiver, he or she probably will scream as though his or her heart will break.

HOW CAN I EASE THE SEPARATION?

There are several things you can do to help your child adjust to being away from you:

- *Time your departures.*   Your child will become more susceptible to separation anxiety when tired, hungry, or sick. If you know you're going to go out, try to schedule your departure so that it occurs after your child has napped and eaten.
- *Don't make a fuss over leaving.*   Instead, have the caregiver create a distraction (a new toy, waving hello to the baby in the mirror, a book). Then say good-bye in an upbeat voice, reassure your child that you'll return later, and leave quickly.
- *Remember that most children will stop crying within minutes of your departure.*   Your child's outbursts are for your benefit, to persuade you to stay. With you out of sight, your child will soon turn his or her attention to the other person. Some children may cry much longer. This may be difficult for caregivers and parents, but eventually the crying does stop.
- *Practice being apart from your baby.*   Invite the babysitter over in advance, so that he or she can spend time with your child while you're in the room. Leave the room for short periods of time so that the baby sees that you come back.
- *Stay upbeat and calm.*   Try not to let your child pick up on any feelings of apprehension. By the second half of a baby's first year, he or she will look to you for emotional cues whenever an ambiguous or uncertain event presents itself—like the appearance of a new caregiver. If you look sad or wary, or if your voice does not

have that same melodic tone while greeting this nanny, the baby will sense that something is not right.

MY TODDLER IS OVER SEPARATION ANXIETY. WILL HE COPE WITH CHANGES IN CAREGIVERS NOW?

New caregivers, no matter how experienced and loving, will present a source of anxiety for your child up until the age of 5 or 6 years. An unknown person who will now have control is a scary prospect.

Children have a need to predict how the adults around them will behave and to anticipate what will happen in daily life. They feel most comfortable with routines and familiar faces. But change will inevitably happen, so children must learn to manage it. Through everyday changes, a child learns whether he or she can adapt, and whether he or she can trust adults to give information and offer support.

Children can adapt well, especially when they have advance preparation. Once a child learns that a change will soon occur, he or she will begin to make emotional adjustments to accommodate the new situation. You have the ability to make the transition to a new caregiver a smooth one, with advance preparation and nurturing of the new child–caregiver relationship. Positive experiences of coping with small daily changes will help your child face the big transitions later. Here are some things you can do to help your child adjust to a new caregiver:

- *Do not hide the fact that you're going out for the day in an effort to delay the tantrum you anticipate.* This will only increase your child's anxiety. The unknown feels much more frightening than the known. Children need a little time to process information, and may have a lot of questions for you. "Is she nice?" "Will I be able to watch Hannah Montana?"

- *Allow your children to make as many of their own decisions as possible when getting accustomed to a new caregiver.* Autonomy offsets anxiety; it reminds children that they have control over some things in life. "You can have mac and cheese and then choose whatever dessert you want. Can't find something? Here is five dollars for you to spend at the ice cream shop."

- *Preschoolers can quickly convert their anxiety into energy if you give them a project to do to prepare them for their caregivers.* For example, have your child create a welcome sign to greet the new caregiver or ask your child to set aside two books that he or she wants the caregiver to read.

- *Create a goodbye ritual.* Read *The Kissing Hand* or *The Good Bye Book.* In *The Kissing Hand,* for example, mother raccoon kisses the palm of her little raccoon so that, whenever he feels lonely, he can put his palm on his cheek to remember that his mother loves him. You might also use a kiss to your child's palm right before you leave, every time you leave, as a positive parting ritual.

- *When you say a pleasant, loving, and firm goodbye, do not linger.* Reassure your child that you'll be back—and explain how long it will take until you return. Use concepts kids will understand (such as "after lunch"). Give your child your full attention when you say goodbye, and when you say you're leaving, mean it; coming back a minute later will only make your child more anxious and teach him or her that crying is the key to getting you to do what he or she wants.

- *Follow through on promises.* It's important to make sure that you return when you have promised to. In this way your child will develop the confidence that he or she can make it through the time apart.
- *Be positive, truthful, and straightforward.* "I am going to work now. I will be back right before supper." If you get that tantrum you expected, act matter-of-factly, while acknowledging your child's unhappiness. Say something like, "Yes, I know you wanted Jenny to come instead of a new babysitter, but Jenny was busy today. I think you will have a great adventure with Tina. I heard that she likes to play beauty shop, and you can style your hair in wild ways."

Eventually, your child will develop the ability to remember that you always return after you leave, and that will be enough comfort while you're gone. This gives kids a chance to develop coping skills and a little independence. In fact, helping a toddler develop a relationship with a new caregiver is a kind of gift—your child learns that the world is full of people who are loving and who can take care of him or her.

HOW DOES TEMPERAMENT AFFECT MY CHILD'S ABILITY TO COPE WITH A CHANGE IN CAREGIVER?

All people have a particular *temperament*; inborn traits that make up our personality. Temperament is neither good nor bad; it is more like having blue eyes or brown ones. Although we can learn to modify our temperamental impulses by how others treat us or by influences in our environment, our basic temperamental makeup remains the same throughout our lives.

Our temperament makes some situations easy for us and other situations difficult. Therefore, some children have an easier time coping with new caregivers while others feel very agitated by the change. Here are some suggestions for a child, like Carrie, who has an emotional and intense temperament and who does not adapt to new situations as well as does Trevor.

- *Use familiar objects to ease anxiety during transitions.* Have your child's favorite stuffed animal or blanket at hand and tell the new caregiver that this will comfort your child.
- *Let your child take part in planning the transition.* Let him or her choose something to do, and tell the caregiver to let the child take the lead.
- *Ease into new activities.* Talk about the new activity, use the caregiver's name frequently, and give your child a few minutes to transition to it.
- *Offer advance notice when an activity will soon end.* "In a few minutes, we will go upstairs for your nap."

For children who adapt more quickly and take changes in stride, parents and caregivers should encourage more exploring and learning opportunities. These children usually prove more flexible and more keen on a change in routine even than their parents:

- *Offer children a variety of new experiences:* visit a new park, take a trip to the library, etc.
- *Remain attentive to your child's signals.* When a child seems easygoing, adults sometimes take for granted that any change is okay.
- *Let children know about the new situation ahead of time, so they can mentally prepare and look forward to it.*
- *Make certain to add one-on-one time to children's daily routines.* As much as they like to get out and about, these children need individual attention, too.

HOW DO I DEAL WITH FEELINGS OF GUILT?

For some parents, leaving their child with another caregiver is a no-win situation. When your child cries and reaches for you, a part of you feels pleased that you and your child have bonded so completely and that you remain the love object and center of your child's life. But, at the same time, you may feel guilty when you must leave him or her.

When a baby or child willingly or happily goes to the nanny or caregiver, initially you may feel relieved. But you also may feel jealous and begin to resent the nanny. Feeling competitive for your child's love and affection creates a very shaky foundation for you and your caregiver.

Parenthood often feels like a roller coaster of emotions, but most child psychologists agree that the message to the child should be 100% unambiguous: you are going to have a fun day with a super playmate. Remember that sharing your child's care with a nanny gives your child an opportunity to learn new things about himself or herself, and about others, that will broaden and enrich your child's life.

WILL MY CHILD LOVE THE NANNY MORE THAN ME?

No, no, no. Attachment theory, as initially described by British psychoanalyst John Bowlby in the 1960s, refers to a secure emotional base, a place from which a child feels safe enough to leave and explore the world around him or her. Children have primary attachment figures—usually mom is first, and then dad—and form unshakable bonds that last a lifetime. A child who feels securely attached to a primary figure will have more ability to form important emotional bonds with other caregivers. The relationship children have with their nannies and babysitters provides children with a sense of security and safety during times when the primary attachment figure is not present.

Therefore, don't feel distressed if your son or daughter still cries as you leave. Again, this normal reaction usually lasts only a few minutes once you walk out the door. If you feel worried, wait half an hour and call home. Most likely, you will hear happy sounds in the background. Likewise, don't feel distressed if your son or daughter jumps happily into the arms of your caregiver. This represents a healthy developmental milestone when your child has learned to trust someone in the outer world, and will lead to healthy relationships throughout his or her life.

HOW DO I BEST PREPARE MY CHILD FOR A NEW CAREGIVER?

It is important for children to have as much consistency and stability in their care arrangements as possible. In the best of all worlds, your nanny will stay until your child goes off to college! Unfortunately, all parents know that even the best-planned childcare arrangements prove fragile and that transitions from one caregiver to another are inevitable.

A first step might be trying to work out any problems that may come up with your nanny, to avoid unnecessary caregiver changes. If the nanny provides excellent care, but has some sloppy habits, think hard about your priorities. Second, if a change is necessary, you should try to make this the only change occurring at this moment in your child's life. Third, if possible, try not to make the change while your child works through the separation anxiety stage. Here are some suggestions for transitioning to a new caregiver:

- In order to maintain consistency and stability, write out your child's schedule of play, nap time, outdoor time, etc., so that the new caregiver sticks to the familiar routine.
- Have your new caregiver meet your child in a calm, relaxed manner—when you do not feel rushed.
- Prepare an emergency phone number list, including friends, neighbors, and pediatrician. List your children's full names and birthdates. Make sure the caregiver knows about allergies and other pertinent medical information.
- Explain to your child why the change in caregiver is necessary, and encourage your child to express feelings about it. Your child may feel sad, angry, frustrated, or frightened. Don't tell your child that he or she will "love" the new nanny or babysitter. Don't tell your child he or she is "silly" to make such a fuss. Do tell your child that you know change is not easy, but the new nanny seems very nice and loves to play.
- Act positively. Your child will look to you for emotional signals. If you seem genuinely happy and enthusiastic, your child will more likely take the transition in stride. Conversely, if you are anxious about the change, your anxiety will rub off on your child.
- If your child selected a favorite game, toy, book, or stuffed animal to show the new caregiver, make sure the new nanny knows that your child has picked out something very special to show her.
- When you come home, after the nanny leaves, take 10 minutes to give your undivided attention to your child. Research shows that having parents who work or having a nanny has no intrinsic negative impact on children. However, if children feel ignored when tired parents come home and immediately start the dinner rush, negative feelings can develop. Therefore, when you come home, take a few minutes to read, snuggle, or share a hot chocolate together.

SUMMARY

When you leave your unhappy child with a new caregiver, it may seem like your crying, withdrawn, or sulking child feels abandoned or betrayed. But do not fear. Learning to love, count on, accept, and feel safe with a caregiver other than yourself is the best thing you can do for your child. These relationships teach your children trust, and your coming home each time you say you will helps them feel secure.

WHERE TO FIND OUT MORE

Books

Barnet, A., & Barnet, R. (1998). *The youngest minds.* New York: Simon & Schuster.

Gonzalez-Mena, J., & Eyer, D. (1989). *Infants, toddlers and caregivers.* Mountain View, CA: Mayfield Publishing Co.

Lerner, C., & Dombro, L. (2005). *Bringing up baby.* Washington D.C.: Zero to Three Press.

National Research Council. (2000). From neurons to neighborhoods. Washington, D.C.: National Academy Press.

Penn, A. (2006). *The Kissing Hand.* Terre Haute, IN: Tanglewood Press.

Shick, L. (1998). *Understanding temperament.* Seattle: Parenting Press.

Viorst, J. (1988). *The good-bye book.* New York: Aladdin Paperbacks.

Websites

Zero to Three Foundation
   http://www.zerotothree.org

CHAPTER 27

Helping Children Cope with Ethnic, Religious, and Gender Differences

Yo Jackson

Jennifer, an African American, 10-year-old girl, began attending a new school last year, when her parents relocated. She moved from a multiethnic community to a mostly Caucasian neighborhood. Jennifer is the only person of color in her class, and one of only seven students in her school who belong to an ethnic minority group. She has friends in class, but often feels that she has to try harder than her peers to gain acceptance. She notices that she is not often invited on play dates to the home of other kids in the class, and sometimes finds herself sitting alone in the cafeteria.

Nadja, age 14, has just entered high school. As an observant Muslim, she wears a head scarf in public. Although she has special permission to wear a religious head covering, other students have made disparaging comments to Nadja in passing. Although her religious faith has powerful meaning for her, Nadja longs for peer acceptance and at times wishes that she could just blend in like all the other girls in her school.

Ben, age 7, attends karate class at the local community center. Each week, after class, he sees other children coming from the ballet studio next door. Sometimes he watches as the ballet dancers practice, and he asks his parents if he can do ballet too. His parents are unsure how they should respond, as he would be the only boy in the class. His older brother overhears Ben's request and says, "You want to do what? Ballet is for sissies."

It can be hard to adjust to the behavior and reactions of others when a child feels or is perceived as "different" in their peer group or community by virtue of membership in a minority ethnic, religious, or gender group (i.e., Muslim, low-income, or gay/lesbian family). Although being culturally different from others can have its advantages, coming from a culturally dissimilar group makes it more likely that a child will experience discrimination and rejection. The process of understanding what it means to be culturally different unfolds as children pass from childhood through adolescence. The recognition of differences is a normal part of establishing relationships with others. Everyone needs to feel wanted and included. It is easy for children to feel like a part of the group when they are surrounded by those who share cultural similarities. However, when the child's culture represents a minority, or when others do not prize or value the attributes that make the child different, the child is likely to experience stress. This chapter describes the distinctive environmental risk that culturally different youth experience and discusses what you can do to help minimize the negative impact of discrimination on your child's psychological health.

YOUTH FROM ETHNIC MINORITY BACKGROUNDS

The U.S. Census Bureau reports that, by 2023, the majority of children in the United States will have ethnic minority heritage. Learning a new language, being the only child of color in the classroom, and living in a country within the social context of racial or religious prejudice are just a few of the kinds of challenges children regarded as different have to manage. Children of color stand at risk for exposure to a myriad of stressful events including *acculturative stress.* That term refers to challenges people experience when trying to assimilate into a new or different culture. Becoming more acculturated or more like the majority group has both advantages and disadvantages. On the positive side, acculturation provides youth with more access to ideas about how people in the new or majority culture think, which can assist the child in fitting in more effectively with peers. In contrast, attaching to new values sometimes creates tension when the new culture's values seem in opposition to the values of one's culture of origin (i.e., the cultural group determined by birth). Moreover, many youth find that, as they become more acculturated, it becomes harder to relate to more traditional members of their culture of origin. They may come to see traditional ways (and some family members) as simply "old fashioned," and may struggle to figure out in which group they belong.

Children of diverse backgrounds, like all children, experience the common stressors associated with development. For African American children like Jennifer and other children of color, developing a sense of oneself as an ethnic person adds another dimension. Jennifer must not only cope with a new school and adolescence on the horizon, but must also understand herself as a member of the African American minority community. Acquiring such understanding is a process of trial and error, in which the child will seek to find places in both the minority (original culture) and majority culture (new culture) where he or she can feel competent and accepted.

When youth encounter positive images of their culture, the result tends to enhance their self-esteem. Conversely, when youth are exposed to negative images of people who look like members of their cultural group (e.g., criminals in the news, poorly educated, or disrespected people) youth may come to see themselves as part of a "problem group." Although one's sense of ethnic heritage can provide rich positive qualities, such as pride and strength, many children of diverse backgrounds face risk simply by association or stereotype. The result for some is low self-regard and pessimism about the future.

YOUTH FROM RELIGIOUS MINORITY BACKGROUNDS

The United States includes families representing a wide variety of religious and spiritual faiths. When religious or spiritual faith forms a part of the family culture, youth are likely to be exposed to other people who also share their same religious or spiritual background. Inclusion in a faith community provides youth with a significant number of advantages, not the least of which involves the social connection to others and the opportunity for learning from people who hold similar values. Given that Christianity represents the majority of people in the United States (although it is not the most common faith outside of the United States), youth who are not Christians will likely experience some stress when their peer or general community is religiously dissimilar. For example, consider children like Nadja. When religious practices dictate specific dress or behavior, it may prove hard to feel accepted when outside of the faith community. When children learn early on that the way they dress or behave marks them as part of a special group, such as a religious group, it can be hard to understand why others outside the group may ridicule or respond to the child with disrespect.

Feeling different extends well beyond Christian versus non-Christian differences. For example, when Protestant youth attend Catholic school, they may be expected to attend Mass, but due to rules of the Catholic Church, they cannot participate in all of the ceremonial rituals (e.g., Holy Communion). Another way youth may feel stressed by religious or spiritual differences involves religious holidays. Different days of the year qualify as holy for people of different faiths, requiring, among other things, refraining from work (including studying) or required attendance at religious services. Some children may have to reschedule tests and exams, if course requirements fall on the same days as their religious obligations.

HOW CAN I HELP MY CHILD?

Comparing themselves to each other is a normal and expected part of children's development and serves as a way for youth to learn about themselves. Social comparison tends to peak during the preschool and early adolescent years. Most parents want their children to understand and accept differences among others, while at the same time have an appreciation for the qualities in themselves that make them unique and important. Parents of children from cultural minority groups need to pay special attention to their own experiences with prejudice and work through their own issues, so that they can see these events from their child's perspective. When parents carry around their own pain regarding cultural differences, this pain can add to the hurt they feel when their own child is hurt by the comments or teasing of others. The notion that being different is a bad thing is not restricted only to people outside of the family, as prejudices exist even within the same family group. For example, some parents will likely place different expectations or significance on what sons do compared to what daughters do.

To encourage your child to more openly accept differences among others, try the following suggestions:

- *Avoid making derogatory statements.*   Criticizing groups of people, even groups you may belong to, sends a message that it is okay to mock others based on cultural differences.
- *Show children that you value cultural differences.*   One way to do this is by making available materials that are representative of different cultural values and practices.
- *Remain open to your child's feelings.*   Youth need to have a trusted adult to talk to about their feelings, without fear of judgment or correction.
- *Model a positive sense of self-worth.*   Youth prove much more likely to show openness and tolerance of cultural differences when they have a sense of pride in their own culture. Share with your children their history and culture, and teach them to be proud of the differences that make them special.

The following suggestions are some ways you can help your child cope with being different and manage any discrimination and prejudice he or she may face:

- *Think about the ways you manage stress and the kinds of coping methods you use most often.*   Children follow the models parents provide, not only for identifying problems, but also for learning culturally acceptable methods of coping.
- *Remain aware of your own culturally based expectations for your child's behavior.*   Ask yourself, "How do I expect my child to behave in times of emotional distress?" It is important to recognize that your expectations may or may not fit with mainstream expectations.
- *Pay attention to the kinds of stresses your child experiences.*   Talk to other parents and your child's teachers and friends, who can provide a broader picture of the events commonly experienced by today's children.
- *Prepare your child.*   When you know that your child will fall in the cultural minority at a particular setting, take care to prepare your child. Remind your child that other youth may not understand different cultural practices at first and that it may take some time and effort for them to feel comfortable around him or her.
- *Enlist the help of other adults and authority figures in your child's life.*   Having resources in place for children before conflict occurs will prove more useful than trying to find support after a crisis has happened. Helping your child cope effectively with cultural differences is easiest if you have support from a network in the community.
- *Encourage older children to share their experiences with younger ones.*   If your child has an older sibling, it is quite possible that he or she faced the very same kinds of peer group differences that your younger child now faces. Your older child can provide your younger one with some problem-solving solutions.
- *Teach children to choose their battles.*   Often minor cultural differences work themselves out without adult involvement, and parents can help children to understand which cultural conflicts the child should respond to and which events require no response.

- *Talk to your child about his or her feelings.* Most children will internalize or blame themselves after sensing that others do not like them or treat them poorly. Only by sharing their feelings with a trusted adult, who will listen without judging, can youth learn and understand why cultural conflicts occur.
- *Give your child a place to vent.* Youth may feel angry after experiencing rejection by others based on cultural differences. You can help by recognizing these feelings as normal and providing a safe place for your child to vent. After your child has calmed down, help brainstorm possible alternative reactions. By listening and validating feelings, children will feel heard and better able to see more clearly what appropriate reactions might be when others judge them because of their culture.
- *Teach your child how to identify cultural conflicts that are time-limited* (e.g., offensive remarks by a stranger at the supermarket), as well as those that are likely to become chronic (e.g., hostility from a child or adult at the beginning of a new school year). Time-limited conflicts require a more measured response, while those that have the potential to be ongoing should be dealt with immediately. The idea here is to help your child develop a repertoire of responses so that the same reaction does not follow every stressful cultural difference experience the child encounters.

SUMMARY

It is impossible to protect your children from exposure to stressful events triggered by differences in culture. Being different, experiencing unfair treatment, and having to adapt to norms that may differ from the expectations in their culture of origin can be especially challenging for children, and they may require your help. Cultural values often guide people in how one should react to distressing events. How parents from one cultural group manage their child's distress may differ significantly from the expectations that another cultural group may have for the same kind of event, so recognizing customary practices for each particular group becomes important. Remember that simple group membership does not mean that everyone in that group holds the same value system and that many differences exist in any group. Parents can strive to remain as aware as possible of the kinds of stressors their children will likely face, understand that some of these events are typical and happen to all children, and understand that, as parents, they will serve as important role models for how their child will ultimately learn how to manage cultural differences.

WHERE TO FIND OUT MORE

Books

Comer, J.P., & Poussaint, A.F. (1992). *Raising black children.* New York: Penguin.
Diamant, A., & Kushner, K. (2008). *How to raise a Jewish child.* New York: Schocken.
Dwivedi, K.N. (2002). *Meeting the needs of ethnic minority children.* (2nd edition). New York: Jessica Kingsley Publishers.
Goldberger, N.R., & Veroff, J.B. (1995). *The culture and psychology reader.* New York: New York University Press.

Heegaard, M.E. (2003). *Drawing together to accept and respect differences.* Minneapolis: Fairview Press.

Sax, L. (2006). *Why gender matters: What parents and teachers need to know about the emerging science of sex differences.* New York: Broadway.

Tatum, B.D. (2003). *"Why are all the black kids sitting together in the cafeteria?" A psychologist explains the development of racial identity.* New York: Basic Books.

PART FOUR

School Issues

CHAPTER 28

Making Sense of Report Cards

W. Douglas Tynan and Jennifer Shroff Pendley

Karen, now in seventh grade, received an interim report in the middle of the 10-week marking period indicating a failing trajectory in Spanish. Since that time, she has had tutoring twice per week, has shown rapid improvement, and her grades were all Bs on her last three quizzes and tests. However, her report card grade was a low C for the marking period, and she feels very disappointed.

For all parents, and most students, getting a report card can be a stressful event, even if the news from school turns out all good. None of us really enjoy being evaluated or compared to some standard of accomplishment. In the world of schools, we typically use report cards and test scores to track progress, promote to the next grade, or to move a child to a different program or school. So, while we may not like them, schools have relied on report cards for a very long time and do not seem likely to change anytime soon. So, we might as well make use of the report card as an opportunity to learn something about students and help them advance.

WHAT ARE REPORT CARDS?

The term "report card" in our culture generally means a rating of performance, and while it applies to almost any rating system of people or organizations, we all identify the original "report cards" as those that students get from their teachers to share with their parents. Report cards are an essential part of school and have always served as a source of pride, accomplishment, anxiety, and fear or shame depending on the student's performance, the teacher's ratings, and the parent's expectations and responses. The interaction you have with your child around a report card can have positive or negative effects, but ideally it should serve as constructive feedback. A report card is a way for educators to share a student's progress in school with not only the student, but with the student's parents as well. It is important to use this feedback constructively. If your child does well, you will want to maintain that effort and progress. If your child has done poorly, a report card affords an opportunity to make changes to improve performance.

WHAT DOES A REPORT CARD TELL US?

The first thing to recognize involves what a report card actually tells us: how, on average, the student has performed over the last 8 to 12 weeks since the last report card. A lot can happen in that period of time, and you need to keep in mind how your child has performed recently, in the past week or two, versus his or her progress over a longer period of time.

In the example of Karen, at the start of the chapter, you can see that averaging the failing grades in the first 5 weeks of the marking period with the above-average grades in the last 5 weeks, comes out to a C. This student needs to hear that, in this situation, a C grade actually shows very good improvement; last month she seemed close to failing for the term, and if she keeps up the good work, she will probably earn a B next time. The message Karen needs to hear: "Keep up the good work."

HOW DOES THE GRADING SYSTEM WORK?

We all understand familiar letter grades: the universal A for excellent performance; B for very good; C for average basic mastery; D for below average, but still passing; and F for failing grades, with the message that the student might have to take the class over again or repeat the school year. While high schools and colleges routinely use this type of grading, report cards for younger children often use other systems that can confuse parents if not well-explained.

In many North American public and private schools, the grading system used for the primary grades of kindergarten to third grade measure a child's progress toward very specific goals set by the school. In the early grades, the major academic interest of teachers and parents focuses on whether or not the student masters the basic beginning skills of reading, writing, and arithmetic, and the grading system reflects that goal. Indeed, under the federal No Child Left Behind Act of 2001 (Public Law 107-110) and related state regulations, each state has a list of skills that they expect a child to learn at each grade level. This list contains much more extensive material than most parents imagine, and an essential part of the report card asks how many of these skills the child has mastered.

Thus, in most school systems, grades start out as descriptive and tell you how well your child has done compared to the standards developed by educators for each grade. As children get older, they typically receive more traditional numerical or letter grades.

PRIMARY GRADES: KINDERGARTEN TO THIRD GRADE

To measure and rate a child on these skills, many schools use a three-level system of grading that indicates whether the student seems on track and is making expected progress, seems to exceed the standard progress, or appears to be falling behind. Typically, grading in this three-level system includes coding such as:

- O – Outstanding, exceed standards.
- S – Satisfactory, meets standards for the grade.
- N – Needs improvement, or skills are developing.

Some school districts use different letters, but the three-level system applies very commonly; it provides a general description, and most importantly, it rates children against a standard of what they should have learned. This system does not compare children with each other. Recognizing the precise skills also becomes important. For example, in academic areas, separate categories may address different reading skills, such as the ability to sound out words phonetically (often called decoding skills), the ability to comprehend what the child has read, and knowledge of a set of sight words that the child can recognize instantly. Why give three grades in reading? Reading requires a number of distinct skills, and checking the students' progress in all areas enables the school to provide help if particular areas prove weaker. A child might have a good-sized word list for sight reading and can read for meaning, but still have problems sounding out a new word and need help in developing that skill.

Along with academic areas, report cards in primary grades also emphasize social, emotional, and behavioral skills. Learning study and social skills, such as the ability to pay attention, wait one's turn, follow directions, and work and play cooperatively will prove equally or more important than learning academic subjects. Grades in all of these areas qualify as important, and if students do have difficulty in the behavior area, they also may need some help in learning these skills. Future success in school depends on good social, emotional, and behavioral adjustment.

Report cards should not contain unpleasant surprises. As you talk with your children each day about what they have learned and any homework they might have, you should have a good feel for their progress. Communicating with teachers regularly via email or notes can also keep you up to date. As you communicate routinely with your child and the teacher, you will stay on top of the situation, and the report card should provide a quarterly summary of what you know already.

When you review report cards with young children in the primary grades, keep a few things in mind:

- Children this age sometimes think of report cards as just "good" or "bad," and they miss a lot of the details.
- Start by letting your children know that report cards tell how much they have learned and how hard they have worked.
- Talk about children's skills; the subjects they find easy, those that are harder, and things they have learned and have just started to learn.
- One of the best ways to keep up your child's motivation is to remind them of what they could do 2 months ago and what they can do now. For example, "Remember,

when school started you could read a sentence, and now you can read a whole page without help."

Very clear examples of what children have learned help them understand that a report card is meant to measure progress.

INTERMEDIATE SCHOOL TO MIDDLE SCHOOL: GRADES 4–8

If we think of the primary grades as a time when children learn the basic skills of learning, the intermediate grades (starting at fourth grade) mark the point at which they start to use their skills to learn about other subjects. These years include subjects such as history, geography, science, and social studies, along with reading, writing and mathematics. New skills such as note taking and extracting key ideas from reading become important components of the educational program.

In many school districts and in private schools, a change usually occurs in grading at some time during this 5-year period from the three-level system discussed earlier to a letter or numerical grade in the more familiar A, B, C, D, F format that most of us know well. This shift usually occurs in middle school. In most schools, while the grading system changes, it still usually measures whether the student shows progress according to school, district, or state standards. As the number of subjects students study increases, ratings or grades for behavior, social, and emotional skills decrease and tend to play a smaller role.

Another change that occurs during these years involves a shift from having one teacher grading the student in all areas to having several teachers, each grading a different subject. In some systems, students may have as many as six or seven teachers by the end of middle school. The report card now represents the composite work of a much larger group, with all of the accompanying complexities in communication. Many teachers use online grade reports, so that parents can access their child's grades anytime in the marking period and can keep up with their child's progress. However, sometimes, even if you have tried to keep up with the homework and the progress, you still may not know all of your child's teachers or have as much familiarity with all of the assignments as you did in your child's earlier grades. As a result, report cards may become your major source of information for some subjects in these years, and grade surprises may become more common. Your child probably has a very good idea of his or her progress, and you want to have conversations about the report card. The best way to do that may involve starting with open-ended questions, rather than questions that the child can easily answer with a yes, no, or some other single word (e.g., Mom: "How are you doing in math?" Billy: "Good."). Students of this age often wait for parental reaction to the report card, but getting your child's reaction first may help guide you. Here are some suggestions for discussing report cards with middle school students:

- *Start by asking your children how they think that they did.*   This allows for some conversation about what went well and what problem areas may exist.
- *Lead with praise.*   Find at least three things that you can say something positive about before addressing problem areas.

- *Offer specific praise.*   Say things like, "you worked hard to bring your English grade up this time."
- *Comment on effort you noticed at home.*   "I remember I saw you working on math problems a lot the past few weeks."
- *Praise good behaviors.*   Pay attention and comment about behaviors that you want to see more of, such as doing homework, reading, and working on projects.
- *Focus on improvement.*   When you do talk about problem areas, focus on a way to do better. Find out why a grade came in low, and make a plan to address that problem.

Sometimes, a student consistently has a very good report card and parents forget to seize the moment to praise their child. If your child has done well, review his or her report card and comment specifically on the best items. Ignoring good performance may make it seem unimportant or undervalued.

Review all of the subjects, praise hard work, effort, and achievement, and make a plan for improvement if needed. Focus on the effort and the work, and not the person. Try to separate your child from his or her grades; if your child earns a poor grade, you might say, "You're a great kid, but we need to work on improving this grade. Can I help in some way?" Try to identify the problem (e.g., test grades, homework completion, etc.) and then work together with your child to create a plan for improvement.

HIGH SCHOOL: GRADES 9–12

By the time students get to ninth grade, they have a very good sense of which subjects come easily and which are more difficult. They can readily identify favorite subjects—as well as requirements that they can't stand. Students enter high school with a variety of goals. Some simply want to graduate and go to work, some would like to move on to a community college or vocational training, and some want to go on to a 4-year college and beyond. Since the academic expectations vary so widely for different groups of students, grades can become harder to figure out, and teens may prove less likely to want to share the information.

Grades and Grade-Point Averages

Many high schools interchange letter and number grades, and then determine a grade point. To make sense out of a high school report card, you first need to know both the grading standards and the requirements for promotion and graduation. Most states have very specific requirements, including number of completed credits (1-year courses), required courses, and even state-wide achievement testing. If you have moved from another state or transferred school districts, make sure the school's advisors account for required courses in helping your child track progress toward graduation. If students fall behind in required courses, they may have an unpleasant surprise when they get their final report cards and find out that they only have enough credits to qualify as juniors when they thought they had become high school seniors. You will want to avoid these surprises by talking with your child and consulting with the school's guidance counselor.

The next key piece of information to consider involves the level of the courses taken. Has your child enrolled in general-level courses, intended for students who may go straight to work after graduation? Do the courses fall into a college-preparatory, honors, or advanced-placement (AP) track? AP courses can yield college credit, if the student takes and passes the AP examination at a certain level. A good choice of courses should fit the ability and interests of the student in high school, as well as meet the school system requirements. Level of course also becomes important when you review a report card. One student may get a B in an AP course she finds difficult, while another student may get an A in an easier course. Know what type of courses in which your teen has enrolled, and keep that level in mind when you review the report card. Some schools "weight" more difficult courses in their overall determination of a grade point average (GPA). So, in some schools, if one takes an AP course and gets an A that might be equal to a 5.0 for the grade point instead of the usual 4.0. If your child's school reports "weighted" GPAs, find out how they calculate them. If you are not sure, ask the counselor to explain it to you.

The key in helping you work with your high school student involves setting a collaborative tone. At this age, help the student focus on his or her personal goals and how these grades relate to these goals.

- *Ask your child how he or she did, and don't settle for one-word answers.* What does your child feel satisfied or dissatisfied about?
- *Ask how these grades will help your child achieve his or her goals.*
- *Ask if your child wants help.* If there is room for improvement, ask your child if he or she has an interest in doing better or feels satisfied with what he or she has learned. If your child wants to do better, then you can give advice or discuss the issues.

Remember to praise effort as well as accomplishment. Unpraised effort can cause motivation to fade away.

SUMMARY

Consider report cards as quarterly summaries of how your child does in school. If you keep up with your child's work every day and stay in contact with teachers, report cards usually do not present any surprises. In addition, doing so conveys to both your child and his or her teacher that you have a strong interest in education and your child's success at school. In early grades, most report cards rate the student compared to standards of what the curriculum expects of the child in that grade. In later grades, usually sometime after fourth grade, schools use letter or number grades, also linked to standards, but inviting comparison between students. For all students, the best strategy for using the report card involves identifying both strengths and areas needing improvement, making plans to improve performance if necessary and using the opportunity as a time to praise effort.

WHERE TO FIND OUT MORE

Websites

Education.com
Kindergarten Report Cards
   http://www.education.com/magazine/article/Kindergarten_Report_Cards/
Talking over your child's report card
   http://www.education.com/magazine/article/Dealing_with_Report_Cards/
Education Resources Information Center – ERIC Digest
High school report cards
   http://www.eric.ed.gov/ERICDocs/data/ericdocs2sql/content_storage_01/
   0000019b/80/1b/80/37.pdf
Family Education
Talking to your child about report cards
   http://school.familyeducation.com/report-cards/parents-and-school/38368.html
National Association for the Education of Young Children
Your child's first report card
   http://www.education.com/reference/article/Ref_Your_Childs_First/

CHAPTER 29

Starting a New School

Jennifer Shroff Pendley and W. Douglas Tynan

Six-year-old Ben felt excited about the chance to start a new school. He eagerly began riding the school bus like his older brother. He felt a little nervous about meeting his new teacher, but voiced excitement about meeting lots of new friends.

Thirteen-year-old Caroline seemed less thrilled about the prospect of going to a new school. Because her parent's job required moving to a new city, Caroline would have to adjust to a new neighborhood, as well as a new school. Changing school mid-year added to her worries because she feared she would have difficulty fitting in or that she might fall behind her peers academically.

Whether a child is starting a new school within their familiar school district or moving to a completely new community, transitioning to a new school can present difficulties. Changes can be exciting, but also provoke anxiety. This chapter focuses on strategies you can use to help your children adjust to a new school setting. These strategies can be used with children of all ages, from preschoolers to high school students.

HOW CAN I PREPARE MY CHILD FOR THE TRANSITION?

From the very beginning, communicate openly with your child. If relocation includes moving to a new community, explain the reasons and necessities. Although you may have the urge to reassure and try to "talk away" feelings of anxiety or worry, make sure to take the time to listen to and validate your child's feelings. First, listen carefully and acknowledge that the transition may feel scary. Help your child label his or her feelings, as these feelings can become confusing. Often what a child wants most of all is for someone to listen; try to avoid the temptation to immediately offer advice and problem-solve.

Instead, reflect upon what your child says. For example, you may respond by saying something like, "I hear you saying that you feel worried about meeting new friends and that you have concerns you might miss the soccer tryouts for your new school team. It sounds like you feel sad about moving too." Once children know that you understand and accept their concerns, they may more readily begin to problem-solve. After listening, ask your child if he or she would like to discuss ways to make the move easier. If your child seems ready, then take a few minutes to brainstorm together. First, gather as many ideas as possible without evaluating them. Next, decide which suggestions could work for both of you, and then choose one or two to try. Decide on a time to check in to evaluate the effectiveness of the solution. Problem-solving will help empower your child and likely result in your child feeling more control over the situation.

A calendar can also provide a very useful tool to help address the uncertainly about the transition. Young children do not always have a strong concept of time, but respond well to visual cues such as calendars with special dates highlighted. Similarly, adolescents appreciate knowing important dates in advance.

If possible, visit the new school before the first day. If you have a shy child, consider first visiting when the school is empty and having a staff member give a personal tour. Older children may appreciate the opportunity to shadow a current student for a morning. Show your child the school's website, if there is one, and check out some of the extracurricular activities ahead of time. If your child has some special medical, emotional, or learning needs, schedule a meeting with the school nurse, counselor, learning specialist, or psychologist.

Become familiar with school rules and routines. Plan for any dress code and involve your child in shopping. Make sure to have all the appropriate school supplies and health forms ready. Learn about the school's policies on things such as tardiness, using cell phones, and carrying back-packs between classes.

Get off to a good start! Make sure your child has a good night sleep and has time to eat breakfast. Prepare the back-pack the night before. Involve your child in packing his or her lunch. If your child wants to buy lunch, discuss the different options.

If you remain concerned about your child's adjustment after the first week or two, contact your child's teacher or counselor. Email communication may work much more easily than trying to make contact by telephone. Regardless, let the teacher or counselor know your concerns.

DEVELOPMENTAL ISSUES

Taking a developmental perspective may help in understanding your child's particular challenges to adjusting to a new school. Some specific developmental transition challenges come up in each of the preschool, early elementary, upper elementary, middle school, and high school years. For example, preschool may mark the first time that some children experience prolonged separation from their parents, interact and share toys with a large group of children, and need to show sustained attention to academic materials. Focusing on these changes may help the transition. For example, if prior to starting kindergarten, your child has not experienced many separations from you, schedule a play date with a trusted friend or enroll in a week of summer day camp before kindergarten begins. As children transition to lower and upper elementary schools, they experience increased independence and academic demands. Middle school can become a particularly challenging time, with vast changes in school structure coupled with changes in social and physical development. Thus, particular attention should focus on the social aspects of adjusting to a new school during this time period. Furthermore, pubertal changes and associated emotional ups and downs may make your child may seem more sensitive than usual and may require more attention if a transition to a new school occurs at this time.

STARTING SCHOOL FOR THE FIRST TIME

The following are some suggestions for helping your child get ready for the first day of school.

- *Visit the school.*   Prior to the first day, try to provide multiple opportunities for your child to visit the school. Visit the playground several times, if possible. Becoming familiar and comfortable with the school can reduce first-day jitters. The more your children visit the school and play on the playground, the more "ownership" they may have regarding the school.
- *Discuss differences.*   Communicate clearly to your child what might seem different about this school, remembering that you and your child will likely focus on different aspects. For example, if your child will ride the bus, discuss how that might feel. Have your child ride the bus the first day, so that he or she will have the experience of riding with all the other new students. Although it may seem tempting to drive your child the first few days, delaying use of the bus may heighten his or her anxiety.
- *Don't worry if your child shows some separation anxiety or becomes tearful on the first day of school.*   These developmentally appropriate reactions will typically go away after a few days. If your child cries when you leave, remain calm and positive, expressing confidence in your child's ability to succeed. Enlist the teacher for support, and do not linger in the classroom. Children can sense their parents' anxiety which in turn, increases their own distress.
- *Arrange play dates with new classmates.*   Your child's teacher may have suggestions regarding certain peers with whom your child has connected. Play dates can help accelerate your child's feelings of social connectedness.

MIDDLE SCHOOL

Middle school can present especially difficult challenges, due to the numerous changes a child will experience. In middle school, the daily schedule becomes more complicated as children start changing classes six or seven times a day and organizational demands greatly increase. Grade accountability also increases, and the workload frequently becomes harder. Students are assigned longer and more demanding homework assignments, as well as long-term projects. You may also find middle school teachers to be less accessible, and more independence is expected from the student. You may also notice that your child seems more emotionally affected or encounters more pressure to conform to social norms. Although these changes present extra challenges in this transition period, you can take steps to ensure this transition goes as smoothly as possible:

- *Foster organizational skills.*   Because of the increased academic demands, your child may need help developing a system to keep track of classwork and homework assignments. Help your child organize and label class folders so that work does not get lost.
- *Encourage extracurricular activities.*   Try to find one or two activities that your child will enjoy. However, avoid overscheduling, as this may increase stress. Help your child keep track of dates for tryouts or sign-ups for sports teams or clubs.
- *Dress for success.*   For the first day, make sure your child picks out an outfit that he or she really likes and that adheres to the dress code. Children who feel good will feel more confident.
- *Practice locker combinations.*   Have your child write down the combination and put it in a safe place (not inside the locker!), so that he or she has access to it in a moment of panic.
- *Keep track of class schedules.*   Many middle schools and high schools use a rotating schedule (i.e., classes occur at different times each day of the week). Whereas this schedule can seem quite confusing, particularly for parents, students typically catch on to the rhythm of the classes rather quickly. Nonetheless, keep a copy of the schedule at home so that you can refer to it if your child loses the schedule or becomes confused.

STARTING SCHOOL AFTER A MOVE

Adjusting to a new school and new city can pose particular challenges, but again, specific strategies can help with this transition.

There are pros and cons regarding the best time to move. Many professionals feel that summer is ideal, as it gives children a chance to settle into their new locale and then start the school year at the same time as other peers. However, with no local friends, a child may feel isolated during that summer. In contrast, when starting mid-year, children can jump right into activities and possibly connect more quickly with new friends. Yet, mid-year transitions can also add stresses, particularly for teenagers. Trying to enter well-established social groups will often prove difficult.

Before moving, have your children learn about the new community. Visit several times if possible. Videotape and/or take pictures of the new home, and discuss with your children how they want to decorate their rooms. For younger children, decorating their new rooms similarly to their old rooms can offer reassurance. However, teenagers may welcome the chance for a room makeover.

Reassure your children that they can stay in touch with old friends. Emailing, instant messaging, and text messaging (with parental permission and monitoring, of course) provide easy ways to stay connected. Schedule a visit or two back to the old neighborhood, so your children have something specific to anticipate.

Try to allow enough time to get the house settled before jumping into a new routine. Having a cluttered and disorganized room may make it more difficult to get organized for school.

Meet with the school counselors before starting. Let them know of any specific concerns that you may have. Ask if the school implements a buddy system whereby your child would have a peer buddy for the first few days to help with orientation. School lunches often become a source of stress for new students. Ask the counselor if a buddy could help your child negotiate the lunch system and sit with her at lunch. Also, ask for a name of student who lives nearby, rides the same bus, and who may willingly sit with your child on the first few bus rides.

Stay in touch with the new teachers. If possible, schedule a conference a few weeks after your child has transitioned. A conference will help ensure that any difficulties are identified early and subsequently addressed.

HOW DO I HELP MY CHILD MANAGE ANXIETY?

Some anxiety and worries are normal; however, if these worries escalate or do not dissipate as your child begins attending the new school, you may need more intervention. Try to achieve a balance between talking about your child's feelings and overreacting by dwelling on the negative. Often, setting aside a specific time to talk and check in each day proves helpful. When problems arise, listen and then utilize your problem-solving skills.

- *Find extra support.*   Contact your child's guidance counselor or school psychologist and ask them to check in with your child.
- *Reinforce coping strategies.*   Encourage your child to exercise, contact friends, and engage in other activities that have reduced stress in the past.
- *Consider volunteering.*   For younger children, sometimes seeing their parents volunteer in the classroom or school can be reassuring. If, however, your presence seems to increase distress, volunteering in the library or other area of the school can still reassure your child of your involvement.
- *Know when to get help.*   If these strategies do not seem to work or if you see major changes in your child's emotional well-being, you may wish to contact a professional, such as a child psychologist.

SUMMARY

Starting a new school can be exciting, but it can also make children anxious, as they will have to navigate a new and unfamiliar environment on their own. If your family has just relocated and your child is anxious about attending a new school, there are several strategies you can use to help your child manage the transition. Communicate openly with your child about his or her concerns and, if possible, schedule a visit to the school before classes begin. Familiarize yourself with your child's teachers and the school's schedule and rules (e.g., dress code). Give your child time to adjust. If, after a couple of weeks, your child is still showing signs of anxiety, you may wish to enlist the help of your child's guidance counselor or school psychologist. If worries escalate, it may be helpful to contact a mental health professional, such as a child psychologist.

WHERE TO FIND OUT MORE

Books

Faber, A., & Mazlish, E. (1999). *How to talk so kids will listen and listen so kids will talk.* New York: HarperCollins.

Huebner, D. (2006). *What to do when you worry too much.* Washington DC: Magination Press.

Martin, T., & Martin, W. (2006). *Big Ernie's new home: A story for children who are moving.* Washington DC: Magination Press.

Ziegler, R.G. (1992). *Homemade books to help kids cope: An easy-to-learn technique for parents and professionals.* Washington DC: Magination Press.

Websites

American Academy of Child and Adolescent Psychiatry
Children and family moves
    http://www.aacap.org/cs/root/facts_for_families/children_and_family_moves

National Association of School Psychologists
    http://www.nasponline.org/families/

Nemours Foundation
What kids who are moving should do
    http://kidshealth.org/kid/feeling/home_family/moving.html

New York University Child Study Center
Transition points: Helping students start, change, and move through the grades
    http://www.education.com/reference/article/Ref_Transition_Points/

CHAPTER 30

Avoidance and School Refusal

Christopher A. Kearney and Courtney Haight

Brandon is a 12-year-old boy who recently entered seventh grade and has difficulty attending classes at his new middle school. Brandon says he feels overwhelmed by his large number of new classes, teachers, peers, and homework assignments. Brandon occasionally had trouble attending elementary school, but his current problems seem more frequent and upsetting to him and his family. Brandon has missed 4 days of school so far this year, has arrived late to school several times, and has skipped some classes. The school vice principal has contacted Brandon's parents to outline legal and other consequences should Brandon continue to miss school.

School avoidance or refusal occurs commonly but proves a difficult issue for many families because the behavior can become so disruptive to parents, siblings, and others. School avoidance or refusal can come in different forms:

- Some children completely miss school for lengthy periods of time.
- Some children completely miss school for short periods of time or skip certain classes, such as physical education.
- Some children, like Brandon, periodically miss school or skip classes.
- Some children repeatedly arrive tardy to school following several misbehaviors in the morning.
- Some children show repeated misbehaviors in the morning in an attempt to miss school.
- Some children attend school regularly, but do so with great hesitation and dread and often ask their parents to keep them home from school.

Many children who avoid school show different problems on different days, as Brandon does. A child may complain about going to school one day, arrive tardy to school the next day, or skip a class or an entire school day later in the week. Children who avoid school often do so for different reasons as well. We describe common reasons for school avoidance and refusal next.

ANXIETY ABOUT SCHOOL

Some children genuinely feel anxious about school. Preschoolers and children in elementary school often show concern about transitions from one part of school to another, such as from the playground to class in the morning. Other sources of anxiety may include the school bus, a particular school official or classmate, or large spaces such as the cafeteria. Many children feel anxious about school, but cannot say exactly what upsets them. These children often have physical complaints, such as stomachaches and headaches, and typically plead with their parents not to send them to school.

Older children and adolescents often express concern about social situations, such as meeting other people, joining a conversation, working with others on a group project, or interacting with adults at school. Brandon had concerns about meeting many people in a short period of time. Older children and adolescents may also have concerns about situations in which they have to perform before others, such as in physical education or math class, recitals, oral presentations, tests, answering a question in class, or using a public restroom. Older children and adolescents like Brandon may skip certain classes that cause them the most anxiety.

ATTENTION FROM OTHERS

Preschoolers and children in elementary school sometimes avoid or refuse school to stay with parents at home or at their workplace. These children may not have particular anxiety about school, although they might, but they usually feel more driven to remain with their parents. Some of these children will attend school if a parent stays in their classroom, but most schools and parents will not consider this option desirable. Such children may have anxiety about separating from parents but often seek attention in other ways as well. An attention-seeking child may also refuse to attend birthday parties, sleep-overs, or extracurricular activities.

Children who avoid or refuse school for attention often display temper tantrums, defiance, crying, and stubborn and manipulative behavior. They may try to contact their parents many times during a school day, seek constant reassurance from their parents, or become disruptive at school or run away from school to arrive home. These children may have physical symptoms, such as headaches and stomachaches, but sometimes children exaggerate symptoms in a bid for attention.

FUN ACTIVITIES OUTSIDE OF SCHOOL

Older children and adolescents sometimes avoid or refuse school simply because staying out of school provides more fun than attending school. These teenagers may enjoy sleeping late, staying home during the day to watch television or play videogames, or spending time with friends who also skip school. These adolescents often skip classes or large parts of the school day (such as an afternoon), fight with parents about their absenteeism, and break curfew or engage in other delinquent activities.

Teenagers who miss substantial amounts of school time will most likely face legal consequences, such as referral to a truancy court. Excessive school avoidance or refusal may become associated with more significant problems as well, such as other illegal activities or permanent school dropout. This type of school avoidance or refusal often proves the most difficult type to address because the absenteeism has lasted a long time and because the absenteeism usually occurs quite secretively.

BROADER REASONS

Other, broader reasons can help explain school avoidance or refusal as well. Threats from peers or complaints about tedious curricula are common school-based reasons that may help explain a child's avoidance of school. We strongly recommend addressing school-based threats from peers or bullying before attempting the other strategies we describe to address the problem. If a child complains of boredom at school, then consider discussions with school officials to increase the novelty or interest of classroom material and projects.

Other broader reasons for absenteeism exist but fall beyond the scope of this chapter. Examples include pregnancy, extreme family turmoil, and a need or desire to obtain a job, among others. Cases of school avoidance or refusal caused by these factors likely require an extensive therapeutic approach. For relatively new or less severe cases, we next describe a first-aid approach.

FIXING A SCHOOL AVOIDANCE OR REFUSAL PROBLEM

We recommend several basic strategies to eliminate a new school avoidance or refusal problem. These practices work best if parents implement them consistently and support each other in doing so. We also recommend that a child receive a full medical examination prior to these practices to rule out or address true physical conditions, especially when the child uses such symptoms as a basis for school refusal.

Reducing Anxiety Through Relaxation and Breathing

A good way to help a child reduce some physical signs of anxiety is appropriate breathing. Teach your child to inhale slowly through his nose while pushing two fingers gently into his diaphragm. He can then exhale slowly through his mouth, perhaps counting slowly while doing so. Your child can repeat this process once or twice or as needed to release physical tension. He can practice this breathing in school situations that cause distress or in the morning before going to school. Other methods of relaxation, such as tensing and releasing different muscle groups, as described in the book *Getting Your Child to Say "Yes" to School: A Guide for Parents of Children with School Refusal Behavior* (Kearney, 2007), can also prove useful. Brandon learned to use proper breathing to reduce stress when giving an oral presentation, taking a test, or meeting someone for the first time.

Gradually Easing a Child Back to School

If your child misses school completely or for most of the day, then gradually easing her back to school is a good option. This can occur in one of several ways:

- Your child attends school for a set time in the morning, such as 9:00–10:00 A.M.; add greater classroom time each day, such as an additional hour per day.
- Your child attends school at 2:00 P.M. and then comes home when school normally ends (e.g., 3:10 P.M.); add greater classroom time in a backward fashion each day, such as starting the next day at 1:30 P.M., then 1:00 P.M., and so forth.
- Your child attends school only for lunch and then comes home; add greater classroom time before and after lunch, such as 30 minutes prior to and after lunch, then add more time each successive day.
- Your child attends school only for her favorite class or time of day; add greater classroom time according to her next favorite classes or time of day.
- Your child attends a place at school other than her classroom, such as the library, counselor's office, or main lobby; add greater school and classroom time over the next several days, perhaps 1 hour per day.

We generally recommend the first approach in case you have difficulty getting your child to school first thing in the morning. You can then continue to urge your child throughout the day to attend school for at least 1 hour, even if this means sitting with your child in the school parking lot or main lobby.

Changing Unreasonable Thoughts

Many adolescents with difficulty attending school have unreasonable thoughts about harm from others. Teenagers normally worry about what others think of them, but some adolescents become so worried that they cannot attend school. Examples of such worries include assuming terrible things will happen, believing they know what others think of them, jumping to false conclusions, and blaming themselves for things not within their control. Brandon believed he would become severely embarrassed by even minor mistakes, such as hesitating during an oral presentation or not knowing what to say during a conversation. He also worried about his competence and potential teasing in physical education class.

We recommend that parents have regular talks with their children about unrealistic (and realistic) worries they have about school. Discover what social or performance situations at school make your child most anxious and what thoughts your child has in these situations. Help your child consider other, more realistic thoughts, and praise him for doing so. If your child's concern is realistic, however, such as regarding a legitimate school-based threat, then address that concern first.

Brandon's parents explored their son's fear of embarrassment in different situations at school. They helped him think of embarrassment as a temporary and manageable condition that happens to everyone sometime and usually does not lead to severe consequences. They also encouraged Brandon to think about whether he really knew what others thought of him, whether he had handled situations such as tests in the past (he had), and whether he knew for sure something terrible would happen to him. Brandon's parents praised their son when he successfully attended school and developed realistic thoughts during anxious situations.

Establishing a Morning Routine

Many families of children with school avoidance problems report hectic mornings, especially children with attention-seeking behavior. We recommend a child rise from bed 90–120 minutes prior to the start of school. The morning routine should then consist of specific times for specific tasks. Brandon's new morning routine consisted of the following:

- 7:00 A.M.–7:20 A.M. (eat breakfast)
- 7:20 A.M.–7:30 A.M. (brush teeth and wash)
- 7:30 A.M.–7:50 A.M. (dress and accessorize for school)
- 7:45 A.M.–8:00 A.M. (make final preparations for school such as getting back-pack ready).

Allow extra time during each of these sections for minor dawdling and noncompliance. Allow extra time between the end of the morning routine and leaving home for school as well. This extra time allows for a reward, if the child completes the morning routine promptly, such as some quick television time. The extra time also serves as a buffer in case your child could not finish on time. In this case, the buffer time allows for finishing the morning routine (with no reward) and yet the child can still attend school on time. Evening routines that include regular homework time may prove helpful as well. If a child remains home from school during the day, we recommend a regular routine that includes academic work and assigned homework.

Rewards and Punishments

A child's school attendance or nonattendance should link to appropriate daily rewards and punishments. These consequences can follow immediately, as when a child completes or fails to complete a set morning routine. The consequences can also occur at night or after school, depending on the child's behavior that morning. A common rule of thumb we use to determine punishment involves doubling the amount of time a child refused school. A child who had a temper tantrum on the school playground for 20 minutes to avoid school, for example, would "owe" his parents 40 minutes of punishment time that night.

Rewards and punishments can be tangible or intangible. Tangible consequences include special privileges or food, time spent with parents or friends, altered bedtime, and money for school attendance with associated home chores. Intangible consequences include praise, ignoring minor complaints about school or noncompliance, and refusing to accommodate unreasonable requests to remain home from school. Brandon earned special activities, such as movies with friends on Friday night, if he successfully attended school during the week.

Increased Supervision

A child with ongoing school avoidance or refusal requires greater supervision from parents and school officials to ensure proper attendance. This becomes especially important if a child runs or slips away from a school campus or skips classes during the day. Increased supervision should include the following:

- *Work with school officials to develop a plan to monitor your child during the school day;* examples include walking your child from class to class, having your child check in with a school official at set times during the day, and asking each teacher to sign an attendance journal brought to him or her by your child.
- *Work with school officials to develop a response plan if your child leaves the school campus;* examples include contacting school or regular police, having school officials contact you so you can find your child, returning your child to school that day if possible, and giving appropriate consequences that night for nonattendance.
- *Inform school officials when your child will be absent on a given day or if he will be late to school.* Brandon's parents and guidance counselor agreed to send a text message to the other if Brandon refused school or was found missing from class.

WHEN TO SEEK PROFESSIONAL HELP

You might want to seek professional help for a child with school avoidance or refusal if one or more of the following conditions apply to your situation:

- Your child's school avoidance has lasted longer than 2 weeks.
- Your child's school avoidance continues to cause substantial distress for family members.
- Your child's school avoidance has led to academic problems, such as declining grades, or legal or financial problems for you.
- Your child has severe medical problems associated with school attendance.
- Your child has other behavior problems, such as attention-deficit hyperactivity disorder, depression, aggression, substance abuse, or other conditions.

In these cases, we recommend you consult a clinical child psychologist who has experience addressing children with school avoidance issues. Check with the psychology department of a nearby university or online directories at www.abct.org or www.apa.org to find a suitable mental health professional near you. We also recommend ongoing discussions with school officials, such as principals, teachers, guidance counselors, and school psychologists, to discuss broader plans to address more severe cases of school avoidance.

SUMMARY

School avoidance or refusal among children is a common but fixable problem. Providing first aid for this problem, however, requires frequent communication and cooperation between parents and school officials. Ongoing vigilance from both parties is also needed to prevent future episodes of absenteeism. Parents must generally expect their child to go to school and adopt an attitude that only major events such as serious illness or family emergency should prevent a child from attending school. Parents should work closely with school officials as well, to ensure that academic curricula are well-tailored to their child's educational needs.

WHERE TO FIND OUT MORE

Books

Eisen, A.R., & Engler, L.B. (2006). *Helping your child overcome separation anxiety or school refusal: A step-by-step guide for parents.* Oakland, CA: New Harbinger.

Heyne, D., Rollings, S., King, N.J., & Tonge, B.J. (2002). *School refusal.* Oxford, UK: Blackwell.

Kearney, C.A. (2007). *Getting your child to say "yes" to school: A guide for parents with school refusal behavior.* New York: Oxford University Press.

Kearney, C.A. (2008). *Helping school-refusing children and their parents: A guide for school-based professionals.* New York: Oxford University Press.

Websites

American Academy of Adolescent and Child Psychiatry
Children who won't go to school (separation anxiety)
   www.aacap.org/cs/root/facts_for_families/children_who_wont_go_to_school_separation_
   anxiety
NYU Child Study Center
Understanding school refusal
   www.aboutourkids.org/articles/understanding_school_refusal
Anxiety Disorders Association of America
   www.adaa.org/GettingHelp/FocusOn/children&Adolescents/sra.asp
eMedicineHealth
School refusal
   www.emedicinehealth.com/school_refusal/article_em.htm

CHAPTER 31

Conflicts with Teachers

Meghan McAuliffe Lines and Jennifer Shroff Pendley

The new school year started 3 weeks ago and Barbara's son, Dan, is having a hard time settling into his new classroom. Today, Dan came home from school visibly upset. He stormed into the house and threw his back-pack on the kitchen floor. Before Barbara had a chance to ask what had happened, Dan cried, "I'm not going to school anymore! Mr. Cooper is so unfair! He's always picking on me. I think he hates me!" Bewildered, Barbara wondered what she could do to make Dan feel better, how to get a good handle on the situation, and how to help her son have a positive experience in second grade after this rocky start to the school year.

This chapter outlines strategies to help children manage conflicts with their teachers. Like Barbara, many parents in similar situations want to help their children manage conflicts with their teachers so they will feel better about themselves and feel less distressed about going to school. There are several other reasons, however, why it is important for children to get along with their teachers.

WHY IS IT IMPORTANT FOR CHILDREN TO GET ALONG WITH THEIR TEACHERS?

Research has shown important benefits to children of having positive relationships with their teachers. For example, having a relationship with a teacher characterized by closeness, warmth, and trust leads to better academic and social performance in children. This idea makes sense, in that students who have good relationships with their teachers most likely find it easier to ask for help in the classroom. Children who have a history of positive relationships with teachers also will likely develop positive values and attitudes related to school, which helps with their continued motivation even beyond that particular teacher's classroom.

Just as children who have positive relationships with their teachers tend to do well in the future, children who have poor relationships with their teachers may have a more difficult school experience. Poor student–teacher relationships in elementary school have been linked to social and behavioral problems, academic failure, and school dropout.

Given all of this information, Barbara has good reason to worry about Dan's relationship with his teacher and his attitude toward school. Barbara realizes that she needs to do something to help Dan, so that his negative feelings about Mr. Cooper won't affect his self-esteem and whole school experience. So, what's a parent to do?

HOW CAN I HELP MY CHILD MANAGE CONFLICT IN THE CLASSROOM?

Parents face a number of issues when thinking about the best way to help their children negotiate these sticky situations. If your child comes home from school feeling as overwhelmed and miserable as Dan did, your first instinct might tell you to run to his rescue and fix the problem yourself. However, this situation presents a great opportunity to help your child develop a sense of independence and build skills in emotion regulation, problem-solving, and perspective-taking. All of these skills will continue to help your child throughout his or her school career and beyond. So, take a deep breath, and consider some of the following suggestions for helping your child to manage this challenging situation.

TIPS FOR PARENTS OF ELEMENTARY AND MIDDLE SCHOOL STUDENTS

Be a Good Listener

How can you help your children learn to act as their own best advocates without undermining the teacher's authority? Because you are not in the classroom to witness the interactions between your child and the teacher, you might feel a temptation to jump in with lots of questions, so that you can get as much information as possible from your child and understand exactly what has happened. However, resist the temptation to start firing questions. Instead, let your child first vent his or her frustrations and then follow that discussion with open-ended questions. In fact, sometimes children really don't want your input or your solutions; rather, they just want someone to listen to them and validate their feelings. If, however, your child seems to need extra support, after you have listened for a while, you can get more details by asking for specific examples. As you are listening, keep in mind several questions. For example, does this teacher have a style that is new to your child (e.g., more or less flexible than last year's teacher) or does it sound like your child feels singled out in some way? Keep in mind that most children can feel singled out even when this has not happened. Does the conflict sound like a personality clash? It happens sometimes! Or, has your child shown some challenging or disruptive behaviors in class? What is the context? What happened first, next, after? Try to stay calm and supportive even if you begin to feel frustrated with the teacher. You can provide a good example for your child by staying calm under pressure.

Use Emotion Coaching

Emotion coaching provides a way for parents to help children develop their emotion regulation and coping skills, and it can become a useful tool to use in helping your children manage difficult situations. In his book, *Raising an Emotionally Intelligent Child,* Dr. John Gottman lists five key steps to emotion coaching:

1. Become aware of your child's emotion. Does your child feel mad, sad, frustrated, or embarrassed?
2. Recognize the emotion as an opportunity for teaching.
3. Listen empathetically and validate your child's feelings (e.g., "I see . . . " or "I know I would feel sad [mad, frustrated, embarrassed . . .] if the same thing happened to me.").
4. Help your child find words to label his or her emotions (e.g., "It sounds like you feel very frustrated by what your teacher said.").
5. Set limits while exploring strategies to solve the problem at hand (e.g., "What can we do to help you feel better or solve the problem?").

Although they can feel very stressful, conflicts with teachers also provide opportunities for you to use these emotion coaching strategies and help your children learn ways to better manage similar situations independently in the future.

Teach Social Problem-Solving Strategies

Helping your children develop their social problem-solving skills provides another way to support your children when they have conflict in the classroom. Because children may encounter social problems with friends, brothers and sisters, and even adults on a regular basis, they can benefit from every opportunity to learn new problem-solving skills. Supporting your children as they develop these skills helps them to communicate better and think for themselves. Having good problem-solving skills will likely help your child handle conflicts in the workplace as an adult. The book *Raising a Thinking Child: Help Your Young Child to Resolve Everyday Conflicts and Get Along with Others* by Dr. Myrna Shure and Theresa DiGeronimo offers great ideas for teaching social problem-solving at home. The basic steps of social problem-solving include the following.

1. Identify a problem (e.g., "I'm having some trouble with my teacher.").
2. Recognize thoughts, feelings, and motives that lead to interpersonal problem situations (e.g., "He's mean . . . I'm not smart . . . I just hate school . . . She's picking on me . . . She's not fair . . . ").
3. Generate alternative solutions to problems. Don't evaluate the solutions—just brainstorm and see how many solutions you and your child can think of (e.g., "I could ask the teacher what the rules are . . . I can tell the teacher I feel confused . . . I could do nothing . . . ").
4. Consider the consequences of these solutions (e.g., "If I ask what the rules are, the teacher might be able to explain them better . . . If I don't do anything, the situation may get even worse . . . ").

5. Try out the solution that seems like the best idea (e.g., "I think I'll try talking to the teacher and asking about the rules again.").

Your child will probably need help brainstorming and evaluating the solutions, which works just fine. Involving your children in the process helps them learn to think independently and, most importantly, gain confidence in their own abilities to manage interpersonal situations.

Communicate with the Teacher

For young children, direct communication with the teacher regarding what he or she sees in the classroom may prove beneficial. By gathering additional information about the situation, you also let the teacher know that you want to help as a concerned and involved parent. You can then decide whether you need a more formal parent–teacher conference. A daily home–school note, or notes written back and forth in your child's agenda book, can provide an excellent way to establish communication with the teacher. Asking the teacher to give you some individual feedback regarding your child's performance on a daily basis could also help to provide some insight regarding the source of conflict. Email communication also provides an easy and convenient way of checking in with many teachers, and avoids putting the child in the role of message carrier. Whichever way you decide to communicate with your child's teachers, strive for objectivity and diplomacy, and show respect for their time.

Meet with the Teacher

If you work with your child on managing the problem and it does not resolve, consider a meeting with the teacher. A few strategies that can make parent–teacher communication as helpful as possible include identifying your child's strengths and challenges as you see them, sharing techniques that you have found useful at home, and creating an action plan with the teacher. Remember, it is important to communicate in a positive, optimistic manner. Additionally, ask objective questions about the specific nature of your child's struggles. Show respect and tact in your communication, replacing statements that a teacher might perceive as criticism or accusations by using I-statements (e.g., "I feel . . . " instead of "You are . . . "). And remember, look at the situation from the teacher's perspective; your child's impressions may differ vastly from what the teacher has experienced.

ADDITIONAL TIPS FOR PARENTS OF HIGH SCHOOL STUDENTS

Do the same suggestions apply for older children? The general guidelines outline can also work with adolescents, but as children mature cognitively and emotionally, it becomes important to encourage them to take a more active role in working out these issues on their own. The following are some tips for helping your older child manage conflict with his or her teacher.

- *Help your adolescent with perspective-taking.* As you discuss the conflict with your teenager, encourage him or her to step back from the problem and view it from the teacher's perspective. Adolescents have the ability to put themselves in another person's shoes, although they may need a little coaching to get there! This may help your teen better understand the problem and generate some appropriate problem-solving strategies.

- *Encourage a student–teacher conference first.*   Most high school students are preparing to go to college or to enter the workforce. With their college professors or their work supervisors, they will need to fight their own battles. So, this affords a good opportunity for your child to get some practice while he or she still has your support. In addition, adolescents may appear more sincere and invested if they approach their teachers on their own rather than having an adult intervene for them.

- *Know when to step in.*   If your son or daughter tries to manage the situation with the teacher and has only limited success, by all means, step in. If it seems appropriate, schedule a meeting with the teacher and have your teen also attend, so that he or she has the opportunity to advocate for himself or herself with your support. You can even role-play the meeting beforehand, so your child has an idea of what to expect.

HELICOPTER PARENTS: CAN PARENTAL INVOLVEMENT BE TOO MUCH OF A GOOD THING?

The term "helicopter parent" has become popular in the media, referring to those parents who become overinvolved in their children's lives, constantly "hovering" and intervening. Can parents become too involved? Some researchers say "yes"; helicopter parents may actually contribute to a child's psychological distress by overprotecting them and not letting them learn to cope with challenges. The 2007 National Survey of Student Engagement showed that students with helicopter parents (defined in the study as those in frequent contact and frequently intervening on their student's behalf) reported higher levels of engagement in learning, but actually had significantly lower grades than students without helicopter parents. If you constantly intervene, then your children will not learn independent coping skills. At some point, when you are no longer available to help, they will lack strong coping skills to fall back upon. Also, helicopter parenting can backfire in the classroom. Teachers may become weary of the parent who constantly brings up minor issues and subsequently, if a more significant concern arises, teachers may not want to take the time to address it.

ADDITIONAL CONSIDERATIONS

- When you listen to your teenager rant about an unfair teacher, realize that you have heard only one side of the story and make sure not to overlook how your child's behavior may have contributed to the situation. In fact, a fair amount of conflict between students and teachers may start with a student's inappropriate behavior. Make sure that you ask the teacher about your child's behavior, and if the behavior seems a source of conflict, work together to develop strategies to improve it. Often, pairing a home-based reward with a home–school note provides an effective means of improving classroom behavior.

- Some conflicts dissipate over time. Perhaps the teacher or your child just had a bad day. Sometimes waiting a day or two before taking action may result in the conflict naturally going away.
- If your child displays changes in behavior or personality or excessive distress regarding the situation with the teacher, you may want to consider consulting with the school counselor or a child psychologist or other licensed mental health professional.

SUMMARY

Conflicts with teachers will inevitably arise. You have many options in supporting your children in handling such conflicts. Active listening and emotion coaching show your children that you are listening to them, and these approaches help children develop coping skills. Social problem- solving skills help children communicate better and become more flexible thinkers. Open and positive communication with teachers can help resolve conflict, and you can act as a good role model when communicating with your child's teachers. However, although you should take an active role in supporting your children, overinvolvement or "helicopter" parenting can result in children not learning to resolve conflicts independently.

WHERE TO FIND OUT MORE

Books

Gottman, J.M. (1997). *Raising an emotionally intelligent child: The heart of parenting.* New York: Fireside.

Pianta, R.C. (1999). *Enhancing relationships between children and teachers.* Washington, DC: American Psychological Association.

Shure, M.B., & DiGeronimo, J.F. (1994). *Raising a thinking child: Help your young child to resolve everyday conflicts and get along with others.* New York: Pocket Books.

Websites

National Survey of Student Engagement (2007).
Experiences that matter: Enhancing student learning and success.
   http://nsse.iub.edu/NSSE_2007_Annual_Report/
Nemours Foundation (2005).
Getting along with your teachers.
   http://kidshealth.org/teen/school_jobs/school/teacher_relationships.html.
Scholastic (2006).
When kids and teachers don't click.
   http://www2.scholastic.com/browse/article.jsp?id=7306
University of Florida Department of Family, Youth, and Community Sciences (2006).
Communicating with your child's teacher.
   http://fycs.ifas.ufl.edu/news/2006/08/communicating-with-your-childs-teacher.html.

CHAPTER 32

Coping with the College Application Process

Julie A. Fulton

Sandra's mother wants to rewrite her 17-year-old's college application essay because, "It reads like a teenager wrote it." Max wants desperately to apply early to Brown University, but his parents want him to apply early to Yale, "because Brown isn't really impressive enough." Ryan's mother is frustrated, because her son has let all the early application deadlines slip by without getting his "act together" to submit an essay and application.

The stress of college applications can shine a light on many things one would rather not see. For some families, it aggravates tension barely corralled under normal circumstances. For others, the frayed nerves created by the process of applying to college creates conflicts where none seemed to exist before. Adolescents and parents experience some stresses in tandem: the challenge of a handling a new and confusing process, the feeling that there is no room for error, the sorting through all of the information and misinformation, and the exhaustion and expense of campus visits.

Then there are stressors that adolescents and parents feel independently of one another. Adolescents may worry about taking such a big developmental step. They might feel inundated by an unforgiving social culture at school, where details about SAT scores and college preparation are too freely shared. They probably worry about not getting into a school they like, or about getting everything finished on time. And this all hits at the busiest time in their lives, balancing the toughest academic schedule they have faced, along with the most demanding extracurricular responsibilities.

Even though parents are not the ones filling out the college applications (usually), they feel no less taxed. They share the stress of watching their son or daughter go through sleepless nights or burst into tears over the semester's challenges. They have reservations about their 17-year-old's ability to remember and meet all of the deadlines. They wonder if it's possible for their already overextended teenager to manage the difficult balance of making sure that everything gets finished without nagging. Most parents also face concerns about how to pay for 4 years of tuition and living expenses. And don't forget the less tangibles: An overall malaise in anticipation of changing household dynamics, and the impending sense of having to let go and not feeling quite sure how to do it.

The college application process raises constant questions and forces families to make important decisions amid uncertainty. Adolescents who stand in the best position to get into college, who have done "all the right things," paradoxically can find themselves the most challenged. For students (and parents) who have learned the rules at their high schools and know exactly what it takes to succeed there, this might be one of the first times that an outcome feels so uncertain. And, what's more, it can feel very personal.

College administrators have coined a number of terms to describe some of the parental reactions they commonly observe:

- *Helicopter parents* seem to hover over their children, seldom out of reach, overly involved with their children's experiences and problems. Such parents rush to protect their adolescent from any potential harm or failure, sometimes even contrary to the adolescent's wishes, and will not let them learn from their own mistakes.
- *Black Hawk parents*, a term adapted from the military's combat helicopter, move from emotional hovering to more zealous excesses of combative or unethical behavior, such as writing college admission essays for their adolescent.
- *Lawnmower parents* describe mothers and fathers who try to smooth out and mow down all obstacles their adolescent faces; sometimes even interfering at the graduate school or post-college employment setting.
- *Curling parents* describe parents who attempt to sweep all obstacles out of the paths of their children, as with a curling broom.

As with any new endeavor, the best way to handle the unknowns is to be proactive and gather the appropriate information. Applying to college may feel convoluted and strange, but understanding the process becomes easier with the right information. Seek answers from trusted authorities. The following are some commonly asked questions, to help you begin.

WHEN SHOULD MY FAMILY START PREPARING FOR THE APPLICATION PROCESS?

Consider this a two-part question: When should *you* start preparing for the process, and when should your son or daughter begin preparing? Parents can never start the process too early. Resources abound: articles, books, blogs, experts, etc. (see Where to Find Out More). However, exposing your son or daughter to the stresses of applying too early can prove harmful. Most parents consider age and maturity when it comes to talking to their children about other life issues. The same approach should hold true for the college application process. If you push too soon, it could easily backfire with passive resistance or a rebellion against applying at all. Early high school usually proves an appropriate age to start having some general family conversations about college and academic goals. Your might enjoy visiting some schools as a way to explore campus life at this age, but hold off on the temptation to put together a specific list of schools. You can bring up college as a motivator for academic effort, but rather than pressuring your child with "If you don't start getting A's you can forget school X," instead consider saying, "Putting in time and effort now will give you the most options later."

Keep in mind, however, that some things related to the college application process—like the SATs—do come up earlier, while students are underclassmen. To see year-specific recommendations for the college application process, visit the National Association for College Admission Counseling (NACAC) website (www.nacacnet.org/).

TO HOW MANY SCHOOLS SHOULD MY CHILD APPLY?

There is no right or wrong number, but most students will have a list of about 8–12 schools. While some students choose to apply to 20 or more schools, that is often not beneficial. It is an expensive undertaking and a huge amount of work. Applying to so many schools usually means that the teen doesn't want to do the work of scaling down the list ahead of time. It is better to create a narrow, but balanced list (i.e., with schools that seem likely to offer admission, some with a 50/50 chance of acceptance, and some realistically just out of reach), spending more time making those applications as strong as possible.

HOW CAN I HELP MY CHILD COME UP WITH AN APPROPRIATE LIST?

With over 3,000 schools out there, deciding on a short list is not an easy task. Using a process of elimination can make things easier. A small liberal arts college feels very different from a large research university. Even if teens know that they want to attend a school out of state, your family should still visit local campuses. The more schools your adolescent visits, the more he or she will get an instinct for what feels right. Beyond the campus size, other questions can help narrow the list: Does the school offer the right majors? Does a sports culture matter? Does a Greek-life option matter? Is the school in an urban or rural setting? Are there enough options for majors so that your child won't have a problem if he or she decides to change the course of his or her studies?

No student can visit every school, but websites offer many resources. College guides like Fiske detail hundreds of schools. Guidance and college counselors can offer advice. Keep an open mind. Just because you have never heard of a school does not mean that it is a less-respected institution. Brand name recognition can be misleading when it comes to finding the right fit.

HOW MUCH HELP SHOULD I GIVE MY CHILD?

Do some thinking about your family dynamic before crunch time. Does your child generally seem receptive to your help and advice? Does your child tend to push back when you remind him or her to get things done? Is your child highly independent and responsible, or, like most adolescents, inclined not to pay close attention to details and deadlines? And remember to think about how these familial roles play out during stressful times, not just when things are good.

Have a family conversation about the process. Some students will clearly tell you how much help they do or do not want. They may feel very organized, but will want you to help review essay drafts. Others will need a parent to focus on the deadlines and to give them reminders. When students do not want parents closely involved but lack the organizational ability needed to take charge of their own process, you may want to consider involving a favorite teacher or hiring a third party to act as a go-between. Often having that independent and objective voice can help put everyone's mind at ease.

SHOULD WE WORK WITH AN INDEPENDENT COLLEGE COUNSELOR?

If you do decide to hire an independent college counselor, think about how exactly you would like him or her to help, and ask about the counselor's years of experience and professional background. For example, it doesn't necessarily take high school counseling or college admissions experience to look over essays, but if you think you will have questions along the way about schools or the process, look for someone with experience working in those arenas. Also consider the consultant's philosophy. Some will share your family values and some will not. Does it seem like they will listen to your priorities, or will they assert their own bias?

Try to ascertain how effectively an independent counselor would work within the parameters of your high school counseling office. Most high school counselors serve a large number of students, and independent counselors can fill gaps of time and attention. They should not, however, overstep their bounds and authority in ways that cause problems. The high school counselor will have responsibility for the most direct contact with the colleges and the letters of recommendation. Working with someone who does not defer to the high school counselor serves no one in the end.

WHAT EXACTLY NEEDS TO GET DONE?

For better or worse, students actually complete much of the work required to apply to college before they fill out the applications. Generally, colleges consider grades, course selection, and standardized test scores as the most important factors in determining admittance. The following list of the application components shows when to begin thinking about them:

The Transcript

Almost all schools note that a student's transcript carries the most weight. The transcript tells more of a story than just grades. It alerts colleges to the level of rigor a student has chosen. If a student takes higher-level coursework, Honors, Advanced Placement (AP), or

International Baccalaureate (IB) notations appear on the transcript. Selective colleges regard a student's willingness to take on academic challenge as very important. Students should take on as much challenge as possible without overreaching. A 'B' in an AP class will probably look better to a college than an 'A' in a standard-level class, but students should not attempt AP courses if they tend to get Cs in the higher-level classes. Consult with your teen's school counselor to better understand what courses best match your child's abilities and goals.

Virtually every school will send along a high school profile with the transcript. This explains the transcript in context. For example, a student who took only two AP courses will present differently if they attend a high school offering 16 AP courses versus a school that offers only two. Admission officers want to measure each student's performance against their potential. The profile also explains how the high school calculates grade point average (GPA) and rank, if applicable, and how many students from that particular high school go directly to college. All of this information helps admissions counselors understand a student's record.

Standardized Tests

Colleges recognize that standardized tests like the SAT do not tell the whole story nor provide the best indicator of academic potential. Still, most admission offices regard them as an important tool, as they give data that cut across state, background, or type of school. Grade-point averages and courses, on the other hand, vary from school to school. Most admissions officers understand the need to place test score in context. Standardized tests also prove more difficult for underrepresented minorities, students whose first language is not English, and those with a socioeconomic disadvantage. All students typically get the benefit of the doubt with regard to multiple test sittings. If a student takes the SAT two or three times, most colleges will look at the highest scores in each section, regardless of whether they occurred on the same date.

Most schools require either the SAT or the ACT. The SAT tests a student's analysis and logic. For this reason, questions focus less on higher academic skills and more on applying logic to solve problems. The ACT, on the other hand, has four required sections (English, math, reading, and science) and an optional writing section creating more of a skills-based test. For example, the math section will not seem as "tricky" as the SAT, but will test higher-level math, such as trigonometry. Another difference between the tests involves the quarter-point penalty for marking wrong answers on the SAT, whereas the ACT has no guessing penalty.

Many of the most selective schools will require SAT Subject Tests in addition to the SAT Reasoning Test. Subject Tests assess the content learned in particular courses (e.g., languages or sciences). The best time for a student to take any Subject Test would come in the spring of the year when he or she takes the course at school. Students can perform best on the material of the subject as they prepare for final exams in the corresponding class. Knowing this and signing up to take some of these tests as early as spring of sophomore year puts students in a *much* better position later. Students who get to their senior year without having taken any Subject Tests often find themselves scrambling to score decently on material they may not remember well.

Essays

Like many parents, you may feel as if the essay is the most important part of the application. This may or may not be true, as the weight given essays varies from school to school. Many state universities do not even require essays. The general rule of thumb holds that a great essay will not compensate for a poor record, but in a pile of very qualified applicants, a strong essay may provide a needed edge.

Colleges request essays to both learn more about a candidate and to get a sense of writing ability. Students should write these essays in a style closer to personal narrative, than to formal thesis essays. They should show reflective and creative thinking, sharing unique experiences. Crafting essays for the ubiquitous common application, although designed for ease, can actually prove more challenging. This application, accepted at over 300 schools, asks students for an essay on a "topic of your choice." While it may seem much easier to write about anything, what to write about and how to write it can prove difficult. The essays I read that make the biggest impression do not necessarily focus on big topics. Some of the best involve small events or details. They all, however, have focus, demonstrate a reflective nature, and explore deeper ideas; not just the "what" of an experience but the "why" and the "how." To some students, this kind of writing comes naturally. To others, it seems a foreign exercise. For those students, self-reflecting before putting a pen to paper will prove essential.

Before submitting any writing samples, students should have someone review them for grammar, structure, and spelling. With unlimited time to revise, having awkward sentence construction or grammatical errors will seem sloppy.

Online Applications

Colleges prefer to have everything submitted online. Luckily, as today's high school students grew up using the Internet, completing online forms will feel natural. Ironically, the ease of online completion sometimes leads to problems. Online culture has become very informal. Students tend to drop capital letters and fully spelled-out phrases in favor of online shorthand. Remind your adolescent to treat the official applications formally. In addition, it is good policy to prepare essays off line and then copy and paste them into the application, so that hard work is not lost if there are problems with the "save" function on the application.

If students apply using the common application, many schools will also require supplemental applications submitted at the same time as the general deadline. These school-specific forms should get serious attention. Doing a half-hearted job on a school's supplement sends the message that a student may not have genuine interest. Writing thoughtfully, on the other hand, shows genuine enthusiasm, or "demonstrated interest."

Letters of Recommendation

Many schools require letters of recommendation both from the high school counselor and classroom teachers. Sometimes schools will request that teachers mail these letters of recommendation with forms downloaded from their website. Other schools will give the option to teachers and counselors of submitting all recommendations online, rather than mailing in forms. The student must take responsibility for learning what format each recommender would prefer, and for getting him or her the necessary material. Not all counselors and teachers feel comfortable submitting online, and so students should still find and print the paper forms from the application website. Students should allow enough time to do this. Finding and organizing forms seems a simple enough task, but it can prove logistically taxing.

Students should also remember to behave graciously when asking teachers to write them letters of recommendation. Such references technically fall outside the boundaries of the job that teachers are contracted to do. Thank-you notes go a long way!

Supplemental Materials

Sometimes applications can include supplemental materials like art portfolios, music submissions, resumes, or additional letters of recommendation. Before submitting anything additional, students should talk to representatives in the admission offices. Certain schools will not look at supplemental materials. Even if a school does take supplemental letters of recommendation, this does not necessarily mean one should use that option. Remember that the goal involves focusing the reader's attention for the very short amount of time they have for each application. Only include supplemental recommendations if they add significantly and uniquely to the application. Think about quality over quantity.

Some programs (e.g., in performing arts) will require supplemental materials or auditions. If so, carefully follow specific format guidelines. For example, not every school will ask for the same number of art pieces in a portfolio. Some will want the pieces submitted online, while others may prefer slides.

Many schools offer interviews either on the campus or with local alumni. Schools typically do not require interviews anymore, as it puts too great a demand on staff and volunteers. Instead, admission offices grant them on a first-come, first-served basis. Because colleges cannot guarantee interviews, they typically hold a less-critical role in the decision process. Admission offices understand that an interview's purpose involves educating the student about a school (and hopefully selling the student on its benefits) as much as it does learning more about the student. Students should practice and prepare, but also take comfort that an interview will rarely make or break an applicant.

WHAT SHOULD I DO IF MY CHILD DOES NOT DO WELL ON THE STANDARDIZED TESTS?

Do not give up on the test, even if the first time did not go too well. With sufficient preparation, most students will improve when they retest. Preparation can take the form of a course, private tutoring, or independent work in a book. Whatever the method, improvement only comes with diligent practice and a commitment to putting in the time. If retesting does not help, remember that scores comprise only one component of the complete picture, and lower scores do not necessarily rule out a student's chance at a school if the rest of the picture looks strong. A number of institutions have decided to make standardized tests optional. The National Center for Fair and Open Testing compiles a list of all schools that do not require standardized tests to apply.

HOW DO I TALK TO MY CHILD ABOUT WHAT WE CAN REALISTICALLY AFFORD?

An honest discussion about your concerns when it comes to paying for college is important. Price tags may prove deceiving. Many of the "most expensive" private schools provide the better financial aid when it comes to what you will actually end up paying. Financial aid offices calculate an expected family contribution from financial aid applications, like the government supported Free Application for Federal Student Aid (FAFSA). This calculation determines what the financial aid office determines as a reasonable amount for a family and student to contribute each year. The remaining expenses will round out a financial aid package generally consisting of grants, loans, and work-study options. You may not agree in the end that this package covers your needs. Still, financial aid offices have become more progressive when it comes to financial packages. Some schools offer merit scholarships. Others have begun to replace loans with grant money. Very recently, some of the most selective schools in the nation have decided to charge a percentage of a family's yearly income for college tuition. The bottom line: financial policies shift all the time, and you will need to do some research before assuming that you cannot afford a school.

WHAT ABOUT SCHOLARSHIPS?

Ask your school's administration if the high school or the community offers any scholarship competitions. Check in with groups or organizations with which you have affiliations (churches, synagogues, Rotary clubs, community centers, etc.). It's easier to pin down a scholarship when the pool is smaller and local. Beyond that, investigate scholarships offered by private corporations or nonprofit organizations. The website FastWeb is a good starting place to filter through the hundreds of available scholarships. Watch out for scams! You should never have to pay to get consideration for a scholarship, and you should never give out bank information or social security numbers to websites claiming to offer scholarships.

WHAT HAPPENS WHEN THE LETTERS COME BACK?

Decisions come in three categories: an acceptance, a denial, or a waitlist invitation. Obviously, everyone prefers an acceptance, but almost everyone faces at least one rejection letter.

The waitlist equals admission purgatory. Colleges typically admit students from the waitlist when a higher percentage of the accepted students go elsewhere and they under-enroll. If a student wants to stay on a school's waitlist, he or she will need to inform the school and then put down a deposit somewhere else. One should always send a follow-up letter to the "waitlist school" expressing continued interest and providing any positive updates in the applicant's qualifications since submitting the application.

If it's a rejection letter in the end, try to keep perspective. For the student, the application process is deeply personal, but for the college the decision is not. Decisions often come down to what the school community needs, not the competency of the applicant. You can help your teenager work through the feeling of rejection by reminding him or her that each school offers exceptional educational opportunities. While students might have preferences, the favorite school on their list represents one selected out of thousands of institutions. If, for some reason, a "second-best" school does not end up meeting expectations, transferring is always an option. More often, however, students enroll in their second, third, or last choice college and end up saying that they can't imagine having gone anywhere else. So, encourage your child not to dwell on the denials, but to instead focus on the acceptances and the exciting 4 years to come.

SUMMARY

Recognize and accept the idea that the college admission process will pose substantial stresses on both you and your teenagers. Understanding where these stresses come from within each of us, and how the resulting feelings can cause problems in the process, will go a long way toward improving coping. Focusing on the process early, understanding how each element of the process fits with the others, setting reasonable deadlines, and keeping a positive perspective will help you to work with your child to optimize his or her success. Gathering information and careful planning can help everyone feel more control over a process that is full of uncertainty. This can serve as a great opportunity for parents to work together with their teenagers to understand the process, establish a plan, and reach a successful outcome.

WHERE TO FIND OUT MORE

Websites

FastWeb
    http://www.fastweb.com/
Free Application for Federal Student Aid
    http://www.fafsa.ed.gov/
National Center for Fair and Open Testing
    http://www.fairtest.org/
National Association for College Admission Counseling
    http://www.nacacnet.org
The Fiske Guide
    http://www.fiskeguide.com/
Mosaic College Prep
    http://www.mosaicprep.com/resources.php
The College Board
    http://www.collegeboard.com/
The ACT Test
    http://www.actstudent.org/index.html

PART FIVE

Anxiety Issues

CHAPTER 33

Fears and Phobias

Wendy K. Silverman

Maria, age 8, is terrified of dogs. Whenever she sees a dog, she starts crying, screaming, and hovering near her mother. She becomes visibly shaken and reports that her heart starts beating faster and that she feels all "shaky." She will not visit the homes of other children or any family friends' homes if she knows that they have a dog. This has led to her missing out on birthday parties and other social events. She is an excellent soccer player, but she quit because she became fearful that a dog might come into the soccer park, even though her mother has assured her that the park forbids animals. Maria's avoidance behavior has become increasingly irritating to her parents because they feel forced to avoid many places and events that they ordinarily would enjoy attending in order to appease Maria.

Fears occur commonly in children. When a child's fear becomes irrational, out of proportion to reality, and leads to excessive avoidance or distress, then the "fear" has become what mental health professionals call a *phobia*. This chapter discusses common fears of childhood and adolescence and the differences between fears and phobias and how parents can address them.

COMMON CHILDHOOD FEARS

At different ages, certain fears are more common than others. For example:

- Infants and toddlers show fears relating to loss of physical support, loud noises, and unfamiliar people. In toddlers, fears relating to separation from parents or other known caretakers occur commonly.
- Preschool children often demonstrate magical thinking in which imaginative play can seem real. They may show fears of imaginary creatures, ghosts, monsters, scary

or even small animals, and the dark. Such fears may become most noticeable at bed-time or other points of separation from protective adults.

- Six- to 12-year-old children begin showing a decrease in fears with imaginary themes and have more realistic fears. These may include school-related fears tied to issues of achievement/failure, separation, fears of bodily injury, and growing social concerns.
- Adolescents may have any of the fears listed, but will increasingly tend to focus on social fears. This includes fears that other people will evaluate them negatively and fear of embarrassment or humiliation.
- Most of the fears mentioned "come and go" during childhood, and the majority of children outgrow these common fears.
- When fears become intense, and so strong that they begin to interfere with children's functioning, then they have progressed past "normal" or developmentally appropriate fears to become phobias.
- When we speak of "interference," we usually mean that the phobia makes it very hard for the child to participate in the types of activities that we usually expect boys and girls to handle easily. This would include activities relating to school, peer groups, and family; it also could lead to the child feeling distressed and upset. To qualify as a phobia, such interference must persist for at least 6 months.
- Unlike fears, children do not necessarily "outgrow" phobias. Many adults with phobias report that their difficulties began as children, and research supports this claim.

There is usually no typical single reason why a child develops excessive fears and phobias. Instead, many reasons typically interact with one another to explain why some children develop a phobia or multiple phobias. But we do not know why other children who have the exact same experiences never develop a problem with excessive fears or phobias. As we discuss the most common reasons for the development of excessive fears and phobias in the following sections, we will refer to them as *specific phobias*. Specific phobias describe fears that are related to certain objects or events, such as a fear of dogs or a fear of needles.

GENETICS

Research suggests that phobias have strong familial components. This means that, unlike many of the other problems discussed in this book, there is a risk that phobias can be "transmitted" within families. Children with specific phobias are more likely to have parents and other family members who also have, or have had, problems with specific phobias. However, just because you have a specific phobia, it doesn't guarantee that your child will develop one as well. It simply means that, compared to other children, your child may have a greater risk than a child whose parent does not have a phobia. Indeed, many children whose parents or other family members have phobias, never develop phobias themselves. The reason why some children develop phobias may be linked in part to genetics, but also to other reasons as well, as discussed in the sections that follow.

DIRECT NEGATIVE EXPERIENCE WITH
A SPECIFIC OBJECT OR EVENT

Some children develop excessive fears or specific phobias because they had a direct negative experience with a specific object or event. For example, a child with a phobia of dogs may have been jumped on or bitten by a dog; a child with a dental phobia may have had a painful dental experience. Research provides evidence for direct negative experiences leading to phobias in children. Interestingly though, the majority of young people with phobias never report having had a negative experience with the specific thing that they now fear. Because of this, we must consider other explanations to help understand why some children develop phobias and others do not.

OBSERVING OTHERS

Children with phobias who have never had a direct, personal negative experience with the object or situation they fear may have seen a bad or scary event happen to another person. This could involve an actual "live" person, such as seeing a sibling or friend bitten by a dog. It could even result from watching a television show or a movie where, for example, a bunch of snakes or rats crawled over one of the characters who then displayed an intense fear reaction. Such a strong fear reaction, when observed by some children, particularly those with some predisposition for phobias, can lead to the development of a phobia.

VERBAL INSTRUCTIONS OR INFORMATION

Some children who develop phobias may have never witnessed a bad or scary event happen to someone else, either live or in the media. Rather, some children may develop excessive fears or phobias because they heard from someone else that a certain object or event leads to a negative consequence. For example, if a child has heard over and over that "dogs bite," then the child may come to believe that all dogs bite.

By now you may feel a bit puzzled. After all, most people have either heard of or have seen bad things happening to others such as insect stings, snake bites, or becoming stuck in an elevator for hours. Yet, relatively few young people develop phobias about these objects. The development of phobias must involve more complexity than simple genetics and exposure to stressful environmental events. Two additional reasons why youth may develop a phobia and why the phobia can stay in place over time involve how the youth thinks about things and/or because of how other people react to the youth's avoidance behavior.

THINKING PROCESSES

Some research shows that children who are prone to developing phobias tend to focus on and think over and over about the possible bad consequence of encountering the object or event that they are afraid of. We call such thinking *rumination*, and this process can inflate or intensify the negative evaluations that children have of the specific objects or events that frighten them. For example, a child who keeps ruminating about the possibility of an elephant stampede in the neighborhood may develop even broader and more frightening concerns about elephants—even when you live far away from any elephants!

HOW OTHERS REACT

If you or other people in your child's life support your child's avoidant behaviors, your child is likely to remain phobic. Of course, you want to protect your child from getting upset or scared, but supporting your child when he or she is afraid of someone or something will only continue the problem. Allowing children to avoid the things they fear prevents them from learning that the scary consequences they think will happen probably won't. Instead, protecting your child from being afraid tends to validate his or her fear and reinforces the sense that "staying away feels good."

HOW DO I PREVENT MY CHILD FROM DEVELOPING A PHOBIA?

We recommend several practices to prevent a child from developing excessive fears or phobia problems in the first place. The sections that follow outline some basic practices in preventing the occurrence of fears and phobias.

Handle Your Own Fears in a Positive Way

Even though some children can learn to become very afraid and even possibly phobic toward certain objects and events by watching others, including their parents, this does not mean that parents must hide their fears from their child. However, it is a good idea to try, as much as you can, to handle your fears in a way that shows your child that you can cope with and handle them. At a minimum, let your child see you actively trying to cope. If your child sees you "freaking out" at the sight of a dog or a spider, your child may likely begin to model such behaviors.

 Remember, whatever it is you fear will have a high visibility in your child's environment. If your own reaction involves "freaking out," it might prove useful to either (1) talk to your child about the problem and admit to your child that your handling of the object or event is not necessarily the best way or (2) seek professional help for your own phobia problem, so that you can learn to serve as a coping model for your child. Serving as a coping model does not necessarily involve acting bravely all the time. Rather, it is about trying your best to handle the situation in a more appropriate way. Some studies compared children who observed models trying to cope with their fears (i.e., showing some fear) with mastery models who didn't show any fears at all. The results show that children will more likely mimic the behavior of the person who attempts to cope with fear. This may happen because the child can better identify with the person who has some fear and tries to manage it, as opposed to a person who doesn't have any fears at all. All the more reason for you to show your children how you cope, rather than putting up a brave front!

Of course, you cannot control everything your child is exposed to, especially outside of the home. Based on what we have talked about here, if your child tells you about having watched or seen someone have a really bad or scary experience with a certain object or event, it is probably a good idea to talk with your child about what happened and make sure your child understands certain ideas, including:

- If the bad thing that happened is an unusual event, explain this to your child. Help your child to understand the distinction between possible events versus probable events. For example, yes—it is possible that dogs bite and carry rabies. But serious dog bites that lead to rabies rarely occur.
- Just because this event happened to this other person does not mean it will happen to your child, especially since the event has a low probability of occurrence.

Talk About Fears in a Helpful Way

The influence of how you behave toward scary objects or events, or what to do if your child witnesses others having bad experiences also applies to the way you talk about things. Avoid emphasizing how dangerous and scary day-to-day objects and events are in daily discussions. Certainly, children need to know about the genuine dangers in their world! We keep our children safe by teaching them to look both ways before crossing the street, to stay away from animals they don't know, and to never talk to strangers, and so on. But talking about such dangers in the world comes across very differently from focusing day in and day out on *all* the possible harmful consequences of objects and events, especially ones with relatively remote consequences.

Given the role of thinking in triggering some anxious feelings, we also recommend that you have regular talks with your child about unrealistic (and realistic) fears that your child may have. By discovering your child's fears, you can offer help and more realistic ways to think about these things. Sometimes, all your child needs is information. For example, maybe your child does not know that the spiders in your yard are not poisonous (if, in fact, they are not!) and that the elevator in your building has a safety button. Going back to the example at the start of the chapter, Maria's parents talked with their daughter about her excessive fear of dogs. They helped her to think of all the dogs they know, and to realize that none of these dogs ever bit anyone or did anything harmful to anyone. They also encouraged Maria to think about how she might better approach some of the dogs they know and how she can start off with the smaller dogs or those less likely to jump on her. Maria's parents praised their daughter when she successfully went to play soccer because she had become able to handle her rumination about dogs.

Encourage Approach Behaviors and Discourage Avoidance

As soon as you begin to notice that your child does not want to do something or go somewhere because of the possibility that a particular scary object may be present, like a dog, we recommend that you accompany your child to that location and let your child see that the situation is "safe." Remember the old adage: if you fall off the bike, get right back on. It seems simple, but it rings true. The more your child stays away from the bike (or feared object) because he or she fell off, or because someone else fell off, or because your child heard about someone falling off, or because your child just keeps thinking over and over about the possibility of falling off, the more likely that your child's fear of bikes will not go away. And, the more your child thinks about the negative possibilities, the more your child's fear will inflate over time. So, we recommend that you get your child back in contact with the situation or object right away.

If your child's fear has already developed to a somewhat excessive level, and your child refuses to come into contact with the object or event, then it might be necessary to break down your child's approach behavior into a series of small steps. With Maria, for example, her parents broke down her approach of dogs into the following steps:

- Go to a neighborhood pet store and look at, from a distance, the little poodles behind the windowed cage.
- Go to the same pet store, and then Mom and Maria both place their hands in the cage to pet a poodle for a couple of seconds.
- Maria pets the poodle in the pet store without mom's hand touching hers.
- Maria goes to a neighbor house and sits on couch with mom and the neighbor's dog.
- Maria sits on the couch alone with the neighbor's dog.
- Maria pets the neighbor's dog while the dog is restrained on a leash.
- Maria walks into the neighbor's house with the dog not on a leash.
- Maria walks into the neighbor's house with the dog not on leash and pets the dog.
- Maria holds the dog.
- Maria goes to a park where there are many dogs roaming around on leashes with their owners.

Provide Rewards

If your child shows excessive avoidance, rewards for approach behavior (e.g., going near the feared object or event) can sometimes prove useful. It is important to offer the reward as soon as your child displays the appropriate behavior, such as going up to a friendly dog or going to a classmate's birthday party. Rewards can range from gifts, such as small toys, games, or stickers, to privileges like extra TV time, a trip to the ice cream shop after dinner, or a sleep-over with friends. Remember, however: do not provide any rewards for your child's avoidance behavior.

WHEN TO SEEK PROFESSIONAL HELP

You might want to seek professional help for a child with excessive fears or phobias if one or more of the following conditions apply to your situation:

- Your child's fear or phobia has lasted for at least 6 months.
- Your child's fear or phobia continues to cause much distress for your child, for you, and/or the rest of the family.

- Your child's avoidance has led to interference with school (e.g., school refusal or declining grades), peers (e.g., refuses to see other children because of fear of encountering the phobic object or event), or extracurricular activities (e.g., Maria no longer played soccer because she was afraid a dog might be in the park).

In these cases, we recommend you consult a mental health professional who has experience in treating phobias using behavioral or cognitive-behavioral procedures. Cognitive-behavioral procedures have the strongest and most consistent research support. Such procedures emphasize the detailed approaches suggested in this chapter—having the child face his or her fears, and addressing how the child thinks about the scary objects or events. Check with the psychology or psychiatry department of a nearby university or online directories at www.abct.org or www.apa.org to find a suitable mental health professional near you.

SUMMARY

All children have fears, and certain fears are more common than others at different ages. However, not all children have fears that become so excessive and so severe that they interfere with a child's functioning. When this happens, a child may show excessive avoidance and irrational thinking about harm befalling him or her upon contact with the phobic object or event; deterioration in school, peer relationships, and family relations also may occur. Such excessive fears, or phobias, are usually not outgrown.

Providing emotional first aid for excessive fears and phobias requires that parents remain aware of how they respond themselves to objects or events that they find fearful, as well as being aware about how they talk about things to their child. Parents also need to notice whether or not their child is beginning to engage in avoidant behaviors. If so, parents must generally expect their child to face the fearful object or event, rather than avoid it. If the problem has become severe, parents may need to break down the child's exposure to the feared object or event into small steps and provide rewards for each step. If the problems worsen, parents might consider seeking the help or consultation of behavioral mental health experts who have worked with children with excessive fears and phobias.

WHERE TO FIND OUT MORE

Books

Bourne, E.J. (2000). *The anxiety and phobia workbook* (3rd edition). Oakland CA: New Harbinger Publications. (This book helps parents with their own anxiety or phobia problems).

Cain, B.S. (1999). *I don't know why…I guess I'm shy: A story about taming imaginary fears.* Washington, DC: Magination Press.

Huebner, D. (2005). *What to do when you worry too much: A kid's guide to overcoming anxiety.* Washington, DC: Magination Press.

Huebner, D. (2008). *What to do when you dread your bed: A kid's guide to overcoming problems with sleep.* Washington, DC: Magination Press.

Last, C.G. (2006). *Help for worried kids: How your child can conquer anxiety and fear.* New York: Guilford Press.

Maier, I. (2005). *When Fuzzy was afraid of big and loud things.* Washington, DC: Magination Press.

Silverman, W.K., & Kurtines, W.M. (1996). *Anxiety and phobic disorders: A pragmatic approach.* New York: Plenum Press.

Websites

Association for Behavioral and Cognitive Therapies
   http://www.abct.org
American Psychological Association
   http://www.apa.org
American Academy of Child and Adolescent Psychiatry
   http://www.aacap.org
Therapy Advisor
   http://www.therapyadvisor.com

CHAPTER 34

Separation Anxiety Disorder

Sasha Aschenbrand and Anne Marie Albano

Eight-year-old Joshua had difficulty separating from his parents in a number of situations. His parents worried that he had great trouble separating from them to go to school and, as a result, they had to physically hand him over to his teacher, rather than simply dropping him off at the school entrance like the other children. Joshua also refused to stay home with a babysitter, could not separate from his father to play with other children at extracurricular activities, acted clingy with his mother at birthday parties, and often followed his parents around the house like a shadow. Several nights a week, Joshua would beg for his mom or dad to lie down with him until he fell asleep, and most nights he wound up climbing into their bed in the middle of the night. Upon anticipation of separation experiences (e.g., his parents going to the store or out to dinner), Joshua would cry and physically cling to his mother or father.

Separation situations caused much upset for Joshua and his parents. At 8 years of age, we'd expect Joshua to be more comfortable when separating from his parents for social and school events. In young children, we normally expect some age-related anxiety about separating from parents, especially prior to the start of kindergarten. Very young children may appropriately feel fearful of strangers or of new and unfamiliar surroundings. Such separation anxiety generally emerges around 9 months of age and peaks around 12–24 months, although the exact age and amount of fear will vary from child to child. Children as old as 3 years will often feel some anxiety when a parent leaves the room or goes out of their sight. It is not unusual for children to cry when first left at daycare or when brought to preschool, but this upset generally subsides as children engage in activities and become accustomed to their teachers, peers, and the school routine. However, when children continue to show unusually high fear in situations involving separation, especially as they age, the problem may involve a separation anxiety disorder (SAD).

IS MY CHILD'S SEPARATION ANXIETY PROBLEMATIC?

Determining if your child's fears qualify as "problematic" or "abnormal" can prove difficult, as some level of separation anxiety occurs normally in children. A key to distinguishing whether your child's separation anxiety warrants concern involves considering whether it interferes in his or her life. Ask yourself the following questions:

- Does my child's anxiety about being away from me stop him or her from doing activities he or she would like to do? Such as attend parties or sleep-overs?
- Does separation anxiety cause my child difficulties with going to school or with school achievement?
- Does my child have trouble falling asleep without my presence or sleeping through the night alone?
- When I leave my child at home (with a sitter, or alone if he or she is older) does he or she constantly call me and want me to come home?
- Does my child socialize less frequently with peers because he or she does not want to leave my side?
- Does my child have trouble staying alone in one area of the house, such as in his or her bedroom or a television room, while I'm in another? Does my child always want to keep me in sight?
- Do I often have to make accommodations at home to prevent my child's distress, or do tantrums/arguments occur if I plan to separate from my child?

If you answered yes to any of these questions, your child might be suffering from too much separation anxiety, and you might want to consider seeking help to overcome it. Most commonly, extreme levels of separation anxiety in children occur between the ages of 7 and 9 years, although this can occur at any time before the age of 18. Signs of separation anxiety differ in children and adolescents; young children tend to report more nightmares with separation themes and extreme distress upon separation, whereas adolescents more often report physical complaints on school days and other separation events, such as when leaving for camp or even for college. Separation anxiety also appears to be more common in girls than in boys. The key feature of separation anxiety is excessive anxiety or distress concerning separation from home or major attachment figures. Children may express this anxiety through recurrent distress in anticipation of or upon separation, a constant need to know the whereabouts of loved ones (usually, but not limited to, parents), and/or extreme homesickness when away from home. When separated from caregivers, children with separation anxiety often seem preoccupied with fears that harm will befall these people (e.g., car accident, getting sick or hurt) or themselves (e.g., getting lost, being kidnapped). As noted, children with separation anxiety have trouble leaving loved ones to attend school or to go to friends' houses, and/or they have difficulty being alone, even in their bedroom or another room in the house. Additionally, children with separation anxiety often avoid sleep-overs, require that a caregiver or loved one sleep next to them at bedtime, and might have nightmares with separation themes. Children with separation anxiety also often exhibit "clingy" behavior, perhaps even following their parents around. In school-aged youth, homesickness is expected when children first go off to a sleep-over or for longer excursions, such as to sleep-away camp or on a school trip. Calls and pleas to be picked up are not unusual the first time or few times that these situations occur. However, the fun of a sleep-over or camp activities usually comes to outweigh the initial separation worries experienced by most children. With time, children become more focused on the positive aspects of separation and settle into the situation. However, some children exhibit ongoing problems with separation anxiety, never seeming to adapt to the situation. In its most severe form, separation anxiety can lead to school refusal behavior.

WHAT ARE THE SIGNS OF PROBLEMATIC SEPARATION ANXIETY?

Physical complaints, such as stomachaches, nausea, and headaches occur commonly when separation occurs or seems likely. Children and teens may respond differently. Younger children with separation anxiety may cry or throw temper tantrums. Older children and teens may tend to seek excessive reassurance from caregivers before separating and/or may require caregivers to "check-in" frequently while separated. Frequent check-in with parents via cell phone or texting, along with frequent requests to return home, complaints of illness to the school nurse without any physical symptoms (e.g., no fever, vomiting), and excuses to the invitation of friends in the absence of a conflicting obligation are all signals that the child or adolescent does not want to be away from home.

HOW CAN I HELP MY CHILD COPE WITH SEPARATION WORRIES?

For most children, some separation anxiety is normal, and parents can use several strategies to help their child cope with his or her separation fears. Some of the effective strategies are also used with more extreme cases of SAD, and are based on a type of talk therapy that focuses on thoughts, feelings, and behaviors, known as *cognitive-behavioral therapy*, or CBT. CBT focuses on teaching children several major skills, including identifying emotions and physical reactions to anxiety, relaxation training, problem-solving and developing a coping plan, and self-evaluation and reward for coping in anxiety-provoking situations. Children are then taught to implement their skills while gradually facing feared situations. We describe each of these strategies in the sections that follow and highlight the important role that you can play in helping your child overcome significant separation anxiety.

Identifying Feelings and Physical Reactions to Anxiety

To know what to do about anxiety, children need to recognize when they feel anxious. Many children have difficulty describing and naming emotions, so this is the first skill that children are taught in CBT. When your child understands a range of feelings and the ways in which they seem similar or different, your child can begin to distinguish his or her own emotional states and will be able to recognize when coping skills are necessary. You can help your child with this skill by showing them pictures (from magazines, books, TV shows) and asking them to identify how each person feels. Pointing out clues provided by facial expressions and body posture is a good way to help children make subtle distinctions between feelings. You can also role-play different feeling states with your child and take turns guessing what emotion the other person is acting out. With older children and adolescents, you can present hypothetical situations and ask your child to identify the emotion someone might feel in that situation.

In addition to recognizing emotions, it can help children to recognize their physical reactions to anxiety. When a child becomes adept at recognizing the physical changes that happen in the body when anxious, he or she can use them as cues to put a coping plan into effect. You can teach your child about these reactions by asking if he or she can recall a cartoon character in an anxiety-provoking situation. Often, such characters show exaggerated reactions when they feel nervous, such as hair standing on end, violent shaking, red faces, etc. This will help your child to begin to think about physical responses to anxiety and will provide an entry point into inquiring about his or her own physical reactions when separated or anticipating separation from you. Common physical responses include increased heart rate, stomachaches, rapid breathing, sweating, and muscle tension. Some children struggle to identify their responses when they do not currently feel worried; in these cases, you can gently point out the physical reactions you notice in your child when an anxious situation does arise.

Deep Breathing and Progressive Muscle Relaxation

In addition to identifying feelings, it helps to teach children strategies for decreasing and/or tolerating these physical feelings. We teach children that it will help them think more clearly and cope more effectively if they can get their bodies to calm down a little bit.

You can use deep breathing or "belly breathing" exercises, teaching your child to use his or her full lung capacity rather than breathing from his or her chest. This enables a slow, deeper breath, which helps with relaxation and managing anxiety. Have your child inhale to a slow count of 1-2-3, while filling up his or her lungs with air. You can use the image of a tube running down the throat, into the abdomen (or "belly" for younger children) where there is an imaginary balloon. With each inhale, instruct your child to picture the balloon inflating, and then exhale slowly to a backward count of 3-2-1 to deflate the balloon. If the child places one hand on the chest and lays one hand on the abdomen, with the pinky finger just above the naval, only the hand on his or her abdomen should move. This indicates that the child is getting a good, full, and deep breath. Sometimes, it is helpful to have the child lie on the floor with a cup or toy on the abdomen that he or she can try to move up and down with each inhalation and exhalation.

Your child might use deep breathing as the first strategy to calm himself or herself when separating from you for school, a play date, or at bedtime. In addition to deep breathing techniques, your child can practice progressive muscle relaxation exercises. These exercises teach the child to tense and relax each major muscle group in the body, helping the child to distinguish between tense and relaxed states, so that he or she may voluntary relax muscles when anxious or stressed. It can help to practice these exercises during a quiet time of the day, such as at bedtime, particularly since sleeping alone is often difficult and anxiety-provoking for children with separation fears. The *I Can Relax! CD for Children* by Donna Pincus features several helpful relaxation exercises for younger children. For older children and adolescents, find downloadable progressive muscle relaxation exercises on popular music-purchasing programs or by using Internet search engines.

Tuning in to Self-Talk and Using Detective Thinking

Children who worry about separation often harbor unrealistic fears about the nature of the world, catastrophizing and overestimating the probability of danger in everyday situations. Children with separation anxiety frequently report worries about harm coming to their parents or to themselves: they might worry that their parents will become grievously ill or injured when they are separated, or perhaps that they themselves will be kidnapped or get lost. Behind these worries lies a view of the world as a dangerous and threatening place. These anxiety-provoking thoughts and beliefs link to feelings of anxiety, which in turn link to anxious behaviors. For example, a child who worries about his or her parent getting into a terrible car accident will feel acute fear when the parent attempts to drive to the store and might cling to the parent, refuse to stay home alone, and/or attempt to prevent the parent from leaving the house. Helping children challenge their unrealistic thoughts can help to control their anxious responses and behaviors. The key is to replace the unrealistic thoughts and beliefs with more realistic ones through a process of evaluating the evidence for worries, not simply to "think positively" or to "brush them off."

Before you can challenge their thoughts, children need to first pinpoint their worries. You can help your child tune into his or her anxious "self-talk" by illustrating the concept with comic strip thought bubbles. Show the child cartoons of situations they fear (e.g., sleeping alone, going to camp, staying home with a babysitter) and ask them to place thoughts in the characters' thought bubbles. Once you have a sense of your child's worries, you can lead him or her through a process of challenging them—in this step, your child can play the detective, evaluating the evidence for their worried thoughts. For example, ask your child, "How many times have I left the house to go shopping? And, how many times have I not come home at all?" You can help by asking whether we know for sure that the feared outcome will come true, what else might happen in that situation, and what has happened before in similar situations. This process will help your child to generate more realistic thoughts that can be used to calm himself or herself down and manage the worry.

Problem-Solving to Develop a Coping Plan

Now that your child is addressing the physical and cognitive components of the separation anxiety, he or she can also work on what to do in anxiety-provoking situations. Children with separation anxiety can sometimes only see one solution to the problem at hand—and their solution focuses on clinging to the parent for dear life! Prepare your child for separation experiences by developing a list of things that he or she can do to ease the anxiety when such situations arise. Perhaps your child can carry a picture of family members or play a favorite game when you go out. Let your child suggest a number of solutions at first, and then help him or her select those that seem most helpful; the trick is to weed out avoidant solutions that will only increase your child's anxiety in the long run, like making repeated cell phone calls, having you come home much earlier than necessary, etc. Once your child has prepared a coping plan, he or she should feel more confident to handle challenging separation situations.

Rewarding Coping with Anxious Situations

Anxious children tend to treat themselves harshly—they often don't reward themselves for their efforts, except for absolute successes. You can help to shape your child's attempts at being brave by praising and attending to his or her efforts at coping. Children can rate how well they coped with a situation and can reward themselves for trying to confront their fears; emphasize that they need to reinforce small steps in the right direction, not just huge leaps. Encourage your child to pat himself or herself on the back, to engage in a favorite activity, or to save a special snack for when he or she has worked at coping with a difficult situation.

Putting Coping Skills into Action

Once your child learns coping skills, he or she can begin to confront anxiety-provoking situations more effectively. Help your children to slowly face their fears, starting with those that are least anxiety-provoking and moving gradually up to those that provoke the most anxiety. Think of this as gradually climbing a fear ladder; you have to step on each successive rung of the ladder before you can climb higher. Collaborate with your child to form a list of difficult separation experiences, and together select which ones to work on first. Let your child work at his or her own pace in moving up the ladder, but gently encourage your child to keep moving, rather than getting stuck at one point. When your child has confronted his or her lesser fears, he or she should begin to feel a sense of mastery and accomplishment and will have better ability to tackle the bigger fears. Reward your child for his or her efforts to ensure that future brave behavior will more likely occur.

PARENTING DO'S AND DON'TS

What to Do

First, model brave behavior! Anxiety tends to run in families and, as we know, children tend to learn behavior by observing their parents. Take advantage of this fact by acting as "coping models" for your children. This does not mean that you should reveal all of the ins and outs of your own anxieties to your kids; however, you can let your children know about situations or things you fear(ed) and how you manage(d) those fears effectively. For example, using Joshua's situation at the beginning of this chapter, his parent might say, "I used to feel very afraid of staying home with a babysitter when I was your age. To help myself, I thought of fun games to play when my mom went out and reminded myself that she always came home. It really helped me feel better when we were away from each other." If you model effectively how to deal with problems, your child will learn to surmount problems and will see them as challenges, rather than as roadblocks. If you feel as though coping modeling might prove difficult, given your own concerns with anxiety, you may wish to consult a professional as a helpful first step.

In addition to coping modeling, you should also make sure to encourage your children's brave behavior. On a day-to-day basis, separation experiences will come up. Your child will face the challenge of going to school without you, to staying on a different floor in the house, to going to sleep alone, etc. Catch instances in which your child demonstrates bravery, even if just slightly so, and pay attention to him or her in those moments. Give labeled praise that addresses the specific behavior you want to see; for example, you might say, "Joshua, you did an excellent job going up to your room by yourself!" Some parents are afraid to pay attention to nonanxious behavior because they think they will jinx it; on the contrary, the more you pay attention to the behavior you want to encourage, the more likely your child will engage in that behavior.

On the other side of the coin, ignore behaviors you do not want to encourage, like crying, whining, clinging, etc. Remember, your attention has a very powerful influence, and focusing on dysfunctional behavior can reward it and make it happen more often! You can also reward your child with small material items or favored activities contingent upon engaging in challenges. Children can earn stickers, small toys, or snacks for their efforts in separating from you. Additionally, you can reward your child with favored activities for showing bravery—spend extra time with your child playing outside, going for ice cream, or playing a favorite board game in response to successful efforts at coping. This way, your child gets to have the time he or she wants with you, but gets it in response to positive behavior, as opposed to simply as a function of his or her anxiety.

In addition to catching your child confronting anxiety-provoking situations, as we mentioned earlier, you can set up small challenges for your child to overcome. Look for opportunities for your child to practice his or her skills—schedule play dates, go out to the store, and encourage your child to try sleeping alone. Reward any efforts you see at coping effectively with these challenges and be sure that rewards (1) remain contingent upon behavior; (2) prove effective—that your child actually likes the reward; and (3) get awarded as immediately as possible following the accomplishment.

On the flip side of encouraging brave behavior, parents can focus on discouraging avoidance. Often, parents have difficulty seeing their child in distress. Therefore, they will permit their child to escape anxious situations in order to decrease their child's anxiety. This actually serves to reinforce the avoidant behavior because the child does not learn that he or she can cope with anxiety, thereby increasing the chances for future anxious reactions. Discouraging avoidance helps the child to realize that the situation does not pose actual danger and that he or she has the skills to cope with and overcome difficult situations. When your child feels confronted with a situation he or she wants to avoid, encourage him or her to use coping skills. Help your child choose appropriate coping mechanisms to put into place, but watch out for providing all of the answers! Scaffold and support your child, rather than doing the task for him or her. Table 34.1 presents a summary of the "do's" described in this section.

TABLE 34.1. Parents' "To Do" List for helping a child with separation fears

- Model brave behavior.
- Praise and reward efforts at coping.
- Help your child face his or her fears in step-like fashion; start with the easy things first.
- Discourage avoidance of anxiety-provoking situations.
- Be empathic; validate emotions, but not necessarily behavior.
- Prepare your child for anxiety-provoking situations in advance—develop a coping plan, so that the child feels prepared to confront the fearful situation.

What Not to Do

Parents will want to avoid several pitfalls when dealing with a child who is anxious about separation. First, take care to avoid providing excessive reassurance for your child. Parents will sometimes tell the fearful child things such as, "Mommy will be fine, nothing bad will happen to me," or "You will always be safe with or without me." Although these statements sound like helpful and natural ways to respond, they can increase your child's anxiety, rather than decrease it. When your child feels fearful, and you provide reassurance that everything will turn out okay, you are giving your child attention for his or her anxious behavior. Because attention is a highly powerful reinforcer, children will come back for more. The more you provide reassurance, the more your child will need. The reassurance only provides a short-term fix for worry; once its effects wear off, your child will return to you once again for help. Instead, encourage your child to use coping skills to come up with his or her own answers, and reward and praise your child for doing so.

Don't rescue your child from anxious situations. It is often tempting to remove your child from a situation that causes him or her distress. This is as a natural parental reaction. However, if you take your child out of the anxiety-provoking situation, you (1) send your child the message that he or she does not have the ability to cope with it; (2) help your child to remember the situation at the height of his or her fear; and (3) prevent opportunities for mastery. In short, rescuing your anxious child will only serve to increase his or her anxiety in the long run.

A similar concept applies to permitting or encouraging a child's avoidant behavior. When you allow your child to decline an invitation to a birthday party or you allow the child to sleep in bed with you because he or she wants to be near you, your child does not get the opportunity to realize the situation is probably not as dangerous as first thought. If you allow avoidant behavior too frequently, your child's anxiety and impairment from anxiety will only increase. Children with anxiety about separation stand at risk for missing out on fun and rewarding activities, given their strong tendency to avoid separation. Encourage and shape efforts at overcoming fears, rather than running away from them.

As mentioned earlier, coping modeling is a good thing to do for your child with separation anxiety. Conversely, modeling anxiety *without* effective coping strategies will not help. Parents who excessively discuss the things that they fear will likely raise fearful children. Children get the message that the world is a dangerous place over which they have no control. If you discuss what makes you afraid, also discuss how you handle that fear in an effective manner.

Last, parents of anxious children sometimes fall into the trap of trying to control situations for them. Under the guise of helping, parents take over and become intrusive. This strategy sometimes develops in reaction to having seen the child fail in similar situations in the past. Nevertheless, when a parent takes over control, the child loses control, further increasing his or her sense of anxiety. Allow your children to make mistakes sometimes; as we know, this provides a way to learn from them. Table 34.2 presents a summary of the "don'ts" described in this section.

WHEN TO SEEK PROFESSIONAL HELP

If your efforts to help your child do not result in a change in behavior, or if your child's separation anxiety continues to intensify over time, your child may have developed a diagnosis of separation anxiety disorder (SAD). SAD is a condition that affects approximately 3%–5% of children and adolescents. To meet criteria for SAD, the separation anxiety must extend beyond what one expects for the child's developmental level, last longer than 4 weeks, begin before age 18 years, and cause significant distress or impairment in the child's social, academic, or other important areas of functioning.

Children exhibiting three or more of the following symptoms for 4 or more continual weeks, accompanied by impairment in their usual activities, might be suffering from SAD:

- Extreme distress when separating from parents and/or loved ones or when away from home
- Excessive worry about harm befalling parents, caregivers, or other family members

TABLE 34.2. Parents' list of "Don'ts" for the child with separation fears

Don't:

- Excessively reassure your child by telling him or her that "nothing bad will happen," "everything will be fine," or "there is nothing to worry about."
- Rescue your child from anxiety-provoking situations (e.g., picking the child up from school early, staying with the child at birthday parties, staying home rather than going out at night).
- Permit or encourage avoidant behavior (e.g., keeping your child out of camp because it seems too stressful, letting your child refuse play dates outside of the home, permitting the child to sleep in bed with you).
- Model anxiety by talking excessively about your own fears and worries and/or avoiding situations that make your anxious.
- Become overly involved—some parents will respond to a child's anxiety by taking over and attempting to direct the situation, rather than encouraging the child to cope with the situation.

- Difficulty sleeping alone at night, attempting to sleep in parents' bed, or requiring that a parent sleep in their room
- Worries about being kidnapped, getting lost, and/or never being able to see parents again
- Trouble being alone; following parents around the house like a shadow
- Complaining of physical symptoms, like stomachaches, headaches, or nausea, when separation occurs or is anticipated
- Needing frequent reassurance about pick-up plans; panicking if a parent is late
- Frequent calls to check in with parent when separated
- Reluctance or refusal to participate in sleep-overs
- Refusal to go to school or camp
- Frequent nightmares about being separated from or harm coming to loved ones

If these symptoms are present, ongoing, and resistant to your intervention, you may wish to consult with your pediatrician or a child and adolescent psychologist or psychiatrist. SAD is highly treatable: CBT, medication, or the combination of the two may be helpful to your child. Recent studies have shown that these treatments, either alone or in combination, are effective in helping children to overcome serious separation anxiety concerns and return to healthy functioning.

SUMMARY

Most children go through brief and expected periods of separation anxiety at key developmental stages, but for some children this anxiety remains fixed and results in distress for the child and parents. Friendships, school attendance, and sleeping through the night may become disrupted by separation anxiety; however, a specific treatment known as cognitive-behavioral therapy has proven to be effective in bringing this anxiety under control for affected children. Children can learn age-appropriate strategies to calm themselves, think rationally and clearly, and overcome their separation anxiety through step-by-step practice in handling scary situations. Getting control over separation anxiety is important for helping children learn effective ways of solving problems and managing their feelings, and the skills learned in managing separation anxiety will help children over the long term as they take on new challenges throughout their development.

WHERE TO FIND OUT MORE

Books

Chansky, T. (2004). *Freeing your child from anxiety*. New York: Broadway Books.
Eisen, A.R., & Engler, L.B. (2006). *Helping your child overcome separation anxiety or school refusal: A step-by-step guide for parents*. Oakland, CA: New Harbinger Publications.
Huebner, D. (2008). *What to do when you dread your bed: A kid's guide to overcoming problems with sleep*. Washington, DC: Magination Press.
Pincus, D. (2007). *I can relax! A relaxation CD for children*. Available from www.childanxiety.net

Rapee, R.M., Wignall, A. Spence, S.H., Cobham, V., & Lyneham, H. (2008). *Helping your anxious child: A step-by-step guide for parents* (2nd edition). Oakland, CA: New Harbinger Publications.

Websites

The Child Anxiety Network
http://www.childanxiety.net
The Anxiety Disorders Association of America
http://www.adaa.org
Society for Clinical Child and Adolescent Psychology
http://sccap.tamu.edu/EST/index_files/Page637.htm

CHAPTER 35

Shyness and Social Anxiety

Deborah C. Beidel, Teresa Marino, and
Lindsay Scharfstein

Jessica is a 9-year-old girl who refuses to read aloud in front of her classmates, write on the blackboard, or answer questions in class. Her teacher feels that she has no choice but to fail Jessica for not completing her oral assignments. Outside of class, Jessica interacts only with her immediate family, cousins, and one friend. She will not go to birthday parties, and refuses to order food in a restaurant. She refused to sing a solo in the spring concert, even though she has a beautiful voice. She tells her mother that she is lonely and sad.

Shyness is a universal emotion, and most people have felt shy at some point in their lives. Most feelings of shyness are temporary, are related to a new or strange situation, and disappear as the child becomes familiar with the new situation or environment. However, like Jessica, about 3%–5% of children and adolescents feel uncomfortable in social situations, and these feelings are excessive, persistent, long-standing, and significantly interfere with academic and social functioning. These children and adolescents suffer from a condition known as *social phobia*.

WHAT ARE THE SIGNS OF SOCIAL PHOBIA?

Although people of all ages suffer from social phobia, not everyone with social phobia has the exact same set of fears. For some children, anxiety-provoking situations are limited to performing in front of a group, also known as *stage fright*. Performance situations that create distress include reading aloud in front of a group, acting in a play, or playing a sport such as basketball. For other children, like Jessica, fears also occur in every-day social interactions—answering questions in class, talking on the telephone, saying hello to an adult, or interacting with peers.

What these different situations share in common is a pervasive pattern of social inhibition—that is, fear of interacting with other people. Children and adolescents worry that they may do or say something embarrassing or humiliating. Young children may not describe their fears, but instead describe physical feelings of nervousness (butterflies in their stomach, feeling nauseous) when asked or invited to interact with someone. When children or adolescents with social phobia are forced to participate in social situations they fear, they may blush, sweat, tremble, or report heart palpitations. Children also express their fears by crying, throwing tantrums, or refusing to speak. Children with social phobia experience great distress in fear-provoking social situations and often try to avoid those situations altogether.

For children and adolescents with social phobia, avoidance behaviors may include withdrawing from social settings (e.g., eating lunch alone), changing appearance (e.g., wearing their hair in front of their eyes), trying to look aloof or busy (e.g., wearing head-phones), refusing to speak, and refusing to attend school (see Chapter 30 on School Refusal). Sometimes, children may exhibit "behavior problems": they may refuse to participate in an activity that causes distress. Like Jessica, some children refuse to speak even when spoken to, and some may even refuse to go to school. Adolescents with social phobia may use alcohol to cope with their distress.

Although children and adolescents with social phobia avoid social situations, they also desire social interactions. They really want to be able to make friends, participate in group activities, and take part in school activities, such as school plays. However, their anxiety is so intense that they cannot force themselves to do these things. Avoiding social situations is not due to a lack of interest, but indicates the severity of their fears.

Children as young as age 8 have been diagnosed with social phobia, although most youth develop social phobia between the ages of 14 and 16. Adolescents often have a more acute and complicated form of social phobia than do younger children, and their fears and avoidance behaviors are more frequent and severe. A common reason for this has to do with the greater maturity of adolescents compared to younger children. For example, all children are expected to make and keep friendships with other children, but adolescents also are expected to participate in age-appropriate activities like attending school dances and dating. Also, parents usually arrange their young children's social interactions (play dates, dancing lessons, and sports team membership), and children usually can't avoid these situations. However, parents are less likely to arrange adolescents' social interactions (because older children tend to take responsibility for their own social lives), thus creating more opportunities for social avoidance.

Social avoidance not only limits opportunities for making and keeping friends, but also prevents a child from learning how to interact with other children or adults. When asked to join a group of children at recess or speak to a new child in the neighborhood, children with social phobia often say, "I don't know how to talk to people. I don't know what to say." Children with social phobia don't know how to interact effectively in social situations. In fact, teaching effective social skills is an important part of treatment for children and adolescents with social phobia.

HOW DO I KNOW IF MY CHILD HAS SOCIAL PHOBIA?

Parents often ask, "How do I know if my child's shyness is 'normal' or a sign of social phobia?" There are four points to consider:

- *Has there been a recent change in your child's life circumstances?* Children who move to a new neighborhood or start a new school, for example, may suddenly feel shy and awkward in social situations. Similarly, a child who has an embarrassing event—such as falling during a skating competition, forgetting a line in the school play, or getting a question wrong in class and being laughed at by the other children—may be reluctant to interact or to get back on stage. In short, if your child previously was comfortable interacting with other children, but now seems afraid, it is likely that negative events play a role.
- *Does the anxiety occur in the presence of other children as well as adults?* Because adults have power and authority over children, many children appear socially shy or awkward around adults, particularly strangers. Thus, a better indicator is how your child interacts with peers. A sure sign of social phobia in children is a fear of interacting with kids their own age.
- *Does the shyness last for more than a few minutes?* Some children are "slow to warm up"— they appear very shy and quiet but, within a few minutes, become socially engaged. Children who are "slow to warm up" are not considered to have social phobia.
- *Is your child significantly distressed, or is your child's behavior severely limited as a result of distress?* The guideline that therapists use to decide if a child is suffering from social phobia is whether the child or adolescent is experiencing significant distress or whether their behavior is severely limited as a result of their distress. Some signs of significant distress (as listed earlier) include: heart palpitations or sweating; difficulty sleeping or nightmares the night before a social event; crying and refusing to get out of the car at the scene of a birthday party; or vomiting before going to school. Some signs of limited behavior (also referred to as functional impairment) include refusing to go to school, not having any friends, or getting poor grades because of refusal to participate in class. Children with social phobia often suffer from other negative feelings, such as depression or general worry, or they engage in negative behaviors such as abusing alcohol or refusing to attend school. They often do not have any friends and do not belong to any school clubs. Finally, they often get poor grades because they refuse to answer questions in class, to ask the teacher when they have a question about a test, or to give a speech in front of a group.

WHAT CAUSES SOCIAL PHOBIA?

Parents often want to know the origin of social phobia, and the simple answer is that its cause is unknown. Most children and adolescents report that they "always felt scared." They cannot point to a specific event that caused them to begin feeling anxious in social situations. As infants or toddlers, some children with social phobia exhibited a behavior pattern known as *behavioral inhibition*. Characteristics of behavioral inhibition include distress when faced with unfamiliar people, objects, or situations; clinging to familiar persons; infrequent or no spontaneous comments; and reluctance to approach and retreat from unfamiliarity. As infants, they are often described as fussy and irritable.

Not every infant who is behaviorally inhibited develops social phobia. Also, there are many children who were never inhibited as infants but who display social fears in childhood or adolescence. This means that genetics or biology alone does not cause social phobia. Environmental factors are most likely involved. In some instances, children with social phobia have parents who also have social phobia. Although many parents think that this indicates a genetic cause, it is also possible that children learn to be shy or socially withdrawn by observing their parents behave that way. This process, called *modeling*, often occurs when a parent exhibits anxious or avoidant behavior in the presence of their children (e.g., while waiting with Johnny for the morning school bus, his mother does not join in the conversation with the other adults). Although not directly told that a social situation is distressful, the child learns by observing the parent.

Parents love their children and will do anything to keep their children from experiencing negative emotions such as fear and anxiety. Unfortunately, sometimes attempts to protect your child from negative feelings can unknowingly play a role in maintaining your child's fears. For example, you may be tempted to modify your child's environment to prevent him or her from coming into contact with what he or she fears (e.g., Johnny's mom decides to not take him to a classmate's birthday party because Johnny seems so nervous in the car on the ride over). By permitting your child to avoid a feared situation, you may actually make your child's fear stronger.

HOW CAN I HELP MY CHILD OVERCOME SOCIAL FEARS?

You can take several steps to help your children overcome social phobia. First, you should consider several important issues:

- *Does my child want to interact with other children?*   Some children (like some adults) do not desire to interact socially with others. They may withdraw from social gatherings or ignore others' social advances. Children with autism, for example, are not interested in social interactions and therefore, do not have social phobia. Children who do not desire social interactions will not benefit from the strategies discussed here.
- *Is my child's distress in this situation something new?*   If your child has always attended and enjoyed schools or parties and now suddenly is reluctant to do so, something may have changed in your child's life that is causing distress. Perhaps your child started a new school and does not know any other children, or your child was assigned to a class where the teacher has a reputation of being "mean." In such situations, allowing your child to adjust to the new situation will probably alleviate social distress. One possible strategy is to ask the teacher to assign a "special buddy" to help your child become accustomed to the new classroom environment.
- *Is my child slow to warm up?*   If your child has some mild anxiety but does not have the significant impairment described earlier, the strategies listed in the sections that follow may help your child become less anxious.

If your child wants to interact with others, is slow to warm up, or seems to have suddenly become fearful in social situations because of a change in life circumstances (death of a family member, divorce, move to a new school or a new neighborhood), then the following suggestions may be helpful.

Arrange Play Dates

If your child appears uncomfortable and anxious around other children, try to arrange a "play date" with other children.

- Start slowly, perhaps with just one other child, and arrange the play date to occur in your home.
- Keep your child at home, in a familiar situation, as that will lessen your child's anxiety.
- Praise your child for approaching and playing with the other child (this is very important!). You may use stickers, small prizes, or verbal praise.
- Tell your child to be brave. Before the play date, tell your child that you know he or she feels shy but it is important to try and be brave. Be specific about what you want your child to do: "Billy is coming over, and you two can play together for an hour. I know that sometimes you feel shy, but I want you to try and play with Billy. If you try, you can earn five stickers." The key is to praise your child's *efforts* to complete the task—in this case, to try and play with Billy, and not (a) whether or not the task was actually completed or (b) completed without feeling anxious. Tell children that "being brave" is what is important; as long as they try, they will get a reward. In Jessica's case, her mother arranged for a neighbor's daughter (about Jessica's age) to come over and play computer games with Jessica. If Jessica sat next to the other girl and tried to play computer games, Jessica earned five stickers. Depending upon the age and sex of your child, a different prize may be more appropriate. Remember, the prize must be something that your child values and wants to earn, otherwise the plan will not succeed.

Increase Social Opportunities with Other Children

Once your child masters the first step, provide more challenging opportunities for social interaction. Once Jessica began to enjoy having a friend visit at her house, Jessica's mother arranged other social interactions. Jessica (a) was invited to her friend's house, (b) invited her friend for a sleep-over, (c) Jessica invited two different friends to come over and play. Sometimes, schools have "friendship groups" that are designed to improve social interaction and these groups may be helpful for children who have mild to moderate levels of shyness. These groups are usually led by guidance counselors or school psychologists. In Jessica's case, she earned praise and stickers for being brave and completing the task even if she felt scared. Eventually, Jessica joined a Girl Scout Troop to provide further opportunities for her to interact with other children.

Provide Opportunities to Interact with Adults

To help your child become more comfortable around adults, you may provide opportunities to interact with familiar or unfamiliar adults. Of course, it is important to consider your child's developmental age and ability to understand "safe" adults and strangers. You do not want to encourage your child to walk up and start talking to strangers. However, you can have your child practice "being brave" by greeting neighbors, the school crossing guard, the school principal, and your adult friends. In Jessica's case, her mother gave her stickers if she (a) said hello to her school principal, school crossing guard, Sunday school teacher; and (b) ordered her own food at a fast food restaurant.

Encourage "Brave" Behavior

Similarly to becoming comfortable in social interactions, arrange and encourage your child to "be brave" when performing in front of others. The key is to choose an activity that your child will likely enjoy. Another factor to consider is that the activity does not need to be extremely competitive or put undue pressure on your child to excel or perform perfectly. Noncompetitive activities such as dancing lessons, karate class, or music lessons are good choices, provided your child will enjoy the activity. Again, reinforce your child for "being brave" and not the end result of the activity. Jessica's mother started her in dance class and after each class they would stop for an ice cream cone on the way home.

WHEN TO SEEK PROFESSIONAL HELP

As noted, these strategies may be helpful for your child if he or she has mild to moderate levels of social anxiety. However, you may need to seek professional help for your child if:

- You have tried the suggested strategies but your child was not able to be brave for even a few minutes.
- Your attempts to help your child be brave resulted in your child being resistant or defiant.
- Your child's anxiety is severe and creates significant physical or emotional distress.
- Your child's fears are interfering with academic achievement, social adjustment (your child does not appear to have any friends, or your child refuses to get involved in typical child activities), or his or her emotional state.
- Your child's social anxiety is not only severe but has existed for a long period of time. In this case, your child would probably benefit from social skills training, which is best conducted in a group setting.
- Your child expresses feelings of depression, as well as feelings of social anxiety.

In these cases, you should seek professional help from a clinical child psychologist who has experience treating children with social phobia. For example, a university that has a department of psychology or a medical school with a department of psychiatry is likely to have professionals trained to treat social phobia. You can also contact the Association for Behavioral and Cognitive Therapies (www.abct.org) or the Anxiety Disorders Association of America (www.adaa.org) for therapist recommendations. In these cases, treatment may need to combine social skills training and arranging for your child to gradually approach the feared situation using the 'being brave" procedures discussed. A therapist will be best able to determine which treatment elements will best help your child and how the different strategies might be best combined to be most effective. Even when a professional is involved, parents are still an important element of the treatment program. Children are often given homework assignments to complete between treatment sessions, and parents often assist and encourage their children in the completion of these tasks.

SUMMARY

For some children and adolescents, social interactions are very enjoyable. Others approach them with mild anxiety, but soon relax and enjoy themselves. For a small percentage of children and adolescents, interacting with others or performing in front of a group creates significant distress and may lead to impaired social or academic functioning. Left untreated, severe cases of social phobia rarely disappear spontaneously. Yet, social phobia is a treatable condition. Fully 60%–70% of children who are treated for this condition are much improved after about 12 weeks of therapy. The key is education and early identification and a commitment by parents to assist their child in overcoming his or her fears.

WHERE TO FIND OUT MORE

Books

Beidel, D.C., & Turner, S.M. (2007). *Shy children, phobic adults: The nature and treatment of social anxiety disorder.* Washington, DC: American Psychological Association.

Eisen, A.R., & Engler, L.B. (2007). *Helping your socially vulnerable child: What to do when your child is shy, socially anxious, withdrawn or bullied.* California: New Harbinger Publications.

Foa, E.B., & Andrews, L.W. (2006). *If your adolescent has an anxiety disorder: An essential resource for parents.* New York: Oxford University Press.

Last, C.G. (2005). *Help for worried kids: How your child can conquer anxiety and fear.* New York: Guilford Press.

Markway, B.G., & Markway, G.P. (2004). *Nurturing the shy child: Practical help for raising confident and socially skilled kids and teens.* New York: Thomas Dunne Books

Websites

Anxiety Disorders Association of America
    http://www.adaa.org
Academy of Behavioral and Cognitive Therapies
    http://www.abct.org

CHAPTER 36

Situational and Performance Anxiety

Kelly A. O'Neil, Courtney L. Benjamin, Sarah A. Crawley, and Philip C. Kendall

As 10-year-old Corey packs away some final items in his bag for his first soccer practice tomorrow, he begins to fret. He has never played on a sports team before and has started asking his mom, "Do I really have to go?" Corey's parents don't understand why he is asking and showing reluctance because they feel confident that he will have a great time at soccer practice. When they ask, "Why don't you want to go?" Corey says, "I'm not going to have any fun, I don't know anyone on this team. Can't I just stay home?"

Ava, age 15, has a big geometry test tomorrow. She has studied during her free time for the past week but her parents have heard her say "I just don't get it!" The morning of the test, Ava wakes and complains to her parents that she has a stomachache and can't go to school. Ava's parents wonder, "What can we do to help?"

These types of situations occur all too often in the lives of children and adolescents—and such situations can promote and/or maintain distressing anxiety. Anxiety can arise as a normal reaction to unfamiliar situations and performance demands, such as joining a sports team for the first time or a school exam on a difficult subject. Everyone experiences anxiety at different points in their lives, and in certain situations anxiety proves adaptive and reasonable. For example, mild anxiety about an upcoming school or athletic performance encourages adequate preparation. However, high levels of anxiety or frequent anxiety can become distressing and interfering to children and adolescents, and may cause children to avoid situations that make them anxious.

Sometimes determining whether your child feels anxious, or whether there's another explanation for your child's behavior, can prove difficult. Knowing some of the typical signs of anxiety can help you better understand and assist your child.

HOW CAN I TELL IF MY CHILD IS ANXIOUS?

The following are some signs that may indicate your child is experiencing anxiety:

- Your child might directly tell you that he or she feels anxious, although he or she may not use the specific term. Children use the words they know to describe how they feel. These may include (but are not limited to): nervous, worried, scared, terrified, jittery, frightened, or afraid.
- Older children and adolescents may have an easier time verbalizing how they feel and what they fear. Younger children may more likely show behavioral changes or complain of physical symptoms.
- Children may not have the ability to express their anxiety, but may instead say that they do not want to (or can't) do something, or that it won't be fun.
- Children may also complain of physical symptoms, such as stomachaches or headaches.
- You may notice behavior changes, such as your normally talkative child becoming quiet or your typically calm child seeming very tense.
- Your child might say that he or she expects something bad to happen.

WHAT SHOULD I DO IF MY CHILD FEELS NERVOUS?

Parents may feel confused or helpless when their child becomes anxious. This may hold particularly true for parents who find it difficult to understand their child's perspective. However, there are several things you can do to help your child cope with anxiety.

- *Show sympathy.* Empathize with your child and do not simply try to dismiss his or her concerns. When parents respond in this way, children come to see them as allies who can, eventually, help them face their fears. Modeling coping skills for your child can help. For example, telling your child about a time when you felt worried or afraid to do something but you faced your fears teaches a coping strategy. Give specifics as to what made it easier for you to cope with your anxiety, in order to model coping, rather than just success. Children often like to hear stories about their parents' childhood. Try to share the experience without acting "teachy."
- *Help identify the problem.* A child's anxiety can feel frustrating to parents, particularly when they don't know for certain the roots of their child's avoidant and distressed behavior. Without interrogating, ask your child what makes the situation difficult, and what he or she fears will happen. Don't dismiss the answers. Having a better sense of what causes your child to feel anxious will help you begin to work together to solve the problem.
- *Problem solve.* Once you have identified the problem, you and your child can collaboratively generate possible solutions. Don't criticize any of your child's ideas.

Focus on encouraging your child to use active coping strategies to face the feared situation, rather than avoid it. Start by brainstorming any and all ideas for facing the situation, even silly or impractical ones. Then narrow down the possibilities and together pick one or two strategies that seem practical and helpful. For example, perhaps Corey would feel better if he brought a snack to share with his new teammates, or Ava would appreciate playing her favorite game with her parents the night before her exam.

- *Challenge anxious thoughts.*   You can help your child to challenge some of his or her anxious thoughts that seem false or irrational. For example, if Ava says to her parents (or to herself), "What if I fail the geometry test? What if I'm stupid?" her parents could acknowledge her concern about the test but remind her that she has studied very hard. Ava's parents might challenge her concern about feeling stupid by pointing out that she's doing well in several subjects and that having difficulty in one subject doesn't mean that she's stupid. Similarly, in response to Corey's concern that he might not have any fun at soccer practice because he won't know anyone, his parents could acknowledge that he doesn't know the other kids yet. But, Corey's parents can gently remind him that at first he didn't know any of the other kids at summer camp last year, but he ended up making several friends. Corey's parents could ask, "Do you think that the same thing could happen at soccer practice?"

- *Provide positive feedback.*   Offer praise for your child's efforts at showing courage and facing his or her fears. Identify your child's successes, and show how proud you feel about him or her for the effort. A reward might seem in order if your child has done something especially challenging. For example, if Ava goes to school on test day, her mom might reward her by allowing her to pick out what the family will make for dinner that evening.

    Note that rewards differ from bribes. For example, Corey's parents might encourage him to attend practice by suggesting that they do something fun to celebrate his bravery when he returns. However, they would not want to bargain with Corey by telling him that he can have the new videogame he's been wanting if he goes to soccer practice.

- *Remain consistent.*   Even if your child becomes upset or begs to get out of a situation or obligation, don't support avoidance or let him or her back out of commitments. It's important for your child to learn that, at times, he or she will have to do things that may feel scary or uncomfortable, and that the feared situations aren't as bad as he or she fears.

- *Seek additional resources.*   Seeking allies in these situations can help your child face fears directly. A school guidance counselor, coach, or teacher might suggest strategies that have helped other children in similar situations. For example, perhaps Corey could arrive early to practice and meet his coach before it's time for his parents to leave and for practice to start.

WHAT NOT TO DO

Even well-intentioned parents sometimes fall prey to less-than-helpful approaches when their children feel anxious. Although it may seem tempting to try some of the following approaches, they unfortunately often backfire: they have the unwanted effect of maintaining (not reducing) anxiety. Although it can seem appealing to try any technique to help your child feel better when he or she feels distressed, it's best to avoid certain approaches, as discussed here:

- *Do not accommodate the anxiety.* Sometimes it might seem easier to allow your child to avoid part of or the entire situation that makes him or her upset or nervous. However, doing so communicates to your child that anxiety leads to danger or harm, and we shouldn't have to do things that feel difficult or scary. Accommodation also reinforces your child's belief that the feared situation will indeed prove dangerous or too difficult, that he or she lacks the ability to cope, and that he or she won't succeed in the situation. In fact, accommodating your child's anxiety makes it more likely that he or she will feel anxious the next time he or she faces a similar situation. Therefore, it becomes important that Corey goes to soccer practice as planned, and that Ava takes her test on time.

- *Do not provide excessive reassurance.* Although it's helpful to offer your child encouragement and support such as by saying things like, "It's okay," or "I know you can do it," overdoing it on the reassurance makes matters worse. Your child may feel even more anxious if you allow him or her to repeatedly ask the same questions about what might happen in the feared situation. Remain clear and supportive. Your child will hear your first response, so it won't help him or her for you to repeat the same answer again and again.

  Do not invalidate the anxiety. It's important that your child knows that you understand that he or she feels anxious or afraid and that you want to help solve the problem. For example, you may not understand why Ava's geometry test feels like such a big deal to her, but denying its importance could make her feel worse. Try saying, "I know this is hard, but I know you can do well," rather than, "The test is no big deal, why are you so nervous?"

- *Do not single your child out.* Let your child know that the anxiety he or she feels is normal by pointing out that most children and even adults could feel nervous in a similar situation. It's best not to compare your child to siblings or peers, or to point out the anxiety in front of others. For example, Ava's parents would not want to point out Ava's anxiety by asking her study group to help her prepare for the test because she's so nervous. Instead, they could ask Ava what she might do to get support from her friends in preparation for the test.

Keep in mind that what will work best for your child may differ based on his or her age and unique characteristics, so you'll need to stay flexible and try different strategies to find those that work best. For example, a younger child might require a great deal of involvement from you and might benefit most from modeling of coping skills. An older child or adolescent can more likely problem-solve on his or her own with your encouragement and feedback. Similarly, an older child or adolescent might effectively challenge his or her own anxious thoughts, but this strategy could prove too sophisticated or complex for a younger child to grasp.

WHEN TO SEEK PROFESSIONAL HELP

Sometimes children's anxiety reaches a level that parents can no longer manage on their own, so it's important to know when to seek professional help. Consult a professional if you notice any of the following in your child:

- Excessive avoidance, such as:
  - Regularly avoiding social situations
  - Avoiding schoolwork for fear of making a mistake
  - Refusing to go to sleep or school for fear of being away from caregiver
- Interference that results in the child not facing developmental challenges, such as:
  - Extreme shyness
  - Isolation
  - Extreme discomfort when the center of attention
  - Often expecting bad things to happen
  - Excessive worry about upsetting others
  - Asking questions (or asking for reassurance) too frequently
  - Perfectionism
  - Excessive worry about failure
  - Lack of self-confidence
  - Excessive distress upon separation from parents or loved ones
  - Worries that something bad will happen to caregivers or themselves when separated from loved ones
- Excessive or frequent physical distress, such as:
  - Trouble catching breath
  - Stomachaches/headaches
  - Complaints of nausea
  - Sweating
  - Dizzy, faint, or light-headed
  - Heart racing or beating faster than normal
  - Shaking or feeling jittery
- Duration: Consistent anxiety that persists for a few months or more may indicate an anxiety disorder. Consult a professional who can evaluate if your child would benefit from treatment and what treatment might prove most appropriate.

SUMMARY

All children and adolescents experience anxiety at some point in their lives. Anxiety can arise as a normal reaction to unfamiliar situations and performance demands. To help your child cope with anxiety, show sensitivity, help him or her to identify the problem, problem-solve with him or her, challenge his or her anxious thoughts, and provide him or her with positive feedback. It's best not to accommodate the anxiety, provide excessive reassurance, invalidate the anxiety, or single your child out. Seek professional help if you notice excessive avoidance, anxiety that interferes with your child meeting developmental challenges, excessive or frequent physical distress, or consistent anxiety that persists for more than a few months.

WHERE TO FIND OUT MORE

Books

Chansky, T.E. (2004). *Freeing your child from anxiety: Powerful, practical solutions to overcome your child's fears, worries, and phobias.* New York: Broadway Books.

Danneberg, J. (2000). *First day jitters.* Watertown, MA: Charlesbridge Publishing.

Dutro, J. (1991). *Night light: A story for children afraid of the dark.* Washington, DC: Magination Press.

Henkes, K. (2000). *Wemberly worried.* New York: HarperCollins.

Manassis, K. (1996). *Keys to parenting an anxious child.* Hauppauge, NY: Barron's Educational Series.

Marcus, I.W., & Marcus, P. (1991). *Scary night visitors: A story for children with bedtime fears.* Washington, DC: Magination Press.

Marcus, I.W., & Marcus, P. (1992). *Into the great forest: A story for children away from parents for the first time.* Washington, DC: Magination Press.

Rapee, R.M., Spence, S.H., Cobham, V., & Wignall, A. (2000). *Helping your anxious child: A step-by-step guide for parents.* Oakland, CA: New Harbinger.

Wagner, A.P. (2005). *Worried no more: Help and hope for anxious children.* Rochester, NY: Lighthouse Press.

Websites

Anxiety Disorders Association of America
  http://www.adaa.org/
New York University Child Study Center
  http://www.aboutourkids.org/
The Child Anxiety Network
  http://www.childanxiety.net/index.htm

CHAPTER 37

Imaginary Companions

Tracy R. Gleason

One day at breakfast, your preschool-aged daughter says, "You know, the Pink House Bears live in a pink house in the city." Used to hearing proclamations out of context at this age, you ask a few follow-up questions and determine that the Pink House Bears are an imaginary family of bears much like your own family. However, their house has a fantastic tunnel that leads to the local bakery, where they often enjoy a muffin (as does your daughter), and they have a playground with swings and a slide (her favorites). In the following weeks, your daughter often reports on the Pink House Bears and their adventures. They acquire details and characteristics; they encounter challenges that sound awfully familiar. Then one day, you realize you have not heard about them in a while, so you ask about the Pink House Bears. "Oh," your daughter blithely says, "they moved away."

If you are like most parents, these imaginary bears strike you as a charming example of your child's emerging imagination, but after a few months of hearing about their adventures, maybe they make you wonder. Did she create the Pink House Bears because of a lack of real friends? Does she realize that they are imaginary? Should I play along with the fantasy? Will her peers reject her if they hear her talk about the Bears? Perhaps her discussion of them sounds a little bit like a complex pack of lies, and you worry that, if she spins such tales regularly, others will begin to doubt her even when she tells the truth.

Most parents do not realize that somewhere between one-half and two-thirds of children create imaginary companions at some point during early to middle childhood. Of course, many parents never know about their children's pretend friends. Some children think about them, and may even play with them, but do not talk to others about them. Sometimes parents only discover them when they overhear their son or daughter conversing with an imaginary companion, or when their child admits to someone else that they have an imaginary friend. Other parents feel that their homes are populated by more imaginary people than real ones. Some children create and talk endlessly about invisible friends, imaginary families, herds of invisible cows, dragons in the basement, and monsters in the closet. Indeed, imaginary companions come in all shapes and sizes, and they may come and go, shift and change as the child develops. No matter their form, these fantastical creations become important to the children who create them and often elicit strong emotions. Consequently, understanding your child's imaginary companions gives you interesting insights into your child's social, cognitive, and emotional development.

WHAT IS AN IMAGINARY COMPANION?

The classic example of an imaginary companion is an invisible friend. Often, children create invisible friends with whom they can play at home, particularly if they do not have siblings or neighborhood children to play with. These invisible friends vary widely—some are completely made up, some seem based on real children, and some originate with fictional characters. Many present as ordinary children, but others may have superhuman powers and change ages and genders periodically as the child sees fit. Some children will create complex worlds populated by imaginary characters, and others will create a series of imaginary friends, one after the other. Children's descriptions of these friends can seem so realistic that occasionally, parents seek to arrange a play date with their child's new best friend from school only to discover with surprise that the friend does not exist.

Invisible companions exist in different ways. Some only become evident through discussion with the child; children may talk about a creation such as the Pink House Bears, or even relay stories of wild adventures that they have had together with their invisible companions, but never actually pretend to interact with them. Other children can be overheard, especially when alone at home, talking to invisible companions, sometimes arguing with them, sometimes making plans for play or travel. Some invisible friends become associated with particular places, such as a spot under a favorite tree or on top of a light fixture in the dining room. When children enjoy sharing details of their imaginary companions' lives with their parents, they may begin to ask adults to accommodate the companions' requests. For example, many children ask to set a place at the table for an invisible friend, or for a parent to hold the door open a little longer for the companion to come in. Some companions take up space; many a parent has accidentally sat on an invisible friend (to a child's great distress), and some children squish themselves into a corner of the bed so as to leave room for the companion to sleep with them.

Researchers describe another kind of imaginary companion as "personified objects," inanimate objects that the child treats as real and living. Usually, these objects include dolls or stuffed animals. However, any object can become personified if the child loves it. In my own work, I have met countless charismatic blankets, spunky toy trains, and once, a friendly 4 oz. can of tomato paste. These objects do not simply provide a source of comfort to the child. Although they may seem comforting since children often carry them around, sleep with them, and bring them on trips, their function extends beyond that of a so-called "transitional object"—an object that represents the safety and security of a primary caregiver. Personified objects exude personality and tend to serve as friends, as co-adventurers, or as babies that the child nurtures and cares for.

A third form of imaginative play closely related to the creation of an imaginary companion involves adoption of a pretend identity. Some children take on personas that they may retain for weeks or even months. The children will insist on being called by a different name, and sometimes they don an article of clothing (e.g., a cape) to signify their alternate identity. This form of play does not necessarily involve an imaginary companion, as the pretend identity is not separate from the child, and no relationship exists between the child and the pretend identity. However, a few children who engage in this form of play will go back and forth between playing with the pretend identity as a separate person and enacting the role of the identity themselves. Usually, the child will assume the role of the pretend identity during play if the pretend identity is attractive and powerful, like a superhero.

Invisible imaginary companions, personified objects, and pretend identities have several features in common. First, all three phenomena involve the same kind of thinking: the creation and maintenance of an imaginary other who differs from the self in significant ways. In the case of the pretend identity, the child acts out the role of the other. In the case of the personified object, the child projects the other onto an inanimate object, and in the case of the invisible companion, the other may project into space but have no concrete existence. In each of these situations, the child thinks about his or her own thoughts, feelings, and beliefs, while simultaneously imagining the thoughts, feelings, and beliefs of the other person. Adolescents and adults can easily entertain both perspectives, but such a task is much more difficult for a young child. Not surprisingly, preschool children who engage in these activities generally seem a little ahead of their peers in understanding that others' perspectives may differ from their own. Those children who create invisible companions or personify objects may also exceed their peers in understanding the nature of social relationships and the differences between relationships with different people in their social networks.

WHO CREATES AN IMAGINARY COMPANION AND WHY?

One of the most interesting and perplexing facts about imaginary companions is the *lack* of differences between children who do and do not create them. Over the years, researchers have looked for differences between these groups in intelligence, creativity, number of friends, family constellation, social networks, and temperament and have found little to help predict which child might have a pretend friend. In the early 20th century, many clinicians put forth the idea that children created imaginary companions as a result of some deficiency in their lives, especially within the realm of social relationships, such as a lack of friendships. However, the belief that shy, lonely, and friendless children create imaginary companions has no support in the extensive research conducted in the past few decades.

The few differences that separate children with and without imaginary companions paint a rather rosy picture of imaginative activities in early childhood. For example, children who create imaginary companions tend to show *less* shyness than their peers who do not have such friends, and show greater cooperation with both adults and other children. They also prove slightly better than their peers at focusing their attention on a task and, as mentioned previously, understanding other people's perspectives. Of course, some of these characteristics may promote the development of imaginary companions, and some may result from having such a friend. The causes versus the consequences of this kind of imaginative activity are difficult to differentiate; however, pretending about imaginary others seems to go along with these abilities.

Some evidence suggests that imaginary companions will more likely appear in only children or in children with few siblings far apart in age, and they may develop slightly more commonly in girls during the preschool period. These differences have not shown up in every study, and when they do emerge, the differences are usually small. The studies imply however, that one factor distinguishes children with imaginary companions from those without: sociability. Children who create imaginary companions tend to have high sociability, having great interest in social interactions and relationships. In essence, they love people, so when no real others are available, why not make someone up? This possibility leads to the other factor that separates the creators of pretend friends from the noncreators: a predilection for fantasy. Even from late infancy and early toddlerhood, children who later go on to create imaginary companions appear to show more interest in fantasy-related toys and activities than their peers do. The combination, then, of sociability and a love of fantasy may provide the key to predicting who may or may not create an imaginary companion.

Another factor that may contribute to the formation of imaginary companions is the environment provided by important adults in the child's life. Parents who generally support fantasy may foster the creation of imaginary companions in children who love fantasy and crave social interaction. Nevertheless, several examples demonstrate that supportive parents prove neither necessary nor sufficient for these imaginative activities. Pretend friends appear even in cultures in which parents disapprove of fantasy play of any kind. These imaginary companions may remain secret, with children playing with and thinking about them only when alone.

IMAGINARY COMPANIONS ACROSS DEVELOPMENT

Imaginary companions occur mostly in early childhood, but they often exist at older ages, too. Unlike their preschool counterparts, children in middle childhood do not tend to talk to others extensively about their imaginary companions, but rather keep them as a private fantasy. Parents of children in this age group are unlikely to know if their child has an imaginary companion. However, whether imaginary companions of middle childhood qualify as the same phenomenon as imaginary companions in the preschool period is unclear. For example, research on the creation of imaginary companions in middle childhood shows no sex difference; boys and girls are equally as likely to create pretend friends during this period. Also, creation of imaginary companions during this time is linked to heightened creativity, which is a connection that does not appear to exist for preschool children. In addition, in a few studies, children with invisible imaginary companions scored higher on measures of anxiety than their peers without such companions. Even so, their anxiety scores fall well within the normal range. Perhaps imaginary companions help school-age children cope with anxiety, but do not serve such a function in early childhood.

Even in adolescence, imaginary companions do occur in age-appropriate forms. For example, many adolescents keep diaries that they address to imaginary others, as Anne Frank did to her imaginary friend, Kitty. These imaginary companions seem associated with the developmental tasks of adolescence, such as identity formation and the development of autonomy. Similar to the findings for imaginary companions at younger ages, writers of these diaries tended toward adolescents who readily engaged in daydreaming and enjoyed fantasy. Research has yet to determine if the children who create imaginary companions in preschool become the adolescents who write diaries to imaginary others, but using imaginary others in this way may be indicative of a particular developmental pathway followed by sociable people who enjoy fantasy. In support of this idea, professional fiction writers have reported memories of imaginary companions in their childhoods more often than have people in other professions.

SHOULD I WORRY THAT MY CHILD HAS AN IMAGINARY COMPANION?

When parents worry about their children's imaginary companions, their concerns usually center on their child's grasp of reality. Rest assured, having an imaginary companion in childhood by itself almost never indicates a psychological problem. Children whose imaginary companions relate to emotional disturbance almost always show a whole host of other issues and complaints, as well as histories of trauma or abuse. Even in these cases, a skilled clinician can tell the difference between an imaginary companion resulting from psychopathology and one simply created for companionship. Some of the differences include:

- Imaginary companions related to psychological problems may play a frightening or protective role for the child, telling the child what to do and occasionally getting angry. Most typical imaginary companions are associated with play and positive emotions. An important caveat: some imaginary enemies exist in the play of typical children, and mentally healthy children do get angry with their imaginary companions at times. In these cases, the quality of the interaction might seem conflict-ridden and antagonistic, but the companion rarely frightens the child.
- Imaginary companions associated with emotional disturbance have an unbidden quality; they may appear at random times, or at times when the child does not want them. These children do not have a sense of control over their companions. In contrast, normative imaginary companions typically appear when the child wants them around and will go away if the child asks them to.
- Even the youngest children with normal imaginary companions know that they are not real. When pushed, they will acknowledge that their friend is made up, but they may not want to admit it for fear of spoiling the fun of the fantasy. Children with psychological issues, however, may not be sure if their friend is real or not.

HOW DO I MANAGE MY CHILD'S IMAGINARY COMPANION?

Imaginary companions, when they appear, almost universally fit as part of typical development. Figuring out how to parent a child with a pretend friend involves the same sorts of decisions as every other child behavior that proves appropriate in some situations and inappropriate in others. If your child has an imaginary companion or pretend identity, you may be struggling with setting limits on the times and places where your child can play with the friend or act as the character he or she created.

Parents differ in the extent to which they participate and indulge in their children's fantasies. One family might not welcome an imaginary companion to join them for dinner, but another might willingly provide a place at the table. Still other families might wait for a large enough table at a restaurant to seat a family of imaginary companions, but draw a line at ordering them food. Children often delight in their parents' interests in the imaginary companion, and use it as a way to initiate or participate in adult conversation. The following few simple rules can help you manage your child's imaginary companion:

- *Encourage or gently curb the behavior as you see fit.*   The request to buckle a stuffed animal in the car might qualify as trivial, but cooking for imaginary companions might not. Asking invisible people to eat invisible food is perfectly reasonable.
- *Respect your child's expertise with respect to the imaginary companion.*   Part of the fun of having a pretend friend involves acting as the expert on the friend's likes and dislikes, activities, and feelings. In addition, some children seek the positive social interaction with real people that they can obtain when talking about imaginary people. Using the companion as a parenting tool to get your child to do what you want (e.g., "Your invisible friend wants you to go to bed") might seem tempting, but if you co-opt your child's pretend friend's thoughts or feelings, your child may feel robbed of this expertise and its associated joy. Moreover, your child will not likely comply with your request and will then abandon his or her friend.
- *Negative emotions or even death of a companion should not sound a warning of some kind of psychological problem.*   Expressing anger toward an imaginary friend provides your child with a way to feel negative emotions without having to worry about social ramifications. Overcoming disappointment caused by an imaginary companion is easier than overcoming disappointment caused by someone real, like a parent or friend. Also, your child may "kill off" his or her imaginary friend as a way of exploring the concept of death only to "resurrect" the friend the next day.

If you outright disapprove of an imaginary companion, it may disappear, or your child may keep the companion but simply not talk about it anymore. Either way, the companion will no longer serve as a source of conflict in your relationship with your child. If, on the other hand, you act neutrally or supportive, pretend friends can provide an interesting window into the issues your child is currently thinking about. Children figuring out the terms of compromise in friendship might engage in lots of negotiation with their imaginary companions, and children struggling to assert their independence may enjoy acting as the parent to a personified baby doll. Waxing poetic about the life and times of the Pink House Bears may enable a child to catch the attention of a delighted parent and provide a chance for control over a tiny corner of an otherwise externally controlled world. And, of course, sometimes an imaginary companion is simply a playmate who will never say no to an invitation for adventure.

SUMMARY

Imaginary companions are a charming part of the lives of over half of children in early childhood, and they may appear in varied forms at older ages as well. Children who do and do not create such friends differ in few ways, but those who do may take particular delight in social relationships and fantasy. Rarely associated with psychological problems or emotional disturbances, imaginary companions come in all shapes and sizes, and may become a part of a child's or a family's life for weeks, months, or even years. As in all aspects of pretense, parents who know about their children's pretend friends play an important, but not controlling, role in the friends' existence and can set limits on this imaginative activity as they see fit. In general, allowing your child to act as the expert on the imaginary companion gives your child a rare opportunity to exercise control in a safe and supportive setting, at a time in his or her life when parents and other adults dictate almost everything your child does.

WHERE TO FIND OUT MORE

Books

Caughey, J. (1984). *Imaginary social worlds.* Lincoln, NE: University of Nebraska Press.
Harris, P. (2000). *The work of the imagination.* Oxford: Blackwell.
Singer, D., & Singer, J. (1990). *The house of make believe.* Cambridge: Harvard University Press.
Taylor, M. (1999). *Imaginary companions and the children who create them.* New York: Oxford University Press.

Websites

Family Resource
http://www.familyresource.com/parenting/character-development/imaginary-friends-should-you-be-concerned

PART SIX

Sexuality

CHAPTER 38

Sexuality and Preschool- and School-aged Children

Jeanne Swickard Hoffman

Mom stands at the kitchen sink washing dishes and keeping an eye on Aaron and his friend Dallas, who sit playing with their trucks in the sandbox in the back yard. Dallas, from Aaron's preschool class, has come over for a play date. At one point, Mom hears giggling and looks up to see that both boys have taken off their clothes and Aaron is touching Dallas' penis. While feeling like screaming and running out, she instead makes herself walk out and calmly ask what they are doing. They both answer cheerfully that they are looking at their pee-pees. When told to put their shorts on, they easily comply and ask if they can have a snack.

Tiffany's father gets a call to come to school immediately to speak with her teacher and the counselor. The other children in her fourth-grade class have complained that when they go for their bathroom breaks, she wants to watch them use the toilet and today Tiffany attempted to "hump" a second grader. Tiffany feels angry and embarrassed and denies these behaviors. The other children later tell the teacher that Tiffany has bragged about watching her dad's DVDs that show people "humping."

On the way home from school, Malia asks her mom about what she heard in school today. "JJ said that babies get in your tummy when you 'do it.' What does that mean?" Mom takes a big breath. She hadn't thought she would have to have this talk with a first grader.

One thing all these parents have in common is that they hoped they wouldn't have to deal with issues of sexuality until "The Big Talk." They each also worry that their child may have experienced sexual abuse. But these parents first have to know what constitutes normal children's sexual behaviors. In fact, every parent needs to know this information.

WHAT IS NORMAL SEXUAL BEHAVIOR IN CHILDREN?

Sexual behaviors develop just like other behaviors. And, like other behaviors, they show themselves in children's play as a form of exploration. The question of what's normal depends on the age and developmental stage of the child. Children are curious and want to learn about themselves and their world, they are curious about their bodies, and they are curious about others. Normal sexual behaviors are not only playful and explorative, but they also occur spontaneously and intermittently, in the same way that children engage in various activities and play with different toys during the day.

Studying children's sexual behaviors proves somewhat difficult. Scientists can try to observe these behaviors; they can ask parents or teachers; they can ask college students and adults what they remember. Each of these methods has problems based on the unreliability of memory and other factors, but right now it's the best we have, and the information does give us a consistent picture. So, what do we know about normal sexual behaviors in toddlers to preteens?

Preschoolers

The following characteristics are typical of very young children. Preschoolers:

- Explore their own bodies
- May masturbate not only by touching but by rubbing against objects (usually for pleasure or soothing, rather than for sexual arousal)
- Are interested in looking at others' private parts
- Are interested in the differences between boys and girls and mommies and daddies, and may comment on or question these differences
- May want to touch the private parts of others, including familiar adults
- May show others their private parts
- Associate genitals with urination
- May want to watch others using the bathroom
- Play doctor
- Play house, exploring the roles of mommy and daddy
- Usually act lighthearted and silly during such play, which may occur in public without shame
- May insert something in their genitals or rectum once out of curiosity or exploration
- Respond to prohibitions about sexual behaviors

School-aged Children

The following characteristics are typical of children in school (grade school through early adolescence). School-aged children:

- Become more covert with their sexual behaviors as they learn about cultural taboos; typically, they will masturbate in private and engage in sexual play behind closed doors

- Seek more information about genitals and intercourse
- May use "dirty words" for elimination, sexual behaviors, and private parts. Children will more often use these words with their friends and tell "dirty jokes" that focus on bathroom humor
- May show others their private parts; compare genitals with friends
- Play doctor
- Play house, exploring gender roles
- Talk about sex with friends
- Begin to want privacy when using the bathroom or when changing clothes
- May draw sexual parts on figures
- Distance themselves from other gender during play

Certain other behaviors are more characteristic of one gender than another. For example:

- Boys become conscious and sensitive about having erections.
- Boys' sexual verbalization and interest in sexuality increases.
- Girls' play increasingly explores sexuality through relationships and sex roles.

In summary, normal sexual play in children:

- Is typically exploratory and spontaneous
- Occurs intermittently
- Does not involve coercion
- Typically involves children of the same age or developmental level
- Usually takes place among participants who know each other well
- Is playful, occasionally silly, and without anxiety or emotional distress
- Decreases when adults discourage or prohibit the play

Conversely, problematic sexual play among children:

- Occurs more frequently and may appear compulsive
- Doesn't decrease with adult disapproval or negative consequences
- May occur between children who don't know each other well
- Involves children who differ in age by more than a year
- Involves coercion, aggressive, or painful activity
- Causes distress to one of the parties

It is important to remain aware, however, that unusual behaviors occur in normal children without sexual behavior problems and who have not experienced abuse. Keep in mind that children's sexual behaviors differ from adult behavior in motivation, arousal, and understanding. Children typically engage in these behaviors because they're curious and it feels good. At their level of cognitive development, what sounds like sexually related talk may simply involve parroting phrases they've heard or mimicking behaviors they've observed.

Environmental factors also play a role in the expression of sexualized behaviors. Children today are exposed to more sexual material than in previous generations.

TV shows have more sexual and sensual content, as does TV advertising (think Victoria's Secret or perfume ads). Children may hear song lyrics with sexual themes, and certainly preteen idols dress and behave in a far more sexualized fashion than a decade ago—for example, Miley Cyrus, Brittany Spears. Sexualized toys such as *Bratz* dolls are marketed to 6- to 10-year-old girls and, until very recently, even *Scholastic Books* sold *Bratz* books to children at school book fairs. Take a look also at the clothing marketed for young girls: tee shirts with sexualized messages, low-cut jeans, and even thong underwear. Unsupervised cable television and Internet use presents opportunities for children to encounter many levels of sexual content, from nudity to pornography. In the course of exploring, children may discover parents' pornographic videos or adult-content magazines.

Other environmental factors affecting sexual behaviors in children may include cultural and family characteristics. Research has shown that more sexual behaviors occur among children in cultures that treat expression of sexual behaviors in children as natural. In families where more nudity occurs within the home, more sexual behaviors also occur.

WHEN TO SEEK PROFESSIONAL HELP

If you are concerned that your child's sexual behaviors seem outside the norm, or worry that abuse may have occurred, you should seek professional advice. Often the family's pediatrician is a trusted resource and usually readily available. If a question of possible abuse seems relevant, a referral to a child psychologist, child psychiatrist, or a clinical social worker for further assessment may follow. Depending on the state, if sufficient concern or a reason to suspect child abuse exists, a report to the state's children's protective services may be made by any professional involved with the child (physicians, medical personnel, psychologists, teachers).

No standard definition of child sexual abuse exists, but most legal definitions include involvement of a child in a sexual activity by an adult or another child. The activity need not involve force or coercion or actual physical contact. But remember, normal sexual play does not equal abuse. No accurate figures about the prevalence of child abuse exist, since we only know about cases reported to the authorities. The American Academy of Pediatrics has estimated that one in four girls and one in eight boys will experience sexual abuse prior to the age of 18.

A number of common misconceptions exist about children with sexual behavior problems and children who have experienced sexual abuse. Here are some of the facts:

Children with Sexual Behavior Problems (SBP)

- Girls as well as boys can show SBPs.
- Some SBPs are associated with impulsivity, such as that seen in attention-deficit hyperactivity disorder and disruptive behavior disorders.
- Only some children with SBPs have histories of abuse:
  - Other factors include family characteristics, poor parenting, exposure to explicit sexual material, neglect, and exposure to family violence.
- A range of severity of SBPs and a range of dangerousness to other children exists.

- These children have a low risk to commit future sexual offenses if they receive appropriate treatment (2%–3%).
- Children with significant SBPs often have other mental health or family problems.
- Children with significant SBPs differ in many ways from adult sexual offenders.

Abused Children

- Sexual abuse does increase the possibility of SBPs, but not all children who have experienced abuse show SBPs, nor have all children with SBPs experienced abuse.
- Not all abused children go on to abuse other children.
- Not all children who have experienced sexual abuse have long-term problems:
  - Effects depend on the type of abuse, relationship to the abuser, and appropriateness of treatment.
- Abused children do not usually get aroused during their abuse nor do they always seek continued sexual arousal.

HOW DO I TALK TO MY CHILD ABOUT "THE BIRDS AND THE BEES"?

While most parents worry about "The Big Talk," they find that they have many "mini talks" with their child over time. Remember, children have considerable curiosity. They want to know about themselves and their world, and will ask many questions. Kids ask about birds—why do they fly? They ask about bees—why do they sting? Kids ask about their belly buttons, and they will ask about the parts that lie further south. They just want to know.

Each family has its own style, and each family has its own values that guide how to discuss sex and sexuality in the family. All parents should prepare for questions.

Some Guidelines

- Answer the question your child asks:
  - If children want more information, they'll ask another question as long as you'll gladly talk with them about such matters.
  - Monitor the reaction and follow-up if your child seems puzzled or disgusted.
- Tailor the answer to your child's developmental age.
- Use the correct term for body parts—penis, vagina, vulva, etc.
- Don't give false information.
- If you don't know the answer, admit it, and consider helping your child find an accurate answer.
- Don't giggle, get angry, or lecture—your child will watch your reactions carefully.
- Find teachable moments.
- Be ready:
  - Think about what your child might ask at various ages.
  - Think about what you want to say.

- Consider having an age-appropriate book or two on sexuality on the family bookshelf.
- Ask family, a friend, your minister, or your pediatrician about preparation for such talks.

Many resources exist for parents, including books and the Internet. Parents can access general information or information tailored for special situations, such as how to discuss sex with a child with disabilities. Conservative Christian, Mormon, or Muslim families can access materials that support their specific religious views. With one of the large bookseller's websites listing nearly 500 books related to sex education for children, a parent can easily find sources that match your family's value system. See Where to Find Out More for a list of resources.

Children can learn about sex and sexuality in many different ways. Their friends often provide a source for information and misinformation. One study asked college students retrospectively where they obtained their sexual knowledge; the most frequently cited source was friends, with parents coming in third after school sex-education programs. Parents who want to become part of their child's learning in this very important area of life need to find a way to become a trusted and accurate resource.

SUMMARY

Sexual behaviors in children become a source of much anxiety for parents. In the past, some authority figures attempted to deny childhood sexuality. As this attitude dies out, the need for parents to have more information about normal and worrisome sexual behaviors increases. With the high level of concern in our society about sexual abuse, all parents have become vigilant—and some hypervigilant. All parents want their children to grow up to have a happy and healthy life, which includes a healthy sex life. By becoming a resource for their children, parents can provide the building blocks for the life they wish for their children.

WHERE TO FIND OUT MORE

Books

Bancroft, B. (Ed.). (2003). *Sexual development in childhood.* Bloomington: Indiana University Press.
Braun, B.B. (2008). *Just tell me what to say.* New York: HarperCollins Publishers.
Johnson, T.C. (1999). *Understanding your child's sexual behavior.* Oakland, CA.: New Harbinger Press.
Sandfort, T.G., & Rademakers, J. (Eds.). (2000). *Childhood sexuality: Normal sexual behavior and development.* New York: The Haworth Press, Inc.

Websites

American Academy of Child and Adolescent Psychiatrists
Facts for families
   http://www.aacap.org/cs/root/facts_for_families/facts_for_families.

American Academy of Pediatrics
Bright futures
   http://www.brightfutures.aap.org.
American Academy of Pediatrics. (2008).
Parenting corner Q & A: Sexual abuse
   http://www.aap.org/publiced/BR_SexAbuse.htm.
American Academy of Pediatrics. (2007).
Parenting corner Q & A: Talking to your young child about sex
   http://www.aap.org/publiced/BR_TalkSexChild.htm
American Psychological Association. (2001).
Understanding child sexual abuse
   http://www.apa.org/releases/sexabuse/
Child Welfare Information Gateway. (2007).
Recognizing child sexual abuse: signs and symptoms
   http://www.childwelfare.gov/pubs/factsheets/signs.cfm.
Nemours Foundation
   http://www.KidsHealth.org.

CHAPTER 39

Masturbation in Young Children

Carolyn S. Schroeder

Nancy is a 3-year-old who masturbates every time she watches TV or gets tired. Although Nancy's mother is not concerned with the fact that her child is masturbating, she is concerned that Nancy often touches herself out in the open in the family room.

At a regular physical check-up, a father reports that his 5-year-old son, Ted, has recently begun to masturbate excessively and will often go to his room to engage in this behavior for long periods of time. Ted's parents recently divorced, and his mother remarried. Ted's father worries that his son's behavior means he has been sexually abused by his step-father.

Masturbation is probably the most common sexual behavior seen in young children. It typically involves touching, rubbing, or playing with genitalia, and can include unusual posturing, grunting, rocking, and sweating. Infants as young as 3 months old engage in such activity and, at times, parents have mistaken the behavior in infants as a seizure disorder. (If you worry that this is the case for your child, videotape your child during the behavior and ask your physician to review it, so that an informed decision can be made without unnecessary testing.) During the first 2 years of life, masturbation is largely related to general curiosity about one's body. Gradually, however, children discover that genital stimulation results in pleasurable sensations.

Although masturbation occurs commonly in children, many parents react negatively to it and may even punish their children if they catch them touching their genitals. Even parents who accept masturbation in their preschool children may become uncomfortable with this behavior as it assumes a more adult sexual quality. Yet, we have no evidence that masturbation proves harmful, and in fact it may qualify as an appropriate and adaptive sexual outlet for many people.

280

Because masturbation feels inherently pleasurable, the key clinical question regarding masturbation among children is not *why* they masturbate, but *how much* and *where* masturbation occurs. Masturbation does not harm the child unless it occurs compulsively, results in irritation, and/or leads to the exclusion of other activities. Whether or not masturbation constitutes a "problem" will in large part reflect family, societal, and cultural attitudes. Professionals agree that the best way to handle childhood masturbation involves teaching the child where and when it is appropriate to engage in this "private" behavior.

HOW DO I STOP MY CHILD FROM MASTURBATING IN PUBLIC?

In the example of Nancy, the issue for her mother was how to teach Nancy when and where it was appropriate to masturbate. If your child is engaging in masturbatory behavior out in the open, the first and most important thing to do is not overreact. Remember that masturbation is a normal behavior. Children commonly self-stimulate when they get tired, during diaper changes, and at bath time. This functions as a comfort measure or simple experimentation. The best reaction is "no reaction," distraction with a toy that requires the use of hands, or teaching your child that this is a "private" behavior. Scolding or punishing your child for masturbation may lead your child to falsely believe that genitals are dirty or bad, and trigger a sense of shame. You may wish to say something like, "I know that it feels good to rub yourself, but that is something we only do in private. You can do it in your room or in the bathroom, but not here in the living room." After being told to go to the bedroom several times, it is likely that a simple look or the presence of someone else in the room will be enough to stop the behavior.

WHAT IS CONSIDERED "NORMAL" SEXUAL DEVELOPMENT AND BEHAVIOR?

Some people worry that children who engage in certain sexual behaviors, including masturbation, have experienced sexual abuse. However, studies show that not *all* children who exhibit these types of behavior have experienced abuse. For example, surveys of nonabused children aged 2–12 years have found children engage in a wide range of sexual behaviors, including the relatively rare behaviors of putting mouth on sex parts, inserting objects in vagina/anus, imitating intercourse, and masturbating with an object. While sexualized behavior, by itself, does not provide proof of child sexual abuse, if the behavior interferes with other age-appropriate activities, it could provide a warning signal that the child may have other problems. If you are concerned about sexual abuse, contact a professional immediately.

In the case of Ted, it turned out that his frequent masturbation was not a consequence of being sexually abused, but rather a reaction to his parent's divorce and his mother's remarriage. Age-appropriate sex education and his parents' agreement to work together led to a decrease in Ted's masturbatory behavior.

Table 39.1 provides a summary of the types of sexual behaviors that often occur at different ages and what children understand about sexuality at these ages. Understanding when

TABLE 39.1. Normal sexual development

Sexual Knowledge	Sexual Behavior
Birth to 2 Years	
• Origins of gender identity • Origins of self-esteem • Learns labels for body parts including genitals • Uses slang labels	• Penile erections and vaginal lubrication • Genital exploration • Experiences genital pleasure • Touches own and other's sex parts • Enjoys nudity, takes clothes off in public
3 to 5 Years	
• Gender permanence is established • Gender differences are recognized • Limited information about pregnancy and childbirth • Knows labels for sexual body parts but uses elimination functions for sexual parts	• Masturbates for pleasure, may experience orgasm • Sex play with peers and siblings: exhibits genitals, exploration of own and other's genitals, attempted intercourse, may insert objects in genitals • Enjoys nudity, takes clothes off in public • Uses "dirty" words, especially with peers
6 to 12 Years	
• Genital basis of gender known • Correct labels for sex parts but uses slang • Sexual aspects of pregnancy known • Increasing knowledge of sexual behavior: masturbation, intercourse • Knowledge of physical aspects of puberty by age 10	• Sex games with peers and siblings: role plays and sex fantasy, kissing, mutual masturbation, simulated intercourse, playing "doctor" • Masturbation in private • Shows modesty, embarrassment: hides sex games and masturbation from adults • Body changes begin: girls may begin menstruation, boys may experience wet dreams • May fantasize or dream about sex • Interested in media sex • Uses sexual language with peers • Tells dirty jokes
13 to 18 Years	
• Sexual intercourse • Contraception • Sexually transmitted diseases • Date rape and sexual exploitation	• Pubertal changes continue: most girls menstruate by age 16, most boys are capable of ejaculation by age 14 • Dating begins • Sexual contacts are common: mutual masturbation, kissing, petting • Sexual fantasy and dreams • Sexual intercourse may occur in up to one-third

This table was previously published in B. N. Gordon and C. S. Schroeder. (1995). *Sexuality: A developmental approach to problems.* New York: Plenum Press. Reprinted with permission.

certain sexual behaviors are developmentally appropriate can help alleviate your concerns about your child's behavior.

HOW CAN I EDUCATE MY CHILD ABOUT HEALTHY SEXUALITY?

It is never too early to teach your children about their bodies. Sex education is a life-long process, and at different ages, children need different information. The opportunity to influence children's attitudes about sexuality is greater during the preschool years than in any other age period. During this period, parents lay the foundation for children's attitudes about sex roles and beliefs about appropriate and inappropriate sexual behavior. Studies show that children who are provided correct information on sexuality from their parents show more responsibility in their sexual behavior and are less likely to become victims of sexual abuse. The following are some tips for teaching your child about sex and sexuality:

- *Think about what you want your children to know about sexuality.* Clarify your own sexual values. Rehearse sexual words and ways of responding to situations, so that you feel prepared to answer their questions. Answer questions in language your child can understand, and keep your answers short, simple, and specific. Don't worry that you are telling your child too much. Children will stop listening when they lose interest or don't understand!
- *Sexuality is about relationships.* Act as a positive role model for your child. When you demonstrate warmth, affection, and support to your child, spouse, or loved ones, it shows your child how to behave in interpersonal relationships. Talk about love and affection, in addition to providing facts about anatomy and sexual functioning.
- *Purchase or borrow good sexuality education resources.* It is good to have at least one age-appropriate children's book that gives information about body parts and functions, reproduction, and birth. Be sure to read the book carefully to determine that the material is acceptable to you and age-appropriate. Read the book with your child. As your child gets older, buy books with more detailed information. It is also good to have a general guidebook to help you understand the developmental progression of sexuality and to provide guidance in ways to share sexuality information. See Where to Find Out More for a list of helpful resources.

SUMMARY

Masturbation in young children can trigger a range of emotions in their parents. The act itself is generally not harmful, but concerned parents should focus on the issues of how often and where the behavior occurs. Educating and redirecting your child about appropriate behaviors, as described earlier, can provide an important start to the child's sex education. If your child's behavior appears to be causing persistent physical irritation of the genitals or causes you concern that he or she may have been sexually abused, seek professional help from your child's pediatrician.

WHERE TO FIND OUT MORE

Books

Annunziata, J., & Nemiroff, M. (2002). *Sex and babies: First facts.* Washington, DC: Magination Press.

Brooks, R.B. (1983). *So that's how I was born!* New York: Little Simon.

Websites

American Academy of Pediatrics
  http//www.aap.org
Mayo Clinic
  http://www.mayoclinic.com/health/sex-education/HQ00547
University of Michigan Health System
  http://www.med.umich.edu/yourchild/topics/masturb.htm
Dr. Greene
  http://www.drgreene.com/qa/masturbation-young-children

CHAPTER 40

Coming Out as Gay or Lesbian

Neena M. Malik and Kristin M. Lindahl

Your teenager has seemed a bit out of sorts lately—avoiding talking to you, at times seeming secretive and sensitive for no good reason, and getting angry with you. On other occasions, your teenager just seems more withdrawn from you, spending more time in his room, or not wanting to tell you who he has seen, or what has gone on in his social life. If you ask him about a date for the prom, he gets very upset, even when you didn't think you said or asked anything that could hurt his feelings. After a few weeks or months of this behavior, he sits you down and tells you, at some point when you least expect it, "Mom, I'm gay." Or, "Dad, I think I might be gay." While his recent behavior suddenly begins to makes some sense, a range of emotions washes over you almost like a tidal wave.

It is never easy for parents to hear that their child is gay or lesbian, or thinks they might be. Even if you feel that you would be completely comfortable accepting your child's sexual orientation, every parent worries about what it will mean for his or her child. And, if you do not feel comfortable with such news, or if your religious beliefs tell you that being gay or lesbian is wrong, then the news can become extremely difficult to manage. In this chapter, we will explain what it means for a child to "come out" as gay or lesbian, and how parents can cope when this happens with their child. We will also describe ways in which families can rely on and strengthen their relationships with each other when a child may be gay or lesbian. Finally, we will talk about some of the ways to help yourself with struggles you may have with the issue, and some ways to help your child, if he or she is also struggling.

WHAT IS YOUR CHILD SAYING TO YOU?

When a child of any age recognizes that he may have a sexual orientation different from heterosexual, it can take quite a while for that child to tell his or her parents. First, the child must recognize and then come to terms with feeling different from most of his or her peers. This process will likely be lengthy and complex, as connecting and identifying with your peers becomes particularly important in adolescence. Once teenagers come to terms with their sexuality for themselves, they usually tell a friend or several friends. This may happen even before a youth feels fully comfortable with himself or herself as a gay person, and he or she may turn to her friends to seek support and assistance.

There are many reasons why young people might feel reluctant or shy about talking with their parents about their sexual orientation. The nature of the topic itself, sexuality, makes many teens and parents uncomfortable, regardless of the teens' sexual orientation. In addition, there is much difference in beliefs and values about sexuality across generations. Youth who suspect or know that they are not heterosexual are often afraid of how their parents will respond. As a consequence, parents often are the last to know about their child's sexuality. When youth talk to parents, they usually tell their mothers first, and then their fathers, although certainly sometimes fathers know before mothers. In addition, the way in which family members communicate with each other also likely has an impact on when children disclose their gay or lesbian sexual orientation to their parents. In families in which talking about feelings comes naturally, quite possibly parents will learn early, rather than last, about their gay or lesbian child's sexual orientation.

This means that, by the time your child tells you, he or she quite likely has gone through a lot of stress and worry related to trying to understand his or her own identity. Your child may still have a lot of worries, fears, and concerns, and may feel very unsure of himself or herself, or fearful of your reactions. The important thing to realize, however, is that if your child has come out to you, he or she wants an honest relationship with you and to share something very private and important with you.

You may feel a bit confused by what your child is telling you. Sometimes it seems very clear; your son tells you that he is sexually attracted exclusively to men, or your daughter tells you that she is attracted exclusively to women. But sometimes the definitions do not come across clearly, and parents who are already struggling with the idea of a potentially gay child can find that very confusing. For example, young people may use several different terms and definitions these days, all falling under the umbrella of "LGBTQ," which means "lesbian, gay, bisexual, transgendered, queer, or questioning." Many youth and researchers these days also use the term "same-sex attracted." Lesbian, gay, bisexual, queer, questioning, or same-sex attracted all refer to an individual who has a sexual orientation that is not exclusively heterosexual, and may or may not include opposite-sex attraction. Transgender has a different definition, which relates to identifying with a gender that does not match your own biological sex.

Definitions of sexuality have become somewhat fluid these days, which probably seems very different from how society viewed such matters when you were growing up. These changes mean that, for many young people, defining their sexuality does not feel as important as being true to themselves and allowing themselves to feel however they want, about men and women alike. In these changing times, many adolescents have become less likely to feel the need to label themselves one way or another. As a parent, however, the sense of panic you may feel once your child reveals same-sex attractions or feelings of being transgendered may become amplified by not really understanding what your child means. Even if your child seems somewhat vague in discussing his or her sexuality, the scientific data indicate that sexuality has strong biological roots and is not a simple choice. Your teenager may not feel nearly as urgent as you do about "deciding" on a sexual orientation. Regardless of how they ultimately define themselves, settling on a definition is not the same thing as making a choice about their sexuality. Although one can choose labels, one cannot choose one's sexuality. All scientific research reported to date shows that sexual orientation is biological in nature, rather than a personal choice.

Eventually, somewhere around 2%–10% of the population will describe themselves, in adulthood, as what we commonly refer to as "gay" or "lesbian." This means that, if your child has a non-heterosexual orientation, he or she is part of a minority. Your child will become part of a minority for whom our society shows growing acceptance, but with a long way to go. Sexual-minority adolescents will doubtless face some stressful experiences going forward, such as taunting by peers, worries about being accepted by friends and family, and fears of discrimination. Your child probably faces problems like figuring out how to have a same-sex boyfriend or girlfriend, or dealing with a crush, or simply dealing with feeling really different from most other kids.

All these reasons may contribute to why your child might feel touchy about a date for the prom. At this moment in his or her life, support from Mom and Dad becomes critically important. The period of "coming out" definitely qualifies as one of those times when parental support is critical.

WHAT DOES "COMING OUT" MEAN, AND WHY IS THIS IMPORTANT FOR MY CHILD?

"Coming out" refers to the process of recognizing and acknowledging same-sex attractions in oneself, and then sharing that information about one's identity with other people. This process can mean different things for different youth. Kids might talk to you, as we just described, about falling anywhere on a continuum from gay to bisexual to heterosexual. Thus, in order to continue communicating well with your child, you will need to try to understand where your child falls on the continuum, based on what he or she tells you, rather than what you think or want to believe. This will not always prove easy to do. Because society's views about homosexuality vary by age, over time, and by region, kids' definitions and experiences will likely vary from yours as a parent.

The teen and early adult years, when same-sex attracted individuals tend to "come out," normally represent a time of great developmental changes. Establishing an identity, both internally for oneself and in terms of a social or public identity, becomes an important developmental task that we all face as we move forward in the process from childhood to adulthood. Some parents might prefer that their children simply not tell them if they believe they are gay or lesbian. They might prefer not to hear things about their children that they feel uncomfortable about or do not agree with, since it may make their relationship with their children complicated.

A child who comes out to a parent does so with the intent to share something important and personal with their parent. Most kids are aware that this will be hard for their parents and are likely ready to help their parents deal with a number of very common questions parents have. The most likely question, or concern, parents have is, "Did I do something to cause this to happen?" The answer to that question, unequivocally, is "No." You did not do anything wrong. In fact, there is nothing you did or could do that would influence your child's sexuality. Sexuality is not considered a choice nor something influenced by the environment.

HOW WORRIED SHOULD I BE?

Even when parents feel "totally cool" or at least "okay" with having a gay son or lesbian daughter, they still generally worry a lot about what might happen to their child. A son who acknowledges same-sex attractions can become subjected to a host of negativity from peers—even heterosexual adolescents who get taunted by peers as gay or lesbian can find the experience very hurtful. When a child truly identifies as gay, the put-downs strike an even deeper sensitivity. They may encounter friends, family members, coaches, teachers, parents of friends, and others who reject them, and those experiences can trigger feelings of despair and isolation. A child who begins to come out can't really predict how people will respond to her when she tells them about her sexual orientation. She will likely feel a mix of both fear and worry about rejection, along with hope for acceptance as she acknowledges her identity and shares it with others.

The media has reported on horrible acts of violence committed against gay youth, and gay men, even more so than lesbians or other groups that fall under the "LGBTQ" category. This does not mean that risk of victimization for LGBTQ kids ranks high on a day-to-day basis, or that they will likely become victims of violent crime. Harassment, such as teasing, proves emotionally difficult but not physically dangerous, and occurs much more commonly than violence.

Some research reports suggest that LGBTQ youth seem more likely to feel depressed, express thoughts of wanting to die, and attempt suicide, because they face so many stressful experiences. Other reports, however, show a tremendous amount of resilience in same-sex attracted youth. One of the deciding factors in how adolescents cope seems to involve how family members cope with their son or daughter coming out. If youth have a supportive and helpful environment at home, and good relationships, even with only one parent, they seem very likely to cope effectively with whatever negativity and bigotry they may face.

Generally, no one knows your child better than you. If you didn't expect your child to disclose a non-heterosexual orientation, you might feel that you do not know your child as well as you thought you did—but in reality, you still know your child very well. Most parents know how their children express fear, stress, or suffering. Even if sexual orientation is an issue between you and your child, you can still help them to be resilient if you pay attention to their day-to-day feelings, help them cope with difficult experiences, and give them opportunities to communicate with you about important positive and negative events. Even if you cannot talk to them about their sexuality, you can still talk to them about all the other important things in their lives. Not withdrawing from your role as a parent is probably one of the most helpful ways to help your child continue to feel cared for and accepted.

HOW CAN I BE SUPPORTIVE?

The following are some suggestions to keep in mind when your child comes out, in terms of ways to help him or her move forward with the newly understood—or at least newly disclosed—sexual identity:

- *Keep lines of communication as open as possible.* This can be a tricky balancing act for parents who want to show acceptance and concern for their LBGTQ child. A youth coming out seeks acceptance, and it may prove difficult for him or her to hear the legitimate concerns or worries you have. Before discussing your concerns, reassure your child that you love, respect, and feel proud of him or her (in whatever ways you can genuinely say this). Your child will feel more open to hearing about your worries, if he or she knows that the two of you still have a solid foundation in your parent–child relationship.
- *Focus on teaching problem-solving and coping skills to your child.* Acceptance of a child's sexual orientation, like "coming out" for teens, unfolds as a process, developing over time. Even if you do not feel completely comfortable with your child's sexuality at the outset, you will want to protect your child and help him or her cope with any rejection or teasing he or she might experience from others. If necessary, try to put your own doubts about sexual orientation aside.
- *Help your child stay safe.* This will prove less of an issue for young women, but for young men, same-sex attraction and sexual activity can carry a risk for HIV and AIDS. Even for young women, one must remain vigilant about sexually transmitted diseases, regardless of sexual orientation, when becoming sexually active. Educate yourself about safe-sex practices and try to communicate the importance of self-confidence and self-protection for when your child may become sexually active.
- *Support your child and suggest ways to cope, if your child has to face harassment or discrimination.* Helping your LGBTQ child feel a sense of self-worth and a sense of self-confidence will become the most important gift you can give your child. Maintaining a solid sense of self and learning ways to cope with difficulty will prove the most protective skills an LGBTQ youth can have as he or she moves forward into adulthood as a gay or lesbian person.
- *Remain aware of your own biases or prejudices.* As much as society has become more accepting of LGBTQ persons in some quarters, prejudice and negative stereotypes still exist, and you may have some in your own mind without even realizing it. Your child wants you to accept him for the person he is and has always been, even though you now know something very different about him that you didn't know before. Your child can feel very sensitive to expressions that make him feel that you now see him differently, with negative connotations. Remain patient with your child, and with yourself, as you adjust to the new information you have learned.

WHAT IF I FEEL I CAN'T BE SUPPORTIVE?

We said before that you are going to have feelings to deal with as your child comes out, and it may prove very, very hard for you. While having supportive parents can make a great and positive difference in the lives of gay youth, the process can prove extremely hard on all of you, especially if you have trouble accepting your child once he or she comes out to you. Consider ideas for how you can understand, acknowledge, and move forward in your own reactions to your child coming out:

- *Try to remain patient with yourself and do not focus on predicting a negative future.* It may seem that you have hit an irreparable impasse with your child over sexuality. Don't focus on that feeling. Instead, focus on understanding why you have such a negative reaction to your LGBTQ child.
- *Don't feel ashamed of feeling ashamed.* So many parents end up believing they have done something wrong for their child to turn against them, or against God, or against their community. They feel they have done something wrong for their child to turn out gay. Your child's sexual orientation began before birth. We do not yet fully understand the underlying science, but try to get beyond the "how" and "why," since we lack clear answers. If you feel ashamed, or you feel you need to keep things secret, allow yourself to have that reaction. The pain you feel will diminish if you take things slowly.
- *If you feel the need to keep your child's sexuality a secret, remember that your child may experience that need as rejection.* Open communication with your child is key. If you can tell your child that your need to keep his or her sexuality a secret is part of your way of dealing with his or her sexuality, and you do not yet feel ready to tell people, but that you are working on acceptance, your child will likely feel more patient and compassionate with you. Your child probably struggled with all those feelings, too, before coming out to you.
- *Don't blame yourself, but don't blame your child, either.* As you struggle through dealing with your child's coming out, taking blame out of the picture makes communication and understanding much easier for you and your child.
- *Recognize that you are not alone.* For generations, parents just like you have struggled with acceptance of their gay children. You may not feel that you can seek out support, but if you can, do so. You can find support from clergy, friends, counselors, colleagues, and support groups. We've listed some of the places you can go in person or anonymously on the Internet to get some support (see Where to Find Out More).

SUMMARY

Whether your child identifies as gay or straight, and whether this is hard for you or not, remember what you provide most as a parent: support of your child as the person he or she needs to become. The strongest emotional bond in the world forms between a parent and a child. Remember that your child, for the longest time, couldn't even survive without you. Despite the strength of your emotional bond, many things may make parents feel very fragile. Feeling as though you don't know your child, or that your child has not become the person you imagined when they were little, can become the most heartbreaking moment in a parent's life. Remember the remarkable truth that no child really ever becomes exactly who their parent imagined, and every parent has to cope at some point with that realization. Having an LGBTQ child may involve more of a departure from parental expectations than you bargained for or than you ever thought you could deal with. But you can. Your child remains your child, and nothing will change that. His sexuality does not define him. Her choice of partner does not mean she has turned her back on you. The greatest gifts parents can give a child remain love and acceptance for who they are. Even if you think you can never get there with a gay or lesbian child, know in your heart that, if you try, you can. Don't give up on them, and don't give up on yourself.

WHERE TO FIND OUT MORE

Books

DeGeneres, B. (1999). *Love, Ellen: A mother/daughter journey*. New York: William Morrow & Company.
McDougall, B. (2006). *My child is gay: How parents react when they hear the news*. Crows Nest NSW, Australia: Allen & Unwin.
Savin-Williams, R. (2008). *The new gay teenager*. Cambridge, MA: Harvard University Press.

Websites

Human Rights Campaign
Coming out
   http://www.hrc.org/issues/coming_out.asp.
PFLAG: Parents, families, and friends of lesbians and gays
   http://community.pflag.org.

PART SEVEN

Adolescent Issues

CHAPTER 41

Dating, Boyfriends/ Girlfriends, Break-ups

Joanne Davila and Sara J. Steinberg

Your 13-year-old daughter Mandy tells you she needs to stay home from school because she is having problems with a friend. Upon further questioning, you find out that she has lost her virginity to a boy you have never heard of, and is fighting with her best friend because this friend likes the same boy. Your daughter tells you that it's "no big deal," and she is not going out with this boy; she just wanted to have sex. You feel devastated and confused. These are not the values you have raised your daughter with, and you have no idea how to handle the situation.

Your 16-year-old son Evan is moping around the house and, when you ask what's wrong, he responds with an angry and dismissive, "Nothing!" You learn from your neighbor, who has a daughter in your son's class, that a girl Evan is interested in told him that she didn't like him and was flirting with other boys. You wish you could help your son deal with this, but you're angry that he's shutting you out and you have no idea how to approach him and talk to him.

One of the biggest events in the lives of adolescents (and in their parents' lives too!) may occur when adolescents begin dating. It opens up a whole new world to teenagers, a world that can prove incredibly exciting, but also very stressful. It's happening earlier and earlier these days, and many parents don't know how to help their adolescent deal with this often emotionally challenging set of experiences. The scenarios of Mandy and Evan are just two examples of the difficulty parents face in helping their teens navigate the adolescent dating world. So, what do parents need to know?

WHAT YOU NEED TO KNOW

First, parents should take adolescent romantic activities seriously. Many people don't recognize how important these first relationships are to teenagers. Although it may be tempting to see them as "puppy love," especially because teen romantic relationships can prove short or fleeting, these experiences play an important role in adolescents' lives. What happens in their romantic lives can trigger lots of emotions, both positive and negative, can affect their self-esteem, and can increase or decrease their risk for feeling depressed or anxious. Their experiences also teach them important and potentially long-lasting lessons about things like how to behave in relationships, what to expect from partners, how to assess their social worth, how to cope with disappointment, and how to cope with peer pressure and social evaluation. So, even though your child's earliest romantic experiences may seem minor to you, helping them negotiate their romantic world will increase the likelihood that they'll take positive lessons forward and become emotionally healthy adults.

Second, parents should learn more about adolescent romantic relationships. What experiences might your adolescent be having? In later adolescence (ages 16–18), teens may have relationships that fit adult ideas about romantic relationships (e.g., two people dating, spending time together, and becoming relatively committed to one another). However, adolescents of all ages, especially younger ones, may have "relationships" without such obvious or identifiable markers. These relationships may exist largely in theory rather than in practice (e.g., your adolescent is interested in someone and the feeling seems reciprocated, but the two of them barely see or talk to each other). Relationships may occur entirely over the Internet or via text messaging or even through relayed communications between friends. Teenagers may "hook-up" with people (i.e., engage in sexual activity) with no interest in or expectation for commitment or for an ongoing relationship. Many types of romantic activities in which teenagers might engage don't fit an adult definition of a relationship.

Given these facts, parents need to stay well-informed, open to learning more, and open to communication with their teenagers. Teenagers can learn a lot from their parents, even if they don't want to admit it! Most teenagers say they prefer to learn about romance and relationships from their friends, and they report turning to friends, rather than parents, for this information. It is typical for teenagers to learn from peers about relationships and what is accepted within their peer group, and also to learn from the media (e.g., Internet, television, movies). Peers can provide a healthy and comfortable way for adolescents to learn, especially when their friendships involve others with stable personalities and good values. But adolescents also learn from their parents—both through talking and through direct observation of parents' relationships. So, it's important that you act as a good role model and remain open to communication.

As indicated earlier, romantic experiences in adolescence can prove challenging. Adolescents have a lot of things to figure out, and a lot of emotions that come along with doing so. Helping adolescents know how to problem-solve and how to cope with their feelings becomes really important. For example, in the example of Mandy, presented at the beginning of this chapter, Mandy's parents may feel tempted to punish her for her choice. However, the event has passed and now Mandy would more likely benefit from support, validation, and an open discussion about the emotional, social, and health consequences of choosing to have sex. Similarly, Evan's parents may be angry that he won't talk to them, but expressing that anger is unlikely to help Evan open up. The more you can stay supportive and available, rather than punitive, and the more you can model healthy relationship behavior for your child, the better your child will do.

TIPS FOR TALKING WITH YOUR TEENAGER ABOUT DATING AND ROMANTIC ACTIVITIES

Having highlighted the importance of understanding adolescent romantic experiences and encouraged getting involved, you probably find yourself wondering, "What do I do with all this information? How do I talk to my teenager?" To help guide you, we address some common questions that parents have about talking with their teenagers and outline tips for doing so.

When Should I Start Talking to My Teenager?

As soon as possible! It's important to talk with teenagers (1) before they become heavily involved in romantic or sexual activities and (2) before they decide that you won't understand and they no longer want anything to do with you! As parents, you should recognize that there comes a time when your child stops idealizing you and begins to think you're the dumbest and most embarrassing person in the world. You want to start talking with them before this happens, so that they move into adolescence knowing that the lines of communication are open. Unfortunately, many parents avoid discussion with their teenagers about dating and sex because it can feel awkward or because they fear raising the issue too early. In reality, your children will learn this information from their friends and the media at a very early age, whether you want them to or not. So, if they're going to get the information in one way or another, having it come from you will prove the healthier way to go. Note that Mandy's parents had no idea that their daughter was even interested in dating, never mind having sex! If you are thinking, "I don't want my teenager doing what I was doing when I was a teenager," you are not alone. You can use your experiences, even those where you wish you had made different choices, to attract your teenager's attention and potentially bond with your teenager.

What Should I Talk About with My teenager?

Everything! We know it can be challenging and anxiety-provoking to do so, but teenagers need information and need to be listened to. Of course, you can't talk about everything all at once, so a good rule of thumb is to get a sense of what stage your teenager is in with regard to his or her interests and activities. This can prove tricky for parents. For instance, in early adolescence (ages 12–14), many teenagers begin "going out," even though they may rarely see each other. For example, adolescents may have met once, go to different schools, and talk only on the phone and online. Alternatively, others may see each other in school only, but not outside of school. So, your teenager may be "going out" with someone for weeks without you even knowing! Other adolescents may show less romantic precociousness. Although they may have crushes or romantic interests, many adolescents may not begin dating until mid to late adolescence, if then. Still others may show particularly precocious behavior and become involved in more "serious" relationships and/or sexual activities. Therefore, you've got to inquire, so that you can remain aware of your teenager's development in these areas. (For example, using a neutral, yet interested tone ask, "Tell me about your friends. What do you like about Jason?")

As you inquire about your adolescent's romantic interests and activities, remember to take a gentle and respectful tone. No teenager wants to feel judged, made fun of, or embarrassed by his or her parents. (For example, teasing your adolescent about "liking someone" may seem harmless, but it can feel invalidating to your teenager.) Dating and sex are serious things in teenagers' lives. Teenagers also want privacy and don't want nosey or intrusive parents. This can prove a hard issue to get around. Conveying interest and care for adolescents rather than judging their behavior can help. Teenagers often assume, like Evan may have done, that their parents will never understand what they're going through, making it even more important to listen with an open, nonjudgmental attitude. (For example, "I'm here if you want to talk.")

Once you have a sense of the stage at which your teenager might be, follow your child's lead on what he or she wants to talk about. This will convey your respect and acceptance, which might help your child to be open with you. Address questions or concerns directly and seriously, but without criticism. Let your child know you can handle these types of discussions, which may feel difficult for parents who are shy or easily embarrassed, or who quickly assume the worst and become easily angered. But this is important, because if your teenager doesn't think you can handle a conversation, your child won't talk to you.

Finally, be prepared with some things that you want to talk about—things that you think your child should know. Just because we recommend following a teenager's lead does not mean that we don't think there are things that parents should convey, regardless of whether the teenager wants to hear them or not. Parents have a right and responsibility to do so. Also, it is important to keep in mind that teenage boys and girls may have different needs and struggles (e.g., girls may be more focused on their physical appearance and on the "romance" aspect of relationships, and boys may be more focused on the sexual aspect of relationships and managing time spent with their male friends versus their dating partner). It is also important to know that parents of the opposite sex can serve as important learning sources by offering their unique experiences and providing insight into differing male and female experience of romance and sexuality. Here are a few ideas for how to talk to your teenager:

- *Emphasize that romantic and sexual feelings are normal and okay.*   Teenagers, particularly younger ones, may feel concerned or embarrassed about romantic or sexual feelings. Emphasize that feelings are just emotions—they're not right or wrong.
- *Talk about how to make decisions about romantic and sexual experiences.*   Help adolescents see that whatever their feelings are, they can make choices about how to behave. Help them think through the consequences of their choices, so that they can make the best decisions for themselves. A good rule of thumb is to help adolescents see which choices will foster healthy self-esteem and be consistent with their values.
- *Talk about your values and expectations as a parent, and encourage teenagers to develop their own values.*   Teenagers will be much more likely to engage in a behavior if it

meets their own goals, rather than if they feel dictated to by a parent. So, help them recognize their goals and values, and help them to identify the emotional consequences of their behavior. (For example, "I want you to think about what having sex means to you, and how you might know when you are ready.") Since adolescent boys may feel ready to become sexually active before girls, it is important to talk with them about respecting the values of the people they become involved with, and to talk with girls about recognizing and asserting their values and boundaries.

- *Talk openly about a wide range of topics related to sexuality* (e.g., anatomy, hormones, STDs, pregnancy, sexual orientation, emotional and physical consequences of sex, etc.). This may be the hardest thing for some parents to do, but teenagers—boys and girls alike—need factual, reliable, nonjudgmental information to help guide them. (For example, "I want to talk with you about making good sexual choices. I think it is important for us to talk about birth control and protection against diseases. I also want to talk with you about emotions that can arise after sex.")
- *Talk about aspects of relationships that are consistent with your teenagers' stage of development.*   For instance, young teenagers may need guidance about how to pursue a relationship, whereas older teenagers may need guidance about how to balance having a relationship with friends, school, and hobbies, and how to negotiate sexual feelings and activities.

WILL TALKING ABOUT DATING AND SEX PUT IDEAS IN MY TEENAGER'S HEAD OR INDICATE THAT I CONDONE CERTAIN THINGS?

Definitely not! Although many parents feel concerned that talking about dating, and particularly about sex, with their teenagers may put ideas into their heads, this belief overlooks the fact that nature has already put such ideas in there. Teenagers who have accurate knowledge about sex will more likely make safe choices, and talking about such choices may even delay sexual initiation. Furthermore, just because you talk about something, doesn't mean that you condone it, and you can make that clear to your adolescent. For example, parents can educate adolescents about the different way to protect themselves from STDs while still conveying a clear message that, as a parent, you support abstinence. The key involves presenting factual information, while sending a clear message about your expectations. (For example, "You know that I do not believe you should be having sex, and I want you to wait. But I also want you to make safe choices and talk to me, even if you decide to go against my wishes.")

HOW DO I HELP MY TEENAGER DEAL WITH RELATIONSHIP PROBLEMS?

Romantic problems abound in the lives of adolescents! In addition to the expected conflicts, arguments, and break-ups that characterize most adolescent relationships, many other daily situations could lead to feelings of rejection or betrayal. These situations include, but are not limited to things such as your adolescent having a romantic interest in someone who does not feel the same, your adolescent feeling betrayed by a friend who goes out with someone your adolescent has an interest in, peers spreading rumors about your adolescent's sexual behavior, engaging in sexual activity with someone who then ignores your adolescent, and so on. Young adolescents experiencing their first romantic rejection may feel particularly vulnerable, and it is especially important for parents to provide support and validation for their feelings. Older teenagers may have more experience, but they need parental support too.

Of course, just as teenagers may not tell their parents that they have begun dating or engaging in sexual activity, they also may not tell their parents that they have encountered problems in their relationships. Therefore, it becomes important for parents to stay attentive to any changes in their teenagers' behavior, and to talk openly about what may be going on in their lives. (For example, "You've seemed a little distant lately. Is everything okay?") Parents may notice common symptoms of relationship problems, such as increased sad mood, isolation from friends and family, or increased irritability. Parents need to approach these situations with the right balance of concern and support. Here are some ideas:

- *Do not get overly alarmed.* Remember, your teenager is most likely having a common reaction to a genuinely difficult situation. Let your teenager know that you understand that.
- *Do not dismiss their experience.*   Relationships are hard for adolescents. Yes, they will get through this, but they don't have to like it. And the "getting through it" part can become a good learning experience if it's handled well.
- *Help them learn how to tolerate their negative emotions.*   Let them know that their feelings are okay, and a natural reaction to their circumstances. Encourage them to engage in activities that can distract them, keep them busy, or help them feel better, even if only for a moment.
- *Help them plan ahead for coping with the ups and downs of dating.*   Talk through possible scenarios with them. Help them think about what they would do in different circumstances.
- *Help them problem-solve.*   Too often, adolescents, especially girls, can get caught up in ruminating about how bad things have become. Help them identify problems, and encourage them to come up with solutions that they can implement. Help them see the difference about what can and cannot be changed, and then help them make whatever changes they can.

WHAT IF MY TEENAGER DOESN'T WANT TO TALK TO ME?

Typically, at around age 12 or 13, many parents often wonder "What happened to my sweet child who always wanted to be around me?" It is normal for young adolescents to begin to separate from their parents, spend more time with their peers, and suddenly answer their parents' questions about their life with, "I don't know." It also becomes normal for adolescents of any age to not want to talk with their parents, particularly about dating and sex, and that's okay. Even if your teenager doesn't want to have a conversation with you, there are things you can do:

- *Let your teenagers know you're there for them.*   The knowledge that you will keep yourself emotionally available and will support them will go a very long way with teenagers, even if they never take you up on the offer.
- *Tell them the things that you want them to know.*   Even if they don't appear to listen, and even if they actively put down what you have to say, it's important that you say it. They'll hear it on some level.
- *Respect that they don't want to talk about some things with you.*   Let them know that you understand why they might not be comfortable doing so (after all, were you completely comfortable talking about these things with your parents?), and try not to take their behavior personally. They still love you, and the more respect you show them, the more they'll come around to valuing you and your opinion, once they've made it through the difficult teenager years. Remember, acting in an overly involved, overly intrusive, or overprotective way can lead teenagers to rebel or lie about their behavior, which is the opposite of what you want.
- *Model what you want them to learn.*   Maybe they don't want to listen to what you have to say, but teenagers are watching how you behave, whether you know it or not. So, strive to have the kind of relationship that you want them to have. Strive to behave in a way that you'd like them to behave.

SUMMARY

Dating and romantic relationships are challenging and important events in the lives of adolescents. Parents should take these activities seriously. You can help your child by recognizing the importance of romantic relationships, learning about adolescent romantic relationships, and keeping lines of communication open with your child. Be supportive and available, and discuss romantic relationships with your children even before they become heavily involved in romantic or sexual activities.

This chapter provided tips on how to talk with your teenager about romantic relationships (e.g., be gentle and respectful, talk about values and expectations, talk openly about topics related to sexuality) and how to help with relationship problems (e.g., do not dismiss their experiences, help them tolerate negative emotions, help them plan and problem-solve). The chapter also provided tips on what to do if your adolescent doesn't want to talk. Parents' respect and support can go a long way in helping adolescents negotiate this important developmental task.

WHERE TO FIND OUT MORE

Websites

Adolescent Romantic Relationships and Experiences, http://www.du.edu/psychology/relationshipcenter/publications/pdfs/Adolescentromanticrelationshipsand.pdf

Act for Youth, http://www.actforyouth.net

Center for Disease Control, Healthy Schools Healthy Youth,
    http://www.cdc.gov/healthyyouth/

National Adolescent Health Information Center, http://nahic.ucsf.edu/

Keep Kids. Healthy, http://www.keepkidshealthy.com/adolescent/adolescent.html

Boys' Town – Parenting.org, http://www.parenting.org/flight/index.asp

Children Now, http://www.talkingwithkids.org/sex.html

American Academy of Child and Adolescent Psychiatry,
    http://www.aacap.org/cs/root/facts_for_families/talking_to_your_kids_about_sex

New York University Child Study Center, http://www.aboutourkids.org/files/articles/june.pdf

CHAPTER 42

Teenage Drivers

Gerald P. Koocher

Your son, Mike, has expressed increasing unbridled excitement as the date approaches when he will be eligible to apply for a learner's permit. You have mixed feelings about this "coming of age" event. Mike is a "good kid," but still a teenager with all the inexperience and occasional impulsiveness that "teenager" implies. You know that a driver's license will give him more independence and free you from having to drive him everywhere.

Beth's parents face the very same issues, plus they recognize that she is often preoccupied with texting on her cell phone and worry that she will text while driving. Beth's parents also know that driving represents a major new responsibility, with a variety of risks, and that having a teenage driver in the household will increase insurance and other vehicle operating costs. What's a parent to do?

Understanding these issues well before a teenager begins to drive can go a long way toward preventive parenting. According to U.S. government statistics, teenagers represent 6.4% of the driving population, but account for 14% of all drivers involved in fatal automobile accidents and 18% of those involved in crashes leading to police reports. The risk of motor vehicle crashes ranks highest among 16- to 19-year-olds compared to any other age group; in fact, this risk is at a level that is four times greater than for older drivers, per mile driven. Among teen drivers, those at greatest risk for motor vehicle accidents include:

- Male adolescents, who average one and a half times the number of accidents experienced by their female counterparts.
- Teens driving with peer passengers: The presence of adolescent passengers increases the crash risk of unsupervised teen drivers, and the risk increases with the number of teen passengers in the vehicle.

- Teens using cell phones or other distractions: For example, the use of cell phones for voice and text messages while driving contributes to motor vehicle accidents.

The other major risk factors affecting young drivers are related to adolescent development and inexperience in comparison with older drivers and include the following facts:

- Teens have a greater tendency to underestimate dangerous situations or not recognize hazardous situations.
- Teens show a greater likelihood of speeding, and they allow less stopping distances between vehicles.
- Teens have the lowest rate of seat belt use, with 12.5% of males and 7.8% of females reporting that they rarely or never wore seat belts in a 2005 survey.
- In the same survey, nearly 30% of teens reported that, within the past month, they had ridden with a driver who had been drinking alcohol.

WHERE DO I START?

Ideally, parents can start preparing their adolescent driver-trainee early by modeling best practices. People learn a great deal by observing how consequences flow from what others do, and children pay particular attention to their parent's behavior during their early adolescent years. Setting a good example behind the wheel and talking aloud about how and why you make particular decisions will hold special attention as children begin to imagine themselves as drivers. You can create and take advantage of teachable moments. Consider these examples:

- Get in the habit of fastening your own seatbelt and then asking whether everyone else has buckled up before starting the car's engine.
- Imagine that your cell phone rings as you drive along, and comment aloud about how you plan to wait until you can safely pull over to take the call or check for a message.
- When offered an alcoholic beverage at a restaurant or family dinner, the designated driver can say aloud, "Not for me, thank you. I'm driving afterward."
- When a media report of a traffic accident airs as the family sits watching television, note aloud whether the reporter mentioned that alcohol, distraction, or speed played a role.

Such responses offered "in the moment" draw attention to important risk factors as they occur, bring the real-life nature of the event to the foreground, and model concern for the issue in the context of driving safety. As adolescents approach the age at which they increasingly begin to think of themselves behind the wheel, this type of situation will definitely catch their attention. An attitude of "thoughtful casualness" will often have more influence on an adolescent than direct emotional pressure, and consistency on the part of parents will help to reinforce the message.

Some readers may have begun to feel a bit uneasy at this point. Perhaps you have chatted on the cell phone while driving, or had an alcoholic drink (just one, of course) before getting behind the wheel. Perhaps you have shouted angrily at the actions of another driver from behind the wheel, made less than a "full stop" at a stop sign, or occasionally drifted well above the speed limit. Your adolescents will notice such behavior and, in so doing, they will become very attuned to inconsistencies.

The single most important thing a parent can do to raise a child who drives safely is to *model the behavior you want them to learn.* The retort, "Do as I say, not as I do," does not effectively influence this age group (or any age group, for that matter). Most adolescents would be more impressed by a parent who says, "I made a mistake doing that, help me remember not to do it again."

- *Invite your 14- to 16-year-olds to observe and "critique" your driving, talk aloud with them about strategies, and invite questions.* Conversations about what thoughts run through your mind as you prepare to enter a traffic circle, turn left in the face of oncoming traffic, or merge from a ramp onto a highway, can help them to recognize all of the anticipation, judgment, and skill that make experienced drivers safer than novices.
- *Encourage your enthusiastic would-be driver to get a copy of the department of motor vehicles "rules of the road" book months before they would qualify to take the written exam.* Read it yourself, and offer to quiz your child or engage in back-and-forth questioning to see whether one of you can stump the other. Few adolescents can pass up an opportunity to "one-up" their parents, and in striving for that goal they will pay closer attention to the road rules.
- *Teach your adolescent about the vehicle they'll be driving.* Show them the location of controls and demonstrate each one; particularly the headlights, windshield washers, hazard lights, and emergency brake. Show them the location of the spare tire and emergency or repair equipment. Explain how to adjust the seats and mirrors, how to tell if the tire pressure is low or the tread is worn, and how to open the hood, trunk, and fuel filler. When something goes wrong or the vehicle needs service, use the event as a teachable moment—how did you notice the problem, what repairs were needed, how was it fixed?
- *Definitely encourage your adolescent to take a "driver's education" course when they qualify for it.* However, also *provide opportunities for more "practice behind the wheel"* as that builds the kind of experience that reduces accidents. Consider letting your adolescent practice driving with you as passenger, once your child has a learner's permit; but only if you can control your anxiety and avoid any premature protective impulses, such as nervous repetitive cautions and audible gasps. If you cannot manage the necessary comfort level, consider allowing your child to gain experience with another trusted adult driver in the passenger seat.

SETTING CONSISTENT ENFORCEABLE RULES

Keeping in mind the risk factors mentioned earlier, *establish consistent enforceable rules for your adolescent once she has earned her license.* Many states have set limits on graduated licenses for junior drivers that restrict the hours permitted for operating a motor vehicle and require the direct supervision of a parent or other authorized person older than 21. Some states also limit the number of passengers under age 21 that a junior driver can transport, unless the passengers qualify as immediate family or an adult over age 21 is present to directly supervise. A few states deny driving licenses to people under age 18 who drop out of high school.

Parents will certainly want to enforce any state law mandates, but also may wish to incorporate similar restrictions even if their state law does not require them. Such policies focus on reducing distractions, avoiding impulsive behavior based on peer pressure, and minimizing the risk that inexperienced drivers will be in control of a vehicle while over-tired.

Parents may also wish to set limits on destinations, routes of travel, or activities, and to set other acceptable driving rules. Rule-setting works best when done in advance, with clear rationales, and specific consequences. Such rules should account for "responsible exceptions," by clearly indicating the policies to follow (e.g., if the need to vary the plan comes up, the adolescent should contact the parent to seek permission or explain the problem, such as when a traffic jam, bad weather, or flat tire seems likely to delay the planned arrival or return). Setting enforceable consequences in advance of any infraction and applying them consistently will prove most effective.

Ideally, consequences for infractions should fit the nature of the violation. Parents can develop a driving contract before or soon after their adolescent earns a license. Involving the adolescent in the rulemaking and penalty-for-infraction setting has two purposes. First, the young driver will ideally feel respected and involved in the rulemaking, with the ability to make his voice heard. Second, the teen will help create and agree to the consequences of infractions before any have occurred. Adolescents will, by nature, test parental limits frequently. Circumstances may come up that require altering or amending rules, but this should not happen without careful discussion. Parents or other supervising adults must back up the agreed-upon rules and not undermine each other, lest the seriousness and consistency of the message become confused.

REWARDING GOOD DECISIONS

People find it far easier to criticize than to give praise. Ironically, psychological research has consistently demonstrated that praising positive behaviors increases the likelihood that the person complimented will behave similarly again. If the situation warrants it, *compliment your adolescent on his driving when you are with him.* Acknowledge your child's responsibility when you learn of a decision she made to follow the household driving rules, even though doing so proved inconvenient. Make a point of praising your child's driving occasionally when nothing at all has happened, such as a week or month of driving without incident. After all, isn't that what all parents want—an uneventful driving record?

Another part of supporting good decision-making involves helping the adolescent driver understand financial responsibility and related decisions. Automobile insurance, fuel, and repair costs all increase with adolescent drivers in the home. Finding some way for them to participate in sharing the expenses can further instill a sense of responsibility and the real costs associated with responsible motor vehicle operation.

As a parent, you will also earn an important reward for your good decision-making. Modeling safe-driving behaviors, engaging your adolescent in preparation for driving, providing plenty of experience, setting clear, well-enforced rules, and making a point of recognizing good driving and appropriate safety habits all contribute to helping your adolescent become the safe and mature driver you hope he or she will be.

SUMMARY

Parents play a critical role in assuring that their children become safe drivers. The example you set will serve as a model for good or unsafe driving practices long before your children are old enough to get behind the wheel. Using teachable moments that naturally occur while in the car with your children will develop an early awareness of driving skills, how the car operates, and road safety. When your child reaches the age to obtain a learner's permit and take driver's lessons, encourage your child to get plenty of practice, but recognize that you may not make the best on-road teacher if your patience runs low and anxiety runs high. Once your child does earn a license, set and enforce safe driving practices and curfews. Remember that rewarding positive behavior, such as following the rules of the road and practicing safety measures like wearing a seatbelt, will usually prove much more effective than nervous criticism as you seek to encourage mature driving habits and responsibility.

WHERE TO FIND OUT MORE

Books

Berardelli, P. (2000). *Safe young drivers: A guide for parents and teens.* Vienna, VA: Nautilus.
Gravelle, K. (2005). *The driving book: Everything new drivers need to know but don't know to ask.* New York: Walker and Company.
Smith, T.C. (2006). *Crashproof your kids: Make your teen a safer, smarter driver.* New York: Fireside.

Websites

eHow
    http://www.ehow.com/how_2311166_teach-child-drive.html
Family Education
    http://life.familyeducation.com/teen-driving/teen/32797.html

CHAPTER 43

Cigarettes, Alcohol, and Drugs

Deborah R. Glasofer and David A. F. Haaga

You are reading the newspaper in the morning before work. Your 15-year old daughter sits across the table from you silently, looking sleepy and unenthusiastic about going to school. You read an item about a teenage movie star arrested for driving under the influence, and you wonder whether this is a good time to go over your rules about riding in a car with anyone who has been drinking or using drugs.

Your 14-year-old son has been testy with you lately and does not tell you much about what is going on in his life, guarding his privacy in all areas. On a Sunday afternoon, when he is out of the house, you put away some laundry in his room. As you go to pick up some clothes he has left on the floor, you realize that his shirt smells of cigarette smoke.

It is inevitable that, at some point in their lives, most adolescents will be exposed to cigarettes, alcohol, and drugs. They might have friends who misuse prescription medications. They might go to parties where their friends are drinking alcohol. They might have classmates who skip class to smoke cigarettes or marijuana. One way or another, the issue of substance use will come up, and parents need to be prepared to help their children cope with it.

WHAT CAN I DO TO HELP PREVENT DRUG/ALCOHOL/ TOBACCO USE BY MY CHILD?

Substance use in adolescence usually begins with some experimental use of tobacco and alcohol when it is available (e.g., at parties with friends), followed by regular use of marijuana (with continued use of tobacco and alcohol), and increasing experimentation with other drugs. Some parents think that adolescent substance use is a rite of passage that will be outgrown. The data are mixed however, and suggest that, while some teens may stop using drugs on their own, there is a 50% or more risk of continued problems with drugs. Age of onset of experimentation, family history of substance abuse, and a teens' general psychological functioning are among the factors that affect the likelihood of problematic substance use.

Given the incidence of drug, alcohol, and tobacco experimentation among youth, it is important for parents to consider their role in preventing substance abuse in their teens from an early age. A number of studies indicate that positive parenting behaviors can protect against adolescent substance use and progression. Positive parenting strategies include *monitoring* and *communicating openly* about your values and expectations. Maintaining these positive parenting practices has been demonstrated to protect against substance use over time.

Poor parental monitoring is a critical family factor in the initiation of early adolescent substance use, as studies indicate that early adolescent drug use often occurs in the adolescent's own home, in the absence of adult supervision. Monitoring substance use can be very similar to monitoring other aspects of your adolescent's behavior. Important features of monitoring include:

- *Know your child's friends.* It is essential to know who your teen socializes with, particularly because some studies indicate that, as teens progress through adolescence, the relative influence of peers on substance-use behaviors increases.
- *Keep in touch with your teen.* Adolescents can be responsible for checking in with parents or guardians at regular intervals. You can help your teen plan for check-ins ahead of time. Provide your child with a cell phone, and set up times for check-in calls. Call your teen periodically if she is going to be at home unsupervised for an extended time.
- *Communicate with other parents.* Compile a list of phone numbers, email addresses, and home addresses of your teen's peer's families, so that you can keep in touch with your teen as needed in case of emergency.
- *Maintain a current calendar of your teen's after-school activities, so that you always know where your child should be.* Many adolescents tend to get into trouble during after-school hours (3:00–6:00 P.M.). Adult-monitored group activities (e.g., sports team, youth group) may be helpful, particularly if they can be balanced with teens having moderate amounts of unstructured downtime with a responsible adult nearby.

Although monitoring your teenager and dealing with the resistance you are bound to be met with when attempting to "keep tabs" on her is challenging, it can be even more difficult to *communicate* effectively with your teen about illicit drugs, alcohol, and tobacco. Consequently, sometimes the information we try to provide our teens doesn't get through. A national study by the Partnership for a Drug-Free America found that, whereas the majority of parents say they have discussed use of drugs, alcohol, and tobacco with their children, only about one-fourth of teens reported that they learn about the risks of these substances at home.

The following are suggestions for ways to start a meaningful dialogue about substance use with your adolescent:

- *Keep in mind that it is not enough to discuss substance use once.* The dangers of alcohol, tobacco, and drugs should be part of an ongoing dialogue with your child.
- *Use current events as a learning moment.* It can be helpful to use current events (TV or newspaper stories), antidrug commercials, television programs or movies referencing substance use, and school discussions (e.g., health education programming on consequences of substance use) to jumpstart the dialogue in a natural, unforced manner.
- *Listen.* When you ask your teen questions, be a good listener by reflecting or paraphrasing answers, asking follow-up questions, and encouraging your child to ask you questions as well.
- *React to questions and comments in a way that will facilitate further conversation.* If your adolescent makes surprising comments, respond calmly.
- *Be honest.* Share what you know about drugs, alcohol, and tobacco use. Look up what you do not know together as a shared activity. Give some thought to what you would like to tell your children about your own history with the use of drugs, alcohol, and tobacco, and how this information can be provided along with a clear message about the risks of substance use.

Not all conversations about drugs, alcohol, and tobacco need to be lengthy. In fact, to keep communication open and ongoing, it is better for the dialogue to be punctuated with brief comments when the subject arises naturally. Brief interactions provide an opportunity to facilitate connectedness in the family. These conversations can also serve to reinforce rules and expectations regarding substance use, monitor your teens, and offer more education about the risks associated with various drugs. Studies indicate that adolescents' perceptions of connectedness with parents (e.g., feeling able to talk to a parent about their problems, valuing parents' opinions of serious situations) are inversely associated with substance use.

WHAT CAN I DO IF MY CHILD IS ALREADY USING ALCOHOL, ILLICIT DRUGS, OR CIGARETTES?

If you learn that your teen may have tried alcohol, drugs, and/or cigarettes, it is important to address the issue promptly, directly, and openly. The issue will not resolve itself on its own.

Approach your child in a nonjudgmental way, and be honest about why you suspect possible experimentation with substances. Tips for beginning this conversation include:

- *Practice ahead of time* (with your spouse or partner, if you have one) to help you stay calm and keep to the point during the dialogue.
- *Reference earlier discussions* you and your adolescent have had about possible negative consequences of substance use.

- *Gather information from your teen* with an ear toward empathizing with factors that may have contributed to the substance use (e.g., peer pressure, boredom, curiosity).
- *Remain firm* with regards to previously established family rules about consequences for substance use.

If your child continues to show evidence of substance use, it is important to acknowledge the issue and take action.

HOW CAN I HELP MY CHILD STOP SMOKING?

There has unfortunately been much less research on quitting smoking among adolescents than among adults, and it is not clear whether some of the treatments commonly used with adults (e.g., nicotine replacement, antidepressant medication) work well for teen smokers. From the research that is available, here are some guidelines for helping your adolescent son or daughter quit smoking:

- *First and foremost, do not smoke yourself.* If you already do smoke, choose now as the time to quit. Research shows that your quitting will make it less likely that your children will ever start smoking, and if they already are smokers, more likely that they will quit.
- *Back up your actions with words by delivering a clear anti-smoking message.* Adolescents are unlikely to sit still for lengthy diatribes on this subject, but take advantage of opportunities that present themselves. For example, express opposition when watching a movie together that depicts cigarette smoking.
- *Ban smoking inside your house or apartment.* Particularly for adolescents who have not yet developed a strong dependence on nicotine, simply making smoking inconvenient can help stop it. Like the government has done by raising cigarette taxes and banning smoking in restaurants and other public places in many cities and counties, you can increase the "cost" of smoking in your home.
- *Problem-solve.* Adolescents' motives for smoking vary, and girls appear to be more inclined to use smoking as a weight-control strategy. It might be especially important to help your daughter prepare for quitting smoking by planning healthy eating strategies and assessing her body image (review Chapter 44 for more information on promoting a healthy body image in your teen).

It is often difficult for teens to stick with formal smoking cessation programs or methods that play out over several months. It may make more sense to look for easily accessible programs that will, at least to some extent, come to your adolescent. Examples include:

- *Programs delivered at school.* In one study of high schools in Massachusetts, a quit-smoking program delivered by school nurses proved to be effective in helping teens quit, with students being six times as likely to quit in those schools that had the program as in those that did not. It may be possible to advocate for funding for such efforts in your child's school.

- *Programs delivered over the Internet.* These are not all created equal, and results have been mixed, but, at least in some cases, adolescents have fared well with web-based smoking-cessation materials. One study of a successful intervention tracked which pages were used the most and found that adolescents were much more likely to use interactive features (chatting with other teens trying to quit smoking) than informational pages with material about health consequences of smoking and the like. Such virtual communities may be a particularly agreeable way to provide the social support that many smokers find helpful as they attempt to quit.

- *Brief interventions aimed at increasing motivation.* These may occur in a number of settings (physician's office, schools, etc.), but the gist is that the focus is less on techniques and methods of quitting and more on eliciting and bolstering the adolescent's desire to quit smoking in the first place. Adolescents can't always relate to some of the motives commonly cited for quitting smoking, like cancer or heart disease, so it is important to supplement these considerations with short-term reasons for quitting that impact teens directly like saving money, smelling better, and being able to play sports.

- *Creative use of rewards.* One of our students quit smoking for good upon being promised a pickup truck from his parents for doing so. This might not be a fit for every family, but you could work with your teen to select some personally meaning-ful reward that she could earn for quitting smoking for, say, 3 months. Along the way to that goal, your child could use the money saved by not buying cigarettes to buy smaller fun rewards.

WHAT SHOULD I LOOK FOR IN A THERAPIST OR TREATMENT PROGRAM FOR DRUGS OR ALCOHOL?

The first step in addressing an alcohol or illicit drug problem is finding a trusted, profes-sional counselor or reputable treatment program. Many communities have established coalitions that can help with referral information, and local contact information can also be found online or through national organizations. Different types of treatment for addressing adolescent substance use are discussed in the sections that follow. Keep in mind that the intervention an adolescent receives should be appropriate to his or her level of involvement with drugs and/or alcohol.

Outpatient Treatment

Outpatient counseling, which includes individual, family, and/or group psychotherapy, is a mainstay of treatment among adolescents with substance-use disorders. It is appropriate for teens who are in need of mental health resources, but who do not require hospitalization. The length of outpatient interventions varies substantially and can often be tailored to the needs of the particular individual. Research indicates that even brief treatments of only a few sessions can have a positive effect in reducing or eliminating illicit drug and alcohol use. However, when considering outpatient psychotherapy, it is important that an adolescent is committed to working on substance-abuse issues, has a strong external support system, and relates well to the outpatient counselor.

Individual therapy methods include motivational interviewing and cognitive-behavioral therapy (CBT). Motivational interviewing aims to help adolescents grapple with their ambivalence about changing substance-use behaviors. Ambivalence about change is viewed as normal and acceptable, and the counseling provides a nonhostile environment in which the teen's thoughts about substance use are acknowledged and explored. The goal of this approach is to increase a teen's awareness and help her make gradual adjustments toward behavior change through improved motivation. Motivational counseling has been demonstrated as effective in reducing drug and alcohol use by adolescents. This intervention appeals to teens because it is typically a brief treatment and is characterized by a nonconfrontational approach.

CBT teaches teens to explore the connections between their thoughts and feelings, and to understand how these affect their behavior. In particular, adolescents are encouraged to identify problematic thinking and emotional triggers that cue their substance use. As treatment progresses, adolescents explore the consequences of their substance use. The ultimate goals are to learn how to identify circumstances that lead to substance use and to either avoid these situations or use healthier coping strategies.

The aim of family psychotherapy is to address a teen's substance use within the context of the family network. This approach stems from research indicating that parents and caretakers play an essential part in treatment, recovery, and relapse-prevention of adolescent drug and alcohol use. Certain kinds of family therapy have been shown to be helpful, particularly those in which parents and guardians effectively monitor their teen's behavior, encourage healthy choices through positive reinforcement and rewards, and consistently use negative consequences for inappropriate or risky behavior.

Group psychotherapy is a commonly used treatment type for adolescent substance-abuse treatment. Twelve-step group programs, such as the model used by Alcoholics Anonymous (AA) and Narcotics Anonymous (NA), are mainstays of adult group treatment programs but have not been as widely researched in adolescents. In contrast, several research studies have compared cognitive-behavioral group psychotherapy (centered on skills training, problem-solving, and role-playing) with broadly defined supportive group psychotherapy (aimed at building trust, support, and providing an environment in which teens can safely share their thoughts and feelings with their peers) for teens with substance abuse. A recent review of multiple outpatient intervention studies determined that non cognitive-behavioral psychotherapy groups (i.e., supportive group psychotherapy) performed unfavorably (e.g., had poorer immediate treatment outcome) when compared to cognitive-behavioral group interventions for the treatment of adolescent substance abuse. Thus, it is either advisable to consider group treatment programs that include a cognitive-behavioral approach or to rely on other types of treatment, such as individual or family psychotherapy, with documented empirical support.

Day Treatment

Day treatment (partial hospitalization) may be appropriate for teens who require more intensive psychotherapy than outpatient treatment and who have a stable and secure home environment to return to each evening. Adolescents typically work with a multi-disciplinary treatment team that can offer a range of therapeutic services, including individual, family, and group psychotherapy. Often, tutoring is provided between sessions. Little data have been gathered on day treatment services, but some studies indicate that teens participating in partial hospitalization have similar rates of program completion and reduction in substance use as compared with teens receiving a higher level of care, such as inpatient hospitalization (discussed next).

Inpatient Treatment

Inpatient treatment options include detoxification, acute residential treatment, and ongoing residential programs. Detoxification programs offer medical monitoring of patients who are experiencing severe withdrawal symptoms. This process is typically accomplished prior to rehabilitation (outpatient or inpatient). Research indicates that detoxification is not an adequate treatment in and of itself for long-term recovery.

Acute residential care is designed to be a short-term placement to defuse crisis situations by providing a safe environment until teens can successfully transition to outpatient treatment. This is typically conceptualized as the start to a treatment process, and may last from a few days to a week.

In contrast, ongoing residential programs offer comprehensive treatment services for an extended period of time. This level of care is most appropriate for adolescents whose substance use has resulted in a substantial disturbance in their functioning at home and in school. These centers provide therapy, schooling, and activities in a structured and supervised environment beneficial to teens who are at greater risk to themselves or others by virtue of their substance abuse.

SUMMARY

Drug use is a complex issue confronted by all parents. Your involvement could at one point be as innocuous as pointing out a discarded cigarette butt on the ground and admonishing your 8-year-old never to start smoking, or at another point as heart-rending as needing to pick out the fifth treatment program to try for an adolescent who has committed burglary to support a heroin habit. But whatever your family's circumstance, your child is likely to fare best if you can stay involved, persistent, connected, and compassionate. Your loving concern, and your wisdom in knowing when to call on professional help, will be your child's best weapon against the perils associated with cigarettes, alcohol, and illicit drug use.

WHERE TO FIND OUT MORE

Treatment Facility Locator
  http://findtreatment.samhsa.gov/
  or call 1-800-662-HELP

Advice and Information for Parents
  http://www.theantidrug.com/
Teen Smoking
How to help your teen quit smoking
  http://www.mayoclinic.com/health/teen-smoking/TN00016
Staying Connected with your Teen program
  http://channing-bete.com/prevention-programs/staying-connected-w-your-teen/?src=em

CHAPTER 44

Body Image and Physical Appearance Concerns

Heather Shaw and Eric Stice

In the middle of a family dinner, your teenage daughter abruptly exclaims, "I can't eat that pasta—I'm already way too fat!" As a parent, you don't know how to respond, other than to say, "That's ridiculous, you look fine, now eat up and stop worrying!" Later, you wonder why your daughter thinks she's too fat, what caused this concern, and how you might respond to her in a better way in the future. You want to help her improve her feelings about her body and overall self-image.

When you pick up your adolescent son after basketball practice, he says, "Mom, I don't think I'll ever be big enough to compete with Max on the court—I just don't have the right build! I wish I weren't so small!" This may seem like an innocuous statement reflecting a physical reality, but it could suggest a deeper discontent your son has with his body that is affecting his life beyond the basketball court. How can you help him feel better about himself?

These scenarios will seem familiar to many American families. As parents, relating to what our adolescents experience can prove a challenge, and our responses to their concerns can seem more emotionally reactive than productive.

During adolescence, girls experience physical changes and social pressures that can make dealing with every-day issues, particularly those surrounding eating and body image, a distressing experience. They find their bodies may be developing in a way that seems different from what our society and their peers define as attractive. They also find others reacting to them in new ways, based on their evolving body shape. It is important to understand how our culture propagates messages about how being thin and attractive contribute to a women's success, so that you will know how to help your daughter navigate this developmental period.

Many boys feel dissatisfied with their bodies, sometimes wishing they were taller and bulkier, rather than skinnier. This discontent reflects the "muscular male" body ideal promoted by our culture. Because body dissatisfaction and eating disorders occur much less often among boys than girls, research has focused more on girls. However, similar to girls, the dissatisfaction many boys feel with their bodies can lead to feelings of inferiority or low self-esteem.

Body dissatisfaction among adolescents is so widespread that we consider it almost normal. Approximately 60% of girls and 30% of boys report wanting to change their body size or shape, and nearly 25% of adolescent girls report significant body dissatisfaction. How does this discontent translate into maladaptive behaviors? An estimated 12% of girls and 5% of boys report using extreme weight-loss strategies (e.g., fasting, use of diet pills, laxative abuse, or vomiting), and an estimated 12% of boys report frequently using or thinking about using food supplements or steroids to gain muscle bulk. Further, body dissatisfaction increases the risk for a variety of problems such as depression, substance use, and eating disorders.

What causes adolescents to harbor negative feelings about their bodies? How can we protect our children against endorsing a cultural standard that defies reality and is very difficult to attain? In this chapter, we will discuss the prevalence of body image concerns, what factors influence body image concerns and thus can be altered to prevent developing negative body image, and strategies that parents can use to help their adolescents overcome negative feelings about their bodies and develop a positive sense of body and self.

THE DEVELOPMENT OF BODY IMAGE

Sociocultural (cultural emphasis on thinness), biological (body size, genetic factors), and psychological (low self-esteem, depression) factors all contribute to body dissatisfaction. Sociocultural factors can foster body dissatisfaction through repeated messages from parents, peers, dating partners, and the media suggesting the universal acceptance of a thinner or bulkier, more attractive ideal to aspire to. These messages arrive directly, such as through a parent or other adult (e.g., sports coaches, ballet instructors, etc.) telling a child that he or she needs to lose or gain weight. They also arrive indirectly by repeated exposure to advertisements showing skinny female models or muscular male models, as well as in ads for diet pills or supplements. These forces can prove very powerful and difficult to fight, especially given that people who fit the narrow standards of beauty created by society are viewed as being more competent, more attractive, and better adjusted. In addition, they generally get treated better than those considered unattractive. These sociocultural forces are particularly damaging for females, as appearance remains central to the female gender role and evaluation of women in Western culture. This is in direct contrast to the traditional male gender role that focuses more on external accomplishments.

During adolescence, when body dissatisfaction emerges, the weight gain typically associated with this developmental period moves girls further away from the thin-ideal body type. Even though girls as young as 7 recognize and endorse the thin-ideal, this does not seem to translate into overall body discontent until adolescence, when they begin to feel intense social pressure to be thin. Similarly, boys' preference for a large and muscular-ideal male body appears to develop between 6 and 7 years of age. Studies have found that boys who reported trying to look like celebrities or sports figures would more likely develop weight concerns and begin altering their diets. In contrast to females however, the strong muscular physique of the male ideal plays out more consistently with their natural development, as boys typically gain both muscle and fat mass during adolescence and thus move closer to the muscular stereotype. This might explain the lower percentage of boys experiencing body dissatisfaction.

Higher body mass or increases in body mass becomes the most reliable biological predictor of body dissatisfaction in girls and boys. Girls who are more overweight than their peers or their ideal cultural standard appear most dissatisfied with their bodies. We know less about the relationship for boys, as this is complicated by the fact that boys appear to split between those wanting to be thinner and those wishing they had bigger muscles. In addition to deviating from the thin-ideal, the heavier girls become, the more pressure they probably receive to lose weight. Body dissatisfaction appears to increase for girls with the onset of puberty and accompanying weight gain. Fortunately, girls appear to become increasingly more satisfied with their bodies as they get older. Interestingly, research suggests that girls feel dissatisfied with their bodies regardless of their objective weight, whereas boys' dissatisfaction focuses more on objective standards of excess weight.

Psychological factors also interact with these sociocultural and biological forces to impact body dissatisfaction. The evidence on how unpleasant emotions affect body dissatisfaction among girls and boys shows mixed results. Some research findings suggest that low self-esteem puts boys at higher risk for endorsing the muscular-ideal and to pursue it through attempts to increase muscle mass. However, because the population of boys shows a split between those wanting to be bigger and those wanting to be smaller, some studies have found that boys who endorse sociocultural standards of appearance attempt to gain weight, and others attempt to lose weight. Other psychological factors, such as social support, play a role in the development and maintenance of body dissatisfaction, although the evidence of this also seems inconsistent. Girls with more social support might report less body dissatisfaction, because friends provide positive feedback on one's attractiveness. However, the relationship could also conceivably operate in reverse, as a strong social network could translate into peer pressure to conform to the thin-ideal and thus lead to greater body dissatisfaction.

This summary suggests that both girls and boys experience high levels of body dissatisfaction, influenced by sociocultural, biological, and psychological forces. In the next section, we present strategies shown to successfully prevent body dissatisfaction and explain how parents can implement these at home.

HOW CAN I IMPROVE MY CHILD'S BODY SATISFACTION?

Several exercises developed to help protect children against sociocultural forces and to improve body satisfaction can easily become a part of family life. These exercises focus on helping children identify ways in which their thoughts about their bodies contribute to negative body image, and how they can learn to think more positively about their bodies.

Healthy weight and exercise changes that can be incorporated into your family's lifestyle are also discussed.

Cognitive Behavioral Therapy

Interventions based on cognitive-behavioral therapy (CBT) can successfully remedy conditions associated with negative body image, such as depression and anxiety, and increase body satisfaction. In these interventions, participants learn ways to challenge errors in their thinking related to body image. Participants are encouraged to gain more self-awareness around thoughts related to their bodies, and to challenge them if they're potentially harmful. You can try some exercises based on these interventions with your children at home:

- Help your child identify thoughts that might reinforce negative body image, and help her challenge these thoughts. For instance, your daughter may think, "Everyone thinks my thighs are fat." However, when you probe her about how she knows this, she can't name one person who has ever said anything that would confirm this.
- To help your child recognize positive physical attributes, have her stand in front of the mirror and list five things she likes about her body.
- Individual behavior challenges also prove helpful for combating body dissatisfaction. These exercises ask adolescents to engage in an activity involving a public display of something physical that they previously avoided because of body image concerns. For example, a teenage girl who avoids wearing shorts because she thinks her legs are fat could challenge herself to wear shorts to a picnic or other social event. A boy who avoids wearing tank tops because he believes his arms are too skinny could work out after school in a tank top for a week. For another teen who had longstanding concerns about the appearance of her ears, this exercise could entail pulling her hair back into a ponytail so that her ears show. These challenges should help adolescents disprove their own negative thoughts about their bodies (e.g., that people will comment on their "flabby" arms) and stop the avoidance that often serves to maintain body image concerns.

Cognitive Dissonance

Cognitive dissonance refers to an uncomfortable set of feelings that get triggered when people acts or thinks in a manner inconsistent with a previously held belief. This leads to a state of dissonance, or mental tension, which can shift their thinking away from their initial beliefs. Psychologists have used this general human tendency by designing programs that strategically induce such tensions to reduce unrealistic or inappropriate body image concerns. *The Body Project* published by Oxford University Press (Stice & Presnell, 2007) is an example of one such intervention. Designed for groups of adolescent and college-aged girls, the program asks participants to complete a series of verbal, written, and behavioral exercises critiquing the thin-ideal. For example, girls take part in role-plays in which they try to counter pro-thin ideal statements. Another exercise asks participants to write a letter to an imaginary girl alerting her to the dangers of pursuing the thin-ideal. We believe that asking boys who have internalized the muscular-ideal to similarly critique this ideal would also promote body acceptance. This same notion could be used at home in the following ways:

- Have your daughter discuss a scenario in which someone engages in "fat talk" (as illustrated in the first case example in the chapter). Have her generate statements to combat this type of talk. For example, a friend mentions to her that she really wants to get down to a size 2 because she feels fat in her size 4 jeans. Have your daughter think of reasons why this is unfounded (e.g., she looks great the way she is, she should not care about what other people think, etc.).
- Have your son think of a scenario when someone engages in talk that reinforces the muscular-ideal. For example, after school, a friend tells him he seems too skinny to make the football team. Have your son generate reasons why he should see that remark as unreasonable (e.g., he has a lean physique that makes it hard to see his muscles, he has agility as an athlete and agility matters more than bulk; he doesn't want to play football anyway!).

These exercises should help your child realize that, often, friends, family, and other adults reinforce the slender and muscular ideals without even being aware that they have done it. It can also prove useful to discuss the costs of pursuing the thin-ideal or muscular-ideal. In addition, you can practice accepting appearance-related compliments, which can help adolescents overcome the shame often associated with recognizing and accepting the positive physical attributes that they possess.

Body Activism

Cognitive dissonance-based programs like The Body Project and Reflections (a program for college women that is available nationwide through a large sorority system) incorporate aspects of CBT, such as addressing and challenging irrational thoughts, and exercises such as *body activism*. Think of body activism as private or public acts of resistance to the thin-ideal. These activities target the sociocultural forces that impact body dissatisfaction on both the individual and structural level.

One good strategy asks adolescents to generate ideas about the top 10 ways to challenge the thin- or muscular-ideal. These exercises often involve confronting advertisers and other direct proponents of thin-ideal messages to suggest alternatives to marketing a beauty standard beyond the reach of most adolescents. For example, an adolescent could write a letter to a company stating that she opposes using only thin models in the company's advertising. Adolescents could also write letters threatening to cancel subscriptions to magazines that include diet ads, or write letters to stores that use only thin mannequins in their displays. Other body activism exercises target the diet industry. One adolescent snuck into several bookstores and inserted Post-its® saying "You look great the way you are" into diet books. Several youth have also hung large signs in school bathrooms with sayings such as "Love your body." Body activism exercises that challenge the social pressures for thinness in the adolescent's microenvironment (schools, dance classes, sports teams) can prove particularly powerful, as they may directly affect change in external pressures for thinness or muscularity.

All of these exercises empower the adolescent to actively challenge damaging messages that contribute to body dissatisfaction. Parents might successfully apply these exercises by incorporating them in a family setting, one-on-one with one's child, or in a more organized fashion, such as a parent-initiated after-school group that could involve multiple adolescents and their families. Some of these ideas could also prove useful in the context of organized sports. Parents and/or coaches could work with groups of young girls and boys to work on these exercises.

Healthy Weight and Exercise Changes

While some adolescents who experience body dissatisfaction have a distorted view of their actual weight (i.e., thinking that they're overweight when they're actually healthy or underweight), some are legitimately overweight or obese. For these adolescents, healthy weight loss is an appropriate strategy for enhancing body image. Moreover, it is important to address weight problems because most obese children and adolescents will become obese adults, and because obesity at even this young age links to serious health problems such as diabetes and high blood pressure. Promising new research on healthy weight interventions suggests that programs encouraging small, gradual changes to diet and exercise can lead to sustainable increases in body satisfaction. For example, people seem able to make gradual healthy dietary changes and gradual physical activity changes to their weekly regimen that, over time, help youth achieve and maintain a healthy weigh and body satisfaction. Some suggestions that can help your child and entire family make healthy changes include:

- *Snack healthy.*   Encourage your child to substitute an unhealthy snack (e.g., potato chips or cookies) with fruit, vegetables, or nuts.
- *Eliminate unhealthy food from your immediate food environment (the home).*   Similarly, try to avoid going to restaurants that serve unhealthy food or buying unhealthy snacks from vending machines.
- *Encourage your child to add strength training to an existing exercise routine,* or to meet a friend twice a week to work out.
- *Add creative exercise to your family's life.*   For example, walk or bike to school, if possible. Park farther away from your destination, and use the stairs rather than the elevator when you can.

This incremental approach to achieving a healthy lifestyle seems more likely to succeed than a traditional approach that requires drastic changes simultaneously. Exercise can improve body satisfaction as it potentially enhances awareness of physical capabilities, while reducing awareness of physical appearance. Broader structural changes also provide an important issue to consider. These might include working to change the content of school vending machines and school lunch offerings, and offering more physical education to students. However, parents have less control over these structural changes, which often fall under the influence of governmental education budgets and school policies. Teaching your children strategies to achieve and maintain healthy bodies through gradual lifestyle changes can be very empowering and lead to higher body satisfaction, and hopefully overall greater well-being.

SUMMARY

Our culture sends conflicting and confusing messages to adolescents that simultaneously espouse the importance of striving to achieve a thin-ideal while bombarding us with advertisements stressing the allure of fast-foods, high-calorie energy drinks, and sugary cereals. Parents often find themselves confused regarding how best to achieve a healthy, active lifestyle in a sustainable way. We have shown how you can help your adolescent question these messages through some simple cognitive exercises and healthy lifestyle changes. We hope this chapter has provided you with some tools to help your adolescent achieve a higher level of body satisfaction and general well-being, and a healthy skepticism of misleading cultural messages that can leave us with a feeling of discontent and powerlessness.

WHERE TO FIND OUT MORE

Books

Brumberg, J.J. (1998). *The Body Project: An intimate history of American girls.* New York: Knopf. Also see http://www.thebodyproject.com/

Chadwick, D. (2009). *You'd be so pretty if...* Philadelphia: DaCapo Press.

Herrin, M., & Matsumoto, N. (2007). *The parent's guide to eating disorders: Supporting self-esteem, healthy eating, and positive body image at home.* New York: Gurze Books.

Lock, J., & le Grange, D. (2004). *Help your teenage beat an eating disorder.* New York: Guilford.

Lonczak, H. (2006). *Mookey the Monkey gets over being teased.* Washington, DC: Magination Press.

Schechter, L.R. (2009). *My big fat secret: How Jenna takes control of her emotions and eating.* Washington, DC: Magination Press.

Websites

American Psychological Association
   http://www.apa.org/topics/eating/index.aspx
Reflections Body Image Program
   http://www.bodyimageprogram.org/
Substance Abuse and Mental Health Services Administration
   http://mentalhealth.samhsa.gov/publications/allpubs/CA-0006/default.asp
The Nemours Foundation
   http://kidshealth.org/parent/emotions/feelings/bdd.html?tracking=P_RelatedArticle
National Association of Social Workers
   http://www.naswdc.org/practice/adolescent_health/ah0204.asp

CHAPTER 45

Suicide Risk and Self-injury

John D. Guerry, Nadja N. Reilly, and Mitchell J. Prinstein

Your 16-year-old daughter, Maria, swallowed 43 pills last night and had to be rushed to the hospital. You had no idea she was depressed, let alone suicidal. You wonder how you missed the signs. On the face of things Maria is a normal, happy girl who does well in school and has many friends. She is outgoing and friendly, but in the days after the attempt she stops eating and sleeping and withdraws from those closest to her.

Your 14-year-old son, Reggie, secretly has been cutting himself on his legs where no one can see the bruise. He does not want to die, but says that he feels a lot better after he cuts himself, especially if he can make himself bleed just a little. Reggie has been having a lot of stress, and has a hard time calming himself down.

For parents few burdens feel as heavy as the fear that their adolescent child may be at risk for suicide. But some comfort may come from knowing that many others share this burden—parents and children alike. It may also come as a comfort for both parents and adolescents to arm themselves with certain fundamental truths about suicide. To begin with, suicide can touch the lives of anyone, regardless of ethnicity, gender, age, or economic circumstance. Moreover, an adolescent's experience of feeling suicidal is fairly common; among high school-aged students, nearly two out of ten girls and more than one of ten boys report that they have seriously contemplated suicide at some point in the past year. Thankfully, in the end, most of these individuals decide to live by coming to realize a life-sustaining truth: Life crises are usually temporary, suicide is always permanent.

Most importantly, *suicide is preventable.* Most suicidal adolescents desperately want to live, but struggle to see alternative solutions to their problems. Additionally, as this chapter addresses in detail, suicide is often not a silent killer, even though an adolescent considering suicide may not directly verbalize the extent of his or her despair to others. Indeed, the majority (~75%) of suicidal individuals give some definite warnings of their intentions to harm themselves to a friend or family member. As is all too often the case, however, important members of an adolescent's social circle seem either unaware of the significance of these signals or do not know how to respond to them. For parents, it is a normal tendency to initially deny that something serious might be occurring, or to attribute a change in your child's emotions or behaviors to "growing pains," or simply due to "adolescence."

In this chapter, we hope to raise a culture of awareness and acuity among significant figures within the adolescent's support system. As with any preventable tragedy, parents and other central caregivers often remain an adolescent's most reliable line of defense. First, we broadly highlight several important facts and figures about adolescent suicide to characterize and contextualize the nature of this public health problem. After all, adolescent self-harm represents not just a personal crisis but a national imperative as well.

Second, we bring the latest in research and clinical expertise to bear on the problem of adolescent self-injury. It is essential for others to learn to recognize and respond appropriately to the list of general risk factors and early warning signs. Third, and most critically, we outline strategies to help prevent a suicide crisis, as well as present several concrete guidelines for how to respond in case one happens. We sincerely hope that this information will provide both parents and adolescents with some level of comfort, clarity, resolve, and, above all, the necessary catalyst for action. Finally, we conclude the chapter by calling attention to the increasing and related problem of adolescent nonsuicidal self-injury.

SUICIDE STATISTICS

According to most recent national estimates, suicide is the fifth leading cause of death among children aged 5–14 years, and the third leading cause of death for adolescents between the ages of 15 and 24, behind only accidents and homicides. To put the seriousness of this epidemic into perspective, each day approximately 12 youths under the age of 25 die by suicide in the United States; this roughly corresponds to one youth suicide every 2 hours and 11 minutes. Alarmingly, for every completed adolescent suicide, between 100 and 200 adolescents attempt to take their own life. According to most recent figures provided by the Centers for Disease Control and Prevention, the overall prevalence of suicide attempts is higher among Black (7.7%) and Hispanic (10.2%) than White (5.6%) high school-aged students.

The American Association of Suicidology, examining research findings and national statistics, concluded that the majority of adolescent suicides occur after school hours, in the teen's home, and are most often precipitated by interpersonal conflicts. Although firearms remain the most commonly used method of youth suicide, contributing to an estimated 49% of all completed suicides among adolescents aged 10–19 years, rates of suicide by suffocation (mostly hanging) (38%) have been increasing within this age group. Statistics on attempted adolescent suicide, however, reveal that drug overdoses are by far the most common method. There also appears to be a fairly striking difference in the patterns of suicidal adolescent girls and boys. Adolescent girls attempt suicide more than twice as often as adolescent boys, but adolescent boys are nearly five times as likely to complete suicide.

SUICIDE, DEPRESSION, AND OTHER MENTAL DISORDERS

Studies overwhelmingly indicate that the single best way to prevent suicide involves early recognition and treatment of mental illnesses. In fact, the vast majority (over 90%) of individuals who die by suicide in the United States had a mental or emotional disorder that was or could have been diagnosed at the time of their death. But tragically, very few of these individuals received adequate treatment.

The two most common diagnostic categories or profiles of adolescents who engage in suicidal behaviors are the *impulsive-aggressive* type and the *depressed-perfectionistic* type.

Impulsive-aggressive adolescents:

- Are often diagnosed with conduct disorder, a disorder characterized by chronic behavior problems. Overall, as many as 30% of adolescents who attempt suicide and 22% of completed suicides involve features of conduct disorder, such as aggression, destruction of property, and school truancy.
- Demonstrate pronounced irritability, extreme sensitivity, and intense reactions to frustration, and an impulsive approach to problem solving.

Depressed-perfectionistic adolescents (like Maria who was described at the beginning of the chapter):

- Often suffer from symptoms of depression, such as persistent feelings of hopelessness, self-defeat, shame, guilt, and loneliness, as well as a tendency to use or abuse alcohol and/or other substances.
- Often possess an ambitious but rigid personality type, and have a high need for approval from others, an exquisite sensitivity to criticism, and typically strong reactions to failure or loss.

Some additional key facts to remember are:

- *Most depressed people do not feel suicidal, but most suicidal people do feel depressed.* Over 60% of all people who die by suicide suffer from major depression; approximately 30% of all clinically depressed individuals attempt suicide, and about half of these people (~15%) will ultimately die by suicide.
- *Today's children are at a higher risk for depression than any previous generation.* As many as 9% of children will experience a major depressive episode by the time they are 14 years old, and 20% will experience a major depressive episode before graduating from high school.
- *Alcohol and drug use, which often accompany depression, increase the risk of suicide.* In one study, approximately 37% of completed adolescent suicides and 12.5% of

adolescents who contemplated or attempted suicide had abused alcohol or other drugs.

While these statistics cause concern, safe and effective treatments are available for most of these adolescents. Treatments include medication, psychotherapy, family therapy, and group therapy. In particular, cognitive-behavioral therapy (CBT) and interpersonal therapy can significantly improve symptoms of youth depression. There are vital lessons, of course, for the role that parents can play in therapy and getting it under way. It is important for parents to become familiar with the various symptoms of depression and pay close attention to signs that your adolescent may be struggling with these or other mental health difficulties.

SUICIDE RISK FACTORS AND WARNING SIGNS

The sections that follow describe general risk factors commonly found among people who attempt suicide, along with certain warning signs that may indicate impending self-injurious behavior (see italics). Parents and others can help prevent adolescent suicide by learning to recognize these features, taking them seriously, and knowing how to respond to them.

- *Mental health disorders.* As previously discussed, the presence of mental health problems puts an adolescent at high risk for suicide. The most serious of these include severe depression; conduct disorder; bipolar disorder; personality disorders, especially borderline or antisocial; certain anxiety disorders, such as post-traumatic stress disorder (PTSD), bulimia, or anorexia nervosa; and schizophrenia. In particular, pay attention to:
  - *Increases in observable signs of depression,* such as unrelenting low mood, pessimism, hopelessness, desperation, irritability, sleep problems, and/or social isolation and withdrawal from friends and family.
  - *Sudden anxiety & agitation.* In younger adolescents, aged 10–14 years, mounting symptoms of depression often link closely to anxiety. These youngsters may seem fearful, nervous, more "clingy" with caretakers, and report physical problems, such as headaches and stomachaches. Older adolescents often continue to have symptoms of anxiety, but they additionally experience more guilt, hopelessness, and increased thoughts of death and suicide.
- *Previous suicide attempts.* Between 20% and 50% of people who ultimately commit suicide have made one or more previous suicide attempts. Those who made more serious, life-threatening attempts, or those who expressed regret that the attempt failed, are at much higher risk for eventually killing themselves.
- *Use of drugs and/or alcohol in excess.* The risk of suicide among those who abuse alcohol or drugs is approximately 50%–70% higher than the general population. *Notice especially any sudden use or increased usage of alcohol and/or drugs.*
- *Impulsive and/or aggressive behavior.* Adolescents who exhibit sudden, unexpected rage, anger, or severe irritability, and/or those who demonstrate a pattern of impulsive behavior are more likely to act on suicidal thoughts and feelings.

- *Recklessness:* increases in impulsiveness and/or unnecessary, risk-taking behaviors; suddenly breaking rules such as skipping school or running away from home.
- *Access to firearms.* As noted previously, guns are used in the majority of adolescent suicides. Of those households containing guns, approximately 83% of gun-related deaths are the result of suicide, often by someone other than the gun owner.
- *Genetic or familial predisposition.* Research has shown that a family history of suicide, suicide attempts, depression, or other psychiatric illnesses significantly raises the risk that an adolescent will self-injure.
- *Past death of a friend or loved one, especially if by suicide.* A recent exposure to another person's suicidal behavior can be particularly dangerous.
- *Suicidal ideation.* Threatening suicide, expressing a strong wish to die, or more generally communicating thoughts of death, dying, or the afterlife. For adolescents, this preoccupation with death may take the form of an interest in death-related music and art.
- *Making various suicide plans.* Writing a suicide note, giving away prized possessions, purchasing a firearm or obtaining/putting into place other means of killing oneself (e.g., poisons, medications, etc.).
- *Feeling trapped.* Exhibiting rigid thinking, such as believing that there are no solutions and nothing will help.
- *Recent stressor(s) or precipitating event.* Presence of stressful life events that are either objectively severe (e.g., loss of a loved one, difficulties related to sexual orientation, unplanned pregnancy) or feel very important to the adolescent (e.g., failing a test, breaking up with a boyfriend/girlfriend, a serious argument with parents).

In addition to behavioral signs, it is important to listen for language that signals increased hopelessness, despair, or thoughts of death. Worrying statements that adolescents may make include, "Nothing matters anymore," "I'd be better off dead," or "I won't be a problem for you much longer."

WHAT CAN I DO IF MY CHILD IS SUICIDAL?

Being confronted with suicidality in a child is one of the most frightening experiences a parent can ever encounter. During a suicide crisis, there are many important things you can do:

- *Be aware.* Trust and listen to your instincts. Learn the warning signs.
- *Get involved.* Be available to your child, both physically and emotionally.
- *Take it seriously.* ALL suicide threats and attempts must be taken seriously.
- *Do not leave your child alone.* Closely monitor your child until help becomes available.
- *Show interest and support; listen and ask questions:*
  - *Don't be afraid to be direct.* Take the initiative to ask what is troubling your child and persist to overcome any reluctance to talk about it. If your child or adolescent is depressed, ask directly if he or she is considering suicide. It is all right to ask if your child has a specific plan or method in mind. *Using the word "suicide" will NOT increase chances that your child will take his or her own life.*

- *Do NOT attempt to "argue" your child out of suicide.* Instead, let your child know you care and understand. Assure your child that he or she is not alone, suicidal feelings are temporary, depression can be treated, problems can be solved, and you will always be there for them.
- *Safeguard the area.* Remove and encourage your child to give up anything he or she could use to hurt themselves(e.g., guns, knives or other sharp objects, pills, etc.). Not only will removing these items potentially reduce the chance of an impulsive suicide, but it will also show your concern and ability to intervene on your child's behalf.
- *Seek professional help.* Take your child for an immediate evaluation in an emergency room. If you believe your child will not be safe during the drive to the hospital, call 911 for an ambulance. You may also consult with the **National Suicide Prevention Lifeline** [http://www.suicidepreventionlifeline.org/] **at 1-800-273-TALK (1-800-273-8255).**
- *Follow-up on treatment.* Take an active role in facilitating your child's access and adherence to treatment. This may entail accompanying your child to therapy or making sure your child is taking medication(s). Pay attention to possible medication side effects, and be sure to notify the physician. Often, alternative medications can be prescribed. Advocate for your child; don't be afraid to push "the system" to make it work.

NONSUICIDAL SELF-INJURY

Another, much less well understood type of adolescent self-injury has been gaining increased attention. Nonsuicidal self-injury (NSSI)—which refers to such nonlethal behaviors as skin cutting, carving, or burning; head banging; or hair pulling—can be defined as deliberately harming oneself in the absence of suicidal intent. Reggie, discussed at the beginning of this chapter, is a good illustration of this problem. NSSI does not include some forms of painful body alteration (e.g., tattoos or body piercings) that are deemed acceptable by society. Although NSSI has been recognized as a widespread public health problem, these behaviors occur most frequently among youth. Research has estimated that 7% of middle school-aged children and nearly 14% of high school-aged adolescents have engaged in NSSI at some point in their lives.

Although, by definition, adolescent NSSI behaviors do not themselves qualify as imminently life-threatening, parents should nonetheless remain alert to them and respond accordingly. First and foremost, the fact that an adolescent has engaged in any kind of self-harm clearly indicates extreme distress. In fact, a majority of individuals perform NSSI as a desperate attempt to alleviate intensely negative feelings. Second, regardless of whether the intention to commit suicide is present, some types of self-injury can sometimes lead to accidental death. Finally, and most troubling, some authorities have warned that the repetitive engagement in NSSI may serve as "suicide training." Individuals who regularly injure themselves, whether consciously or not, may be desensitizing themselves to the physical and psychological repercussions of suicide. Thus, the same essential ingredients (i.e., offering compassionate support, seeking urgent professional help, etc.) outlined for suicidal behaviors should follow in response to an adolescent's nonsuicidal self-harm.

SUMMARY

Many parents are understandably concerned that their adolescent child may be at risk for suicide. In fact, adolescents commonly report that they have seriously contemplated suicide at some point in the past year. However, it is important for parents to know that *suicide is preventable*. The single best way to prevent adolescent suicide is to recognize and obtain treatment for adolescents' mental health problems.

This chapter provided information so that parents might recognize and respond appropriately to general risk factors and early warning signs of adolescent suicide. The chapter also outlined strategies to help prevent a suicide crisis, and provided concrete guidelines for how parents can respond if a crisis should arise. Finally, the chapter called attention to the related problem of adolescent NSSI, and what parents can do to help their adolescent child.

WHERE TO FIND OUT MORE

Books

Beardslee, W.R. (2002). *Out of the darkened room: Protecting the children and strengthening the family when a parent is depressed.* Boston: Little, Brown, and Company.

Ellis, T.E., & Newman, C.F. (1996). *Choosing to live: How to defeat suicide through cognitive therapy.* Oakland, CA: New Harbinger Publications.

Goldsmith, S.K., Pellmar, T.C., Kleinman, A.M., & Bunney, W.E. (Eds.). (2002). *Reducing suicide: A national imperative.* Washington, DC: The National Acamedies Press.

Gordon, S. (2004). *When living hurts: For teenagers, young adults, their parents, leaders, and counselors* (Rev. ed.). New York: URJ Press.

Joiner, T.E. (2005). *Why people die by suicide.* Cambridge, MA: Harvard University Press.

Websites

American Association of Suicidology. (2008a).
Youth Suicide Fact Sheet
   http://www.suicidology.org/associations/1045/files/2005Youth.pdf
American Association of Suicidology. (2008b).
Suicide in the U.S.A.
   http://www.suicidology.org/associations/1045/files/SuicideInTheUS.pdf
American Foundation for Suicide Prevention. (2008a).
When you fear someone may take their life. http://www.afsp.org/index.cfm?fuseaction=home.
   viewpage&page_id=050FEA9F-B064-4092-B1135C3A70DE1FDA
American Foundation for Suicide Prevention. (2008b).
Risk factors for suicide.
http://www.afsp.org/index.cfm?fuseaction=home.viewPage&page_id=05147440-E24E-E376-
   BDF4BF8BA6444E76

American Foundation for Suicide Prevention. (2008c).
Warning signs of suicide.
http://www.afsp.org/index.cfm?fuseaction=home.viewPage&page_id=05147440-E24E-E376-
   BDF4BF8BA6444E76
Centers for Disease Control and Prevention.
Suicide prevention.
   http://www.cdc.gov/violenceprevention/pub/youth_suicide.html

PART EIGHT

Unique Stressors

CHAPTER 46

Grief and Loss in Children and Families

Linda Sayler Gudas

Joey woke up on the morning of his eighth birthday complaining of a "real bad" stomach ache. He said his head felt "funny" and asked to stay home from school. Although Joey did not look ill, his mother felt panicky. Joey's older brother, Sam, died of a brain aneurysm 3 years ago, following a severe headache and vomiting. When she called the pediatrician to describe Joey's symptoms, she recalled a conversation with the psychologist Joey had seen after Sam's death. The psychologist had told her that children's grief reactions can include experiencing physical symptoms similar to those of a dying sibling. Sam had died 1 month after turning 8 years old. Although Joey had been screened for his possibility of an aneurysm, the pediatrician asked to see the boy. After carefully examining Joey's head and stomach, the pediatrician reassured Joey that he was fine and did not have the problem that caused Sam's death. Joey left the office feeling better and went home to enjoy his birthday party.

The onset of Joey's eighth birthday triggered an understandable psychological connection to his brother's death. Such expectable reactions can cause an upsurge or resurfacing of grief. Because the adults in Joey's life (his mother and primary care physician) understood and addressed his anxiety, the child's symptoms quickly abated, and he returned to his regular activities.

WHAT IS "NORMAL" GRIEF?

Grief is a personal, emotional state or an anticipated response to loss. Although often a reaction to the death of a loved one, children and adults also experience such natural pain and suffering when encountering loss and separation in everyday events.

Research demonstrates that bereft people show enormous diversity in their emotional responses. The unique ways in which we experience grief depend on many factors that vary markedly across places, times, ages, groups, beliefs, and cultures. No one sign, symptom, or distinct pattern defines "normal" or "typical" grief in children. Rather, children's responses are influenced by the ways they experience loss and the meaning they attach to it. Parents can play a valuable role in helping their children be resilient. Grief does not have a time frame, and the bereaved individual does not "get over" the loss. Instead, children and adults can incorporate the loss into their lives, learn positive coping skills, adapt to a changed but meaningful life, and move on in age-appropriate tasks and life activities.

WHY TALK ABOUT GRIEF?

All children think about death, encounter death in daily life, and experience worries about separation from loved ones. Questions and concerns about death, dying, and loss are a normal part of growing up, and should be treated as such. You should not wait until the death of an important person or a significant loss in your child's life to begin thinking about how to communicate these issues. Providing children with information about the grief process increases their coping and decreases thoughts and feelings that may contribute to adjustment problems.

WHEN SHOULD WE TALK ABOUT DEATH AND LOSS?

A child's encounters with death and loss may show themselves in several different ways. The most common experience occurs in normal, everyday events. These times create natural "teaching moments" to begin a family discussion with your child. Examples might include a dead animal at the side of the road, ambulances racing past, movies where a loss occurs (e.g., *Bambi, The Sound of Music, The Lion King,*), books (e.g., the Harry Potter series), and commemorative holidays such as Veterans' Day, Memorial Day, or Martin Luther King Day. Opportunities abound to lay a foundation for what death means, to identify feelings of loss, to normalize grief reactions, and to discuss religious, cultural and social responses to death and dying. Such experiences generally do not pose emotional complications because the child has not confronted a personal loss, neither the child nor parent is actively mourning, and the event does not affect the family in an ongoing way.

A related example involves public news accounts of a death or disaster. Through the media, every child and adult in America will at some point witness natural disasters (e.g., a hurricane, tornado) or human-made tragedies (e.g., automobile accidents, terrorist attacks, school shootings) involving death. Children, especially adolescents, may also become involved in "public mourning" for celebrities, television stars, and public figures whom they learned about through media coverage. While children may be upset and genuinely feel sad, such mourning differs from true grief. Emotional reactions to these deaths tend to be short-lived, highly media-driven, dependent upon peer response, and do not affect the child's daily life. At the same time, children and adolescents often do not have the skills needed to cope with such complex loss events on their own.

Parents should supervise children's viewing of such media coverage and ideally remain present to answer their children's questions and address their fears as they attempt to cope with these events.

Children may also experience grief as a result of the loss of a significant person, place, animal, or object. The death of a beloved family member is, inevitably, the most difficult of losses. Should a child experience the simultaneous occurrence of the loss of a loved one and exposure to a disastrous event (e.g., a home fire, a hurricane, a flood), the interplay of grief and trauma can feel overwhelming for a child and family. Parents will find it helpful to consult with a mental health professional in dealing with these complicated grief situations. Examples of other personal losses that trigger similar responses include estrangement of family members as a result of divorce or the loss of neighborhood friends as a result of a geographical move. Non-person losses (e.g., the death of a pet) may be the first significant loss a child experiences, or may reactivate grief from previous losses. Many secondary losses occur as the result of a personal loss (e.g., changing of routines, less emotionally available family members, relocation), which adds disruption and pain for the child and may be unknowingly overlooked by others.

Children may also have concerns about death or loss as a result of their own serious or life-threatening illness. Examples include not only life-shortening illnesses (e.g., AIDS or cystic fibrosis) but also medical trauma (e.g., loss of a limb or paralysis) or chronic illness requiring lifestyle changes (e.g., diabetes). Seriously ill children as young as 5 or 6 years of age have a very real understanding of their condition, and even younger children show reactions to the effects of illness on themselves and their families. And, terminally ill children seem to know innately when they are dying. Ill children are often aware of the tendency of parents, loved ones, and medical personnel to withhold or minimize information. Addressing losses as they occur (e.g., the inability to play a sport) and transitions in the progress of the illness (e.g., the first hospitalization) is critical to helping a child cope. Life will change for a child and family coping with life-threatening conditions, and anticipatory grief occurs. Early consultation with a mental health practitioner in such situations can provide skilled support for parents to help make recommendations for managing stresses and to assist in understanding common psychological reactions.

HOW DO CHILDREN'S DEVELOPMENTAL DIFFERENCES AFFECT GRIEF?

Distinct developmental trends occur in a child's ability and efforts to make sense of and master concepts of death and dying, and these also influence how children adapt in the face of loss and grief. Age and emotional, social, and cognitive development each play a role in shaping the child's response. Children's responses to death and loss also reflect a family's current culture, past heritage, and social environment. Personal experience with illness, trauma, and dying may also aid children's understanding of loss and familiarity with mourning. We know that, for a grieving child, the most common responses reflect age-related concerns about separation from loved ones, physical and emotional pain, and disruption of usual life activities.

Infants and Toddlers

Infants and toddlers cannot understand the permanence of death. However, in infancy, the beginning concepts of separation and loss appear, as demonstrated in games such as "Peek-a-boo" or searching for lost objects. Reactions of protest, despair, separation anxiety, and detachment may occur when nurturing caretakers leave; and a child can feel abandoned. Very young children also respond to observing distress in others. Expressions of loss in this age group include irritability or lethargy or, in severe cases, failure to thrive. A toddler might be better able to understand separation from loved ones, and can show regressive behavior (e.g., clinging, loss of toilet training), especially under traumatic situations. Speech and language development in a toddler is a major milestone, making it possible for a child and parent to communicate directly about feelings of loss.

Preschoolers

In the preschool period, children's thinking is egocentric (self-centered) and circular. Preschool children do not possess logical cause-and-effect reasoning. They typically have magical explanations of death and loss events, and may think of their grief as a direct result of a specific thought or action. For example, a 5-year-old might believe that his friend or neighbor died because he was mad at them. Preschoolers use their own limited and familiar experiences to put events in context. Ideas about what is alive and what is dead are often confused. Thus, they understand death as a changed state, akin to sleep, moving away, or being sick. In attempts to master the finality of death and loss, preschoolers frequently ask unrelenting, repeated questions about the process. Preschoolers cannot yet fully regard death as permanent or irreversible, and they worry most about the length of separation from loved ones that death implies (e.g., "After he finishes being dead, will Grandpa go on vacation with us?" or "If I'm very good, maybe he'll come back."). Young children will express grief intermittently and over brief periods of time. Such responses can feel both frustrating and heartbreaking to parents struggling to manage their own emotions. A full range of emotions may follow a loss, but regression or a return to younger behaviors (e.g., wish to sleep with parents, loss of toilet-training), longing for the deceased person, guilt, self-blame, sadness, denial, and anger all commonly occur. Preschoolers may also experience physical complaints, such as stomach aches and headaches.

School-aged Children

School-aged children, from ages 6 or 7 to 12 years, think more concretely, recognize the permanence and irreversibility of death, and begin to understand the biological functioning of the human body (e.g., "You die if your heart stops working."). They view illness and death by concrete, visible signs (e.g., loss of hair from chemotherapy) and progress to higher-functioning observations (e.g., "Someone who is dead can't think anymore."). Mood and reactions become more stable at this age, but fantasies and fears play an important role in emotional adjustment. Bereaved middle school children, with their understanding of the permanence of death and the reality of their own mortality, tend to experience more anxiety, more obvious symptoms of depression, and more physical complaints than do younger children. As children begin to question any hope of reunion on earth with the deceased or of the ability to undo the loss, they are often left with anger focused on the lost loved person or situation, on those who could not prevent the loss, or on those presumed responsible for the death. The school years are a period of building independence and competency-based activities. These skills are frequently the most vulnerable under stress. Grief responses may show themselves in school or learning problems. Information gathered from the media, peers, and trusted adults form lasting impressions.

Adolescents

At the time of adolescence, children begin to reason abstractly, use symbolic thinking, and analyze "what-if" scenarios. Adolescents realize that "what is" may differ from "what might be"; questions that may not have occurred to younger children become prevalent (e.g., "What happens if the treatments don't work?"). Death and end of life become concepts, rather than events. Teenagers begin to understand complex systems of the body in relationship to both life and death. A developing sense of self and autonomy, coupled with the intense physical changes of this period, gives adolescents an increased bodily interest, a sense of omnipotence, and a focus on themselves. Heightened bodily concerns leave an adolescent vulnerable to physical symptoms as a result of any stress. Responses to grief are no longer limited to those seen in younger children (e.g., stomach-aches); the adolescent may develop highly sophisticated syndromes (e.g., lack of energy, eating disorders). Faced with powerful emotional threats (a death, a break-up of a relationship, a life-altering medical diagnosis), an adolescent may express grief via risk-taking behaviors (e.g., substance abuse, lack of adherence to a medical regimen), resentment, mood swings, or rage, as the teenager seeks answers to questions of values, safety, and fairness. Alternatively, adolescents may seek philosophical explanations or spiritual meaning to ease their sense of loss (e.g., "He is at peace."). Quality of life takes on meaning, as the teenager develops a sense of the future. Fascination with dramatic (e.g., suicide of a peer), sensational (e.g., a school shooting), or romantic deaths (e.g., the movie *Titanic*) often occurs and may find expression in copycat behaviors (e.g., cluster suicides), as well as in competitive behavior ("He was *my* best friend."). Teenagers may demonstrate their grief by constructing spontaneous shrines, such as murals, roadside flowers, or memorial websites as their own personal, emotional links to the deceased.

HOW CAN I HELP MY GRIEVING CHILD?

I recommend five "P's" of *practical strategies* for helping a grieving child or adolescent.

1. Positive Parenting

Constructive goals for parents focus on resiliency, strength, and normalcy of a child's grief, as well as on a child's ability to successfully cope and grow despite emotional difficulties. Children need to feel a sense of consistency, predictability, and security at home, as their loss has just demonstrated that life is not always so. While none of us is ever precisely "the same" after a significant loss, integrating familiar routines, maintaining a healthy lifestyle, and providing consistent discipline remain important.

Your capabilities as a parent may also feel drained because of your own grief. It is important that you take care of yourself in order to care of your children, whether by professional counseling, social and family support, or such practical assistance as seeking help in managing daily affairs. Children benefit from seeing their parents emotionally and physically strong and healthy (e.g., seeing Mom exercise, knowing Dad eats his fruits and vegetables, watching parents return to work). Such role modeling helps a child feel safe and secure in the face of uncertainty.

2. Permission to Talk About and Express Grief

Children have a right to honest, accurate, and developmentally appropriate discussions about their concerns. However, they must feel that they have permission to discuss their grief, communicate feelings, and address cognitive distortions about death and loss. Protecting or shielding children from salient information does not alleviate their anxieties and concerns. By talking openly, we discover what children know and do not know, and offer children a safe environment in which to share and mourn. To help enable discussions with your children, consider the following:

- What has the child been told?
- What has the child understood?
- What questions is the child asking (or not asking)?

Sharing thoughts and feelings may also help normalize your child's grief. For example, "Do you ever worry that you are going to die, too?" or "Sometimes I ask myself why this happened to us. Do you ever wonder that?" Remembering the past while creating a new future can be modeled by comments such as: "Remember when Grammy used to make her apple pies on Thanksgiving? Maybe we can try her recipe this year," or, "I found a really neat tree in the park down the street, just like the one near where Auntie Jane lived before she died. Want to go see?" To show sensitivity to a child or adolescent who may not feel ready to talk, a statement such as, "If you want to talk about the accident, Mom and I are here," may help.

Many children and adolescents raise poignant concerns and ask difficult questions. No question or thought should be considered off limits, no matter how intimidating or how inadequate you may feel in responding. Elaborating on all concerns at one time is not necessary, but discussions should be sensitive, truthful, and relevant. "I don't know how to answer that. Can I think about it for awhile?" is a perfectly acceptable reply, and a response should follow within a reasonable time frame.

3. Participating in Mourning Activities and Rituals

Helping children creatively express their grief helps the mourning process. Families can use art, play, story-writing, and reading as a way to say goodbye. Children can, for example, write and illustrate the story of their loss (e.g., *The Day Fluffy Didn't Come Home, I'm Not a Brother Anymore, I Have a Wicked Bad Disease*). You can provide your child with books, not only those with themes of loss but also of empowerment in tough situations (e.g., *The Little Engine That Could*). An older child might write an essay for the school paper on ways to help other kids cope with loss. Adolescents might create a collage, scrapbook, poem, or song. Safe websites, such as http://www.Kidsaid.com, provide a place for children and adolescents to share grief with others of their age. Together, your family might make a "memory box," write a letter describing memories, create a scholarship, or plant a tree in honor of the deceased.

Anniversary times (birthdays of the deceased, the date of the death) are important to remember, as children and families often feel sad and lonely as they recall memories at these times. Families can acknowledge these dates by sending up a balloon, visiting the cemetery, cooking the deceased's favorite meal, or even having a birthday cake in the deceased's memory. New family rituals can be introduced during holidays (i.e., "Who shall we have read the prayer now?" or "Shall we go skiing instead of the beach for vacation, now that all of us like the cold weather?"), as well as preserving old routines.

In non-person losses, you might help your child find creative ways of sustaining connections, such as donating time or money to an animal shelter in the deceased pet's name.

A child trying to cope with a loss in the community might send a card or note, attend a funeral, offer food or clothing, perform community service, or get involved in fund-raising—all activities that create a supportive social network.

A child coping with a personal loss should also have the choice to participate in mourning rituals. Depending upon the age of the child, family and religious custom, and the child's preferences, age-appropriate involvement helps the child process the loss and stay emotionally connected to other loved ones. Prepare children by explaining what will happen, in order to keep your child involved and to offer an informed choice. For example, "Lots of people will be at the funeral. Some will cry because they feel sad and miss Bobby. A box called a casket will have the body in it. You can come if you would like, and it's okay to change your mind." It can help to have a supportive person (a neighbor, babysitter) ready to assist your child if needed. This person can provide your child with comfort and allow him or her to leave the service or function without disruption. Adaptive alternatives can help a child as well (e.g., picking out the clothes the deceased will wear, having a private showing, choosing a reading for the service).

With your guidance, your child will learn the etiquette of mourning behaviors and cope in a hopeful, active, and constructive manner.

4. Promoting Healthy Adaptation

You can play an active role in helping your bereaved child maintain social and family connections, reinvest in new relationships, restore life's routines, and adapt to a "new normal" life. At the same time, you can help your child sustain a comforting bond with the deceased. Try to spend special time with your child, to remember and hope together. Positive family interactions and activities separate from mourning are valuable in providing a break from grief. Identify events that children can control ("I will ask Uncle Joe to Grandparents' Day at school this year.") rather than those they can't control ("I only want to go with Grampa."). Minimize any additional family or situational stressors to help your child get used to the loss.

5. Preventing Maladaptive Grief Responses

Grief is predictable following a loss and is not, in itself, "pathological." Many children and families do not require professional help following a death. However, grief reactions can become complicated when they create symptoms that interfere with a child's normal activities and that compromise attainment of age-appropriate skills. Just as no one sign or symptom identifies what is "normal" grief, no one sign or cluster identifies the child or family in need of help. However, duration, intensity, and severity of symptoms, in context with a family's culture, can help you identify the need for further assessment. If your child is experiencing grief that you would describe as *unrelenting, intense, intrusive,* or *prolonged,* your child could probably benefit from professional help. Examples of maladaptive grief responses might include persistent complaints of illness without known cause, severe separation distress, talk of suicide, or new problems at school or with peers. Total absence of grieving should also suggest potential problems.

Be sure to make adequate help available, and allow your children to seek such assistance. As with Joey, a visit to the pediatrician (and parents' visits to their primary care doctor) can prove valuable in determining emotional risk factors and provide reassurance that everyone is physically healthy. Schools offer invaluable support for grieving children and are in a prime position to provide information and opportunities for intervention. Psychological services may benefit an entire family or individual members. Resources include support groups or family, couple, and individual counseling. Combinations of approaches may work well for some children. For example, a child might participate in family therapy to deal with the loss of a sibling and also use individual treatment to address issues of personal guilt or anxiety related to the death.

SUMMARY

Grief is an expected reaction to a death or loss and, in most cases, will take a healthy course. However, you can best assist your grieving child by understanding how your child experiences grief, by learning strategies to foster healthy coping skills, and by knowing when your child requires intervention. The presence of a consistent adult, capable of meeting your child's needs and who permits honest and accurate discussion about the loss, is a crucial factor in helping a bereft child. Our responsibility and duty as parents and adults is to see that children do not grieve alone.

WHERE TO FIND OUT MORE

Books

Brown, L.K., & Brown, M.T. (1996). *When dinosaurs die: A guide to understanding death.* Boston: Little, Brown & Co.
Grollman, E. (1993). *Straight talk about death for teenagers.* Boston: Beacon Press.
MacGregor, C. (1999). *Why do people die?* Secaucus, N.J: Carol Publishing Co.
Piper, W. (1986). *The little engine that could.* New York: Platt & Munk.
Smith, D.B. (1988). *A taste of blackberries.* New York: HarperCollins.

Websites

Healthwise. (2007, November 12). *Helping children who are grieving.* http://www.revolutionhealth.com.

Jewett, C. (1997). *Helping children cope with separation and loss.* London: B.T. Batsford Ltd.

Revolution Health Group. (2006, December 5). Talking to children about death. http://www.revolutionhealth.com.

Staywell Custom Communications. (2006, September 8). *Helping your child cope with death.* http://www.revolutionhealth.com

CHAPTER 47

Coping with Disaster, Terrorism, and Other Trauma

Robin H. Gurwitch and Merritt Schreiber

A 5-year-old boy evacuating with his family from New Orleans after Hurricane Katrina anxiously asks, "Will there be hurricanes where we're going?"

Parents express concern that their 4-year-old daughter repeatedly sets up wooden block towers and knocks them down after watching the events of September 11, 2001, unfold.

A 9-year-old is afraid to return to school after a tornado ripped through her community.

An 8-year-old child feels increasingly worried because his father now serves with the military in Afghanistan.

Parents notice their teenager has been spending significantly more time in his room, not wanting to hang out with his friends as usual, following a crisis at his school.

All too often crises and disasters touch the lives of our children. As much as we wish to protect and insulate them from these events, we cannot. First and foremost, in the aftermath, the most important goal is to assure the safety of our children and tend to their basic needs in terms of food, clothing, and shelter. After taking care of these needs, you can more effectively support their recovery by providing emotional or psychological first aid. Knowing how to provide psychological first aid to our children and taking steps to help build their resilience will improve their coping skills and relieve their distress. Before we, as parents or other caregivers, can begin to help our children, we must understand common human reactions that follow a disaster or crisis.

COMMON REACTIONS IN CHILDREN AFTER DISASTER

Children's reactions to a stressful situation typically fall into four different categories: how they feel (emotional), how they act (behavioral), how they think (cognitive), and how their bodies respond (physiological). When considering children's reactions, it is important to take a developmental perspective. Just as 3-year-olds communicate and interact with the world around them differently from 13-year-olds, they also differ in how they express their reactions to disaster or crisis.

Emotional

Children's worries increase following a disaster. Like the boy in the evacuation example, a primary worry will focus on reoccurrence of the event and particularly, separation from parents. For him, this worry will likely increase with any situation that reminds him of the storm, such as heavy rain or even threatening skies. Fears of reoccurrence generally link to sights, smells, and sounds that bring back thoughts of the crisis. Most children have increased worries and fears about their safety and the safety and security of those they care about. As children age, their sphere of worry broadens from family to include friends, schoolmates, community, and eventually their nation or beyond. Many children expressed concerns about those devastated by Hurricane Katrina even when they didn't know anyone directly affected.

Children may have considerable feelings of worry and/or sadness. They may feel guilty and blame themselves for actions they took or did not take that they believe (usually without cause) contributed to the impact of the disaster on others. In adolescence, feelings of hopelessness can become overwhelming, accompanied by thoughts of an uncertain future and a focus on death.

Behavioral

When we hear the following symptoms—problems with attention and concentration, problems with behavioral control, increased irritability, problems with organization, problems completing work at home or school, and problems with peers—the first thing that comes to mind is attention-deficit hyperactivity disorder (ADHD). However, similar behavioral changes also often occur in the aftermath of a disaster or crisis. If these behaviors appeared after a disaster, but were not present before the event, they likely represent a response to the disaster or crisis, rather than ADHD.

Other common behavioral changes include a decrease in enjoyment of extracurricular activities and time with friends, mood swings (especially increased anger outburst in older children and temper tantrums in younger ones), and social withdrawal. Children may avoid people, places, and situations that remind them of the disaster. Very young children may have a regression (or loss of behaviors they had previously mastered), such as toileting accidents after being potty trained, increased demands for help with dressing, or increased baby talk. Older children may respond by showing increased risk-taking behaviors, such as alcohol or drug use, or other high-risk behaviors such as sexual promiscuity or reckless driving. With all of the behavioral changes, a decrease in school performance may often also occur.

A drop in grades, difficulties learning, and trouble completing assignments can feel upsetting to parents and teacher, especially if unanticipated. Some children may also refuse to go to school or seek to come home early from school. Young children will likely become more "clingy" to parents and teachers, becoming upset at times of separation or transition.

Cognitive

Following disasters, children may experience flashbacks or feelings like the event is occurring again. These feel very real to them and can become extremely upsetting and frightening. Children may ask questions about the crisis numerous times, despite having previously gotten answers from adults. In preteens, these questions may seem gruesome in nature and upsetting to adults. Children may repeatedly retell their stories of their experiences during the disaster. Like the child who repeatedly built up and knocked down her blocks, young children may play out the event over and over again. Adults may find such play concerning if it repeats a destructive pattern without any changes, but this may represent the child's attempt to control and master a scary situation.

Physiological

Children's reactions to disaster can also reveal themselves in how their bodies respond. Parents may notice a change in appetite (eating more or less). Children may have difficulty falling asleep or staying asleep, including an increase in nightmares. Unfortunately, when children do not get enough rest or do not eat well, further problems with learning can develop and increase their risk for poor school performance. Children may become more sensitive to sound, startling more easily. They may appear "on alert" for the disaster or crisis to happen again. They may also have more somatic complaints including headaches, stomachaches, fatigue, and other aches and pains. Visits to the doctor usually result in no medical reason for the complaints; however, the symptoms feel very real to the children.

Factors That Can Make a Difference

A number of factors can reduce children's distress reactions. The greater the child's exposure to certain aspects of the event, the more likely he or she may be at risk for significant reactions. Exposure includes becoming trapped or separated from parents or caregivers, seeing others severely injured, finding themselves in a situation where they fear they may be seriously injured or killed, and losing loved ones, including pets.

"Exposure" can also occur by seeing scenes of destruction or the pain of others through the media. Research has not clearly answered the question of whether more anxious children seek out coverage of the event or if watching more coverage makes children more anxious and upset. The bottom line for parents, however, is to limit your child's exposure to news coverage and to monitor your child's exposure to media coverage over time. Particularly in the case of young children, consider avoiding media exposure completely, if realistically possible.

When children become separated from their families in times of crisis, they may experience an increased intensity of the reactions just described. The quicker everyone reunites the better. Disasters and crises disrupt routines, at home and at school. The longer it takes to return to some semblance of a normal routine, the more difficulties children will likely experience. If children had experienced emotional difficulties prior to the event, they remain at increased risk for greater difficulties coping after a disaster.

Perhaps the best predictor of how well children will do in the face of a disaster is how well their parents are coping. Children look to their parents as role models, and will take their cues from them. Families struggling with stressors or life challenges before the disaster or crisis occurred may have greater difficulty providing positive role models for their children in the aftermath of the event. The age and development of the child also effect how the child understands, reacts, and copes with the event.

PSYCHOLOGICAL FIRST AID

Once you are able to recognize the common reactions and factors affecting your children following a disaster or crisis, you can aid their healing through the use of Psychological First Aid (PFA). The American Red Cross defines PFA as "a set of actions that provide immediate support and coping skills to people in distress."

PFA consists of emotional support, information and education, encouraging the practice of positive coping, and recognizing when one needs more help and getting this extra help. The steps to PFA for children involve actions that parents and other caring adults can provide, which can help reduce the stress caused by the disaster or crisis. As you learn about the steps to PFA for children, you may say to yourself, "I do this already." In most cases, that is exactly right! Putting your instinctive actions together with a few new ideas can help your child cope more effectively with disaster-related emotions and stressors.

PFA steps can be accomplished if parents "Listen, Protect, and Connect." In this model, the steps for PFA for children as provided by parents fall under one of these three broad categories.

Listen

- Pay attention to verbal messages and nonverbal behaviors.
- Remain willing to talk.
- Gently correct confusion that can lead to feelings of guilt, shame, and/or blame.
- Ask questions that encourage conversation (try to avoid asking questions that a scared child can answer with only a yes or no).
- Check in with your children on a regular basis.
- Listen for clues about the child's disaster-related experiences.
- Try to remain patient . . . children need a little extra time and attention.

The first—and perhaps the most important step—is listening. Children will communicate with you through words, behaviors, and expression of emotions. Children often become hesitant to discuss difficult situations with their parents or caregivers. They may wait for you to introduce the topic because they are unsure how to bring it up.

Many adults worry that by directly addressing the issues surrounding an extremely stressful situation such as a disaster, they may make children feel worse. The opposite is actually the case. In the example of the 8-year-old whose father serves in the military in Afghanistan, talking about the thoughts and feelings surrounding the deployment can actually help him feel better. By bringing up the topic, your children know that they can talk to you about it now or in the future. Give children opportunities to talk, draw, or play out their feelings and emotions.

Suggestions for starting the conversation:

- "There have been lots of changes since the hurricane. What do you think about what has happened? What do you worry about most?"
- "Tell me what you think about your dad's deployment. How do you think our family will manage?"
- "Because of the tornado, we have to move to a new home. This will mean changes for our family. We will have lots of different feelings because of what has happened. I want you to know that I want to talk to you about what has happened or will happen, and I will answer any questions you have."
- "I notice that you have not wanted to spend time with your friends much since the crisis at your school. Many teens who have encountered similar situations find it hard to spend time around their friends. Know that I will gladly listen, talk to you, and try to answer any of your questions. We can talk now or whenever you would like."

In all cases, it becomes important to listen. *Do not* assume that you know how your child feels or what he or she thinks. Acknowledge and support how your child feels. For example, if your child says that he feels scared that the event will happen again, rather than saying, "Don't be scared, it won't happen again and everything will be fine," say something like, "I know you feel scared. But remember, our family has gotten out together. We can make plans for anything like this that may happen in the future. We can talk about it. I believe that as hard and scary as it feels now, we will get through this together."

Although it seems you answer the same questions children ask repeatedly, each time you provide the same answer confirms to your children that you have listened and that the story has not changed. The same answer provides assurance that you have not held anything back. Your children may take in a little bit more information each time until they develop a clear answer for themselves. Being asked the same questions and providing the same answers over and over again can be stressful, particularly if you too find yourself struggling to cope. Take a deep breath and answer the questions simply and honestly, and at a developmental level that your children can understand. If they persist, consider asking what else they would like to know.

Listen for any nonverbal expressions that may need your support. For example, your child may begin to exhibit changes in his or her behavior, as discussed earlier. Increased social withdrawal and irritability, temper tantrums, angry outbursts, and mood swings indicate that you may need to find extra time to talk and provide support for your child. You may see problems with getting chores or homework completed as before. Take a step back. In providing PFA, talk to your children about how they plan to get these tasks completed. Consider reducing the work into smaller segments that can be completed in stages. Notice and praise your children's efforts and their accomplishments. All of this emotional and physical support will help their coping and resilience.

When your children do talk, listen carefully to what they say. Listen especially for any confusion (things your children incorrectly believe have happened or will happen) that can lead to feelings of guilt, shame, or blame. Sometimes children may believe that their actions or inactions *caused* the crisis. They may think, "If I had paid better attention, I could have collected all the papers my family needed when we evacuated." "When I had a fight with my father, I secretly wished he would get sent away; now he is fighting in Afghanistan because of me." If you hear these types of statements, gently correct their thoughts and give your children accurate information, always at a level that they can understand.

Not every child will talk, even when you bring up the issues. That's okay—*don't force it.* Just letting your children know that you remain willing to talk about all aspects of the disaster or crisis becomes the key to later conversations. Check in periodically. Mealtimes or driving in the car provide wonderful opportunities for these conversations to occur.

Protect

- Maintain a daily routine.
- Monitor media exposure (reduce or avoid unnecessary exposure to disturbing images, conversations, or sights).
- Monitor adult conversations.
- Find ways for your children to feel helpful.

Another important component of PFA for children is protecting them from increased stress, anxiety, fear, and worry that accompany a disaster. Parents and caregivers can provide very important protection through their actions.

A daily schedule or routine can benefit children of all ages. With routine comes an increased sense of security, safety, and control—much of which can be undermined by the uncertainties and unpredictability that often follow crisis situations. As much as possible, keep the routines that your family had before the event. Keep routines around school, homework, bed and mealtimes, and behaviors.

Although you may feel the urge to be more lenient with your children due to what has happened, remember that negative behaviors escalate. So, if you prohibited certain behaviors from your children before the event, you should not allow these behaviors to occur after.

For the young girl who felt afraid to return to school, one concern may involve worry over what will happen if the family becomes separated. In this case, create a family plan for what everyone can do, if separated for any reason. Also encourage children to return to school, and spend a little extra time with them each day. These actions will help children take the first steps toward feeling as if they can cope, and will show them that parents can support and protect them from worries. Such actions can prevent long-term problems of school refusal.

Whenever a disaster strikes, the event will undoubtedly be covered in the media. Children may talk about it at school, during extracurricular activities, and over the Internet. It is important that you monitor what and how much your children are seeing, and that you discuss it with them. You can say, "Tell me what you think about that news story." Or, "What do your friends have to say about the disaster (or the war)?" Again, keep in mind your children's ages and level of development just as you do around other topics.

Remember, all the details that you understand as an adult may prove confusing or upsetting to your children. Just as you monitor what they see related to the media, monitoring adult conversations about a disaster or crisis, including war, also becomes important. Talking about these issues with friends and family happens normally. But remember, your children will listen in . . . even when you don't notice! Again, they may not completely understand what you are saying, and this may confuse or upset your children as they try to make sense of it.

Another important step of providing PFA is to help your children help others. If children can feel that their actions may help others, even when they are reaching out for help themselves, they will cope better and become more resilient. Work with your children to find small ways in which they can help. These may include actions around the house, such as chores or helping a neighbor. Keep "helping actions" to a developmentally appropriate level. For example, young children may help sort laundry by color while older children may shovel a neighbor's walk. Actions may also link to a parent's deployment. Children may help organize a letter-writing campaign to their parent's unit or send clippings from local papers to keep their parents informed about happenings at home. Talk to your children about their ideas for helping and support, as they often have better ideas than what adults can think up!

Connect

- Connect children with family and friends.
- Connect children with supportive activities and services for children at schools, through faith and cultural resources, and in the community.
- Encourage extracurricular activities (community sports, clubs, hobbies, volunteering for the local service organizations).
- Remind children of positive coping skills they used in the past.
- Keep other important adults in your children's lives informed.
- Consider whether additional mental health services for you or your children might help.

An essential component of PFA for children is making sure they feel connected to others. Clearly, the most important connection is with you. Knowing that they can turn to you for support, information, attention, fun, and love will do more for your children's coping than almost anything else. At home, take time each day to check in with your child. This often works more easily with younger children than for older children who may be busy with school, friends, and extracurricular activities. Consider family meals and bedtimes as opportunities to talk.

When a disaster or crisis strikes a community, services sponsored by organizations, schools, and faith- and cultural-based institutions in the community generally start up.

Learn about what may become available for your children. Places to turn for this information include the American Red Cross, local newspapers or television stations, local mental health services, and your children's schools. The more information you have, the better you will be able to choose what may work best for your children. Most military units now have programs specifically to help children and families cope with the stress related to deployments. Connecting your children with services for others who have experienced the crisis increases their sense that others can understand and that they are not alone.

One common reaction after a disaster or crisis involves social withdrawal and a lack of interest in once pleasurable activities. Your children may not want to continue with extracurricular activities (e.g., sports, dance, playing or getting together with friends, or even attending special events like birthday parties). However, continued participation in such activities keeps children connected to others. In the case of the adolescent who shows signs of social withdrawal, a parent may encourage attendance at a soccer game for half the game and then allow the teen to decide if he would rather stay or return home. As children participate in extracurricular events, even when they "do not feel like it," the simple act of attending generally leads to improved mood and decreased stress, and these in turn can lead to increase interest and increased resilience.

Keeping others in children's lives informed about how your children are coping will also prove important. By letting school, coaches, instructors, and others know about any changes, all the adults in your children's lives can better understand any changes in behaviors and support your children. Just as you keep others informed, ask that they keep you informed about school and extracurricular activities that you may not see on a regular basis. Working together, children can receive the PFA support and caring that increases coping and, ultimately, their resilience.

Experiences with disasters and crises fortunately prove rare in the life of each individual child; however, every child has experienced stressful situations. These may include starting a new school or moving from middle to high school, learning to ride a bike, giving an oral report, or completing a large school project. In each instance, with your support and guidance, your children faced the stressor and succeeded in meeting the challenge. Help your children remember what they did to cope. Skills may have involved setting small step-wise goals to accomplish the task, practicing breathing and relaxation, talking to you about what the challenges would involve and problem-solving how to meet them. Help them use the same or similar skills as they face the large challenge of coping with a disaster. Recognize their efforts through praise and positive attention. This will let your children know you care and are supportive.

One important aspect of PFA that parents provide involves considering when extra help may be needed. You can use some simple ideas to help determine if your child may need more assistance. For example, if your children have witnessed death or injury to others, particularly family members, or felt a threat to their own lives, they may need help in addition to your PFA.

WHEN TO SEEK PROFESSIONAL HELP

Just as emergency room physicians use a system to triage or decide about the best medical care for patients, the Listen, Protect and Connect PFA for Children includes a tool to help you identify if you may need to seek additional help for your child from a mental health professional. The risk factors included in the PsySTART Triage System include:

- Loss of a family member, schoolmate, or friend
- Fear for their lives, observing serious injury or the death of another person
- Family members or friends missing after the event
- Getting sick or becoming hurt due to the event
- Home loss, family moves, changes in neighborhoods, changes in schools, or loss of belongings
- Being unable to evacuate quickly
- Past traumatic experiences or losses
- Pet loss
- Past history of post-traumatic stress disorder, anxiety, or mood disorders coupled with any of the above

As you listen to your children, if they express any thoughts about harming themselves, take these seriously and contact someone who can provide extra help or know how to find appropriate help (e.g., school counselor, child's doctor, or mental health specialist). You know your children better than anyone. For most children, reactions will begin to diminish within 1–3 months after the disaster. If they do not, or if you feel that these reactions are significantly interfering with daily functioning at any time, seek out help for your child. Many communities have mental health providers with expertise in helping children after a traumatic event.

SUMMARY

Disasters and crisis come in different sizes. They may involve a single-family house fire or a hurricane that devastates a large region. Many families across the United States face the crisis of parental military deployment. No matter what the event, children need extra time, patience, and attention as they cope. Providing this and following the action steps of PFA can improve their outcome and strengthen your relationship with your children.

Finally, when a disaster or crisis strikes, you also are affected. As you also feel stressed, make sure that you have resources that you can turn to for support, a listening ear, a shoulder, and a break! Taking care of yourself is important. Remember, if you don't take care of yourself, you can't provide the best care for your children.

WHERE TO FIND OUT MORE

Books

American National Red Cross. (2010). *Coping in today's world: Psychological First Aid and resilience for families, friends, and neighbors.* Washington, DC: American National Red Cross.
American National Red Cross. (2009). *Coping with deployments: Psychological First Aid for military families.* Washington, DC: American National Red Cross.

Brooks, R.B., & Goldstein, S. (2001). *Raising resilient children: Fostering strength, hope, and optimism in your child.* Lincolnwood, IL: Contemporary Books.

La Greca, A., Silverman, W., Vernberg, E., & Roberts, M. (Eds.). (2002). *Helping children cope with disasters and terrorism.* Washington, DC: American Psychological Association.

Websites

Schrieber, M., Gurwitch, R.H., & Wong, M. (2008).
Listen, protect, and connect for teachers
  http://www.ready.gov/kids/_downloads/PFA_SchoolCrisis.pdf
Schreiber, M. & Gurwitch, R.H. (2007).
Listen, protect, and connect for parents
  http://www.ready.gov/kids/_downloads/PFA_Parents.pdf
Schreiber, M., Gurwitch, R.H., Wong, M., & Schonfeld, D. (2009).
Listen, protect, and connect (psychological first aid after natural disasters)
  http://www.cincinnatichildrens.org/svc/alpha/s/school-crisis/psych-aid.htm

CHAPTER 48

How to Recognize When Your Child May Need Professional Help

Gerald P. Koocher and Annette M. La Greca

Freddy, age 4, completed toilet training a year ago but began wetting his bed intermittently following the birth of his sister a few weeks ago.

Emma, age 6, seems shy around unfamiliar adults and has an imaginary playmate named Polly. Emma insists that her parents set a place for Polly at mealtime and seeks to incorporate Polly in most family activities.

Jack, age 10, who never seemed very emotionally expressive, has recently gotten in trouble for setting a number of small outdoor fires in his neighborhood. He seems to enjoy teasing the family's dog, and the neighbors complained that he picked up their cat and threw it over a fence after it wandered into his family's yard. When asked about these events, Jack denies responsibility or simply shrugs.

Nancy, age 15, has caused increasing concern to her parents after they noticed scratch marks on the underside of her wrists caused by some type of sharp object. Nancy also has cut off relationships with some of her long-time school friends, and when asked about these issues, she simply storms off to her room.

All children will experience both physical and psychological bumps and bruises on their way to adolescence and adulthood. Parents naturally want the best for their children, and do not like to see their children in distress. Parents also worry when their child or teenager has difficulty coping, feels sad or moody, can't sleep, has difficulty getting along with family or friends, or becomes involved with alcohol or drugs. Parents are usually among the first to recognize when their child has a behavioral or emotional problem. Even so, the decision to seek professional help can prove difficult or painful.

The main purpose of this book is to provide parents with advice and recommendations for addressing the most common psychological problems children and adolescents typically confront in the normal course of development. As the chapters illustrate, anticipation and prevention of problems can play a key role in helping you successfully negotiate the predictably difficult periods or stressors in your child's life. When implementing psychological first-aid a positive first step generally involves efforts to communicate openly about the problem and the feelings that it stirs up.

But, what if the first-aid measures do not seem to help or resolve the problem? The decision to seek professional help should flow from the *nature, intensity,* and *duration* of the problem, and from whether or not the problem is seriously *interfering with your child's day-to-day functioning.* (Is it adversely affecting school performance? Friendships? Family relationships?) For example, Freddy's bedwetting follows a family stress related to the birth of a sibling and it occurred well after he had completed toilet training. This is not unusual after the birth of a sibling, and if the bedwetting becomes less frequent or resolves in response to some of the strategies described in this book, he will have no need of professional follow-up. However, persistent bedwetting that does not respond to normal interventions may reflect medical or more significant emotional issues that warrant evaluation.

Emma's imaginary playmate does not signal the need for professional help, but if it leads to persistent disruption of family life accompanied by tantrums and emotional outbursts, it could signal a more significant problem. And, if having an imaginary playmate prevents Emma from making "real friends" in her school or neighborhood, it can interfere with her social development. Problems in family or social adjustment that result from having an imaginary friend might signal the need for professional help.

Behaviors that pose a danger to others or involve intentional violence toward people or animals, as exhibited by Jack, suggest a need for prompt expert evaluation. This holds particularly true when such behaviors occur repeatedly or involve serious harm.

Although every teenager feels frustrated and/or depressed at times, Nancy's parents should not overlook her self-injury and social withdrawal behaviors. Self-injurious behavior, or any expression of suicidal ideation, warrant prompt evaluation by a mental health professional whenever they occur.

GUIDELINES FOR PRESCHOOL- AND SCHOOL-AGED CHILDREN

Keeping in mind the nature, intensity, and duration of the behavior or feelings as the three critical factors, you should consider seeking professional guidance in any of the following cases:

- A significant decline in school performance:
  - A sudden, marked drop in the quality of your child's school work
  - Earning poor grades despite seemingly trying very hard
  - New-onset or significant escalation in behavior problems at school

- Severe worry or anxiety, as reflected by:
  - Persistent school refusal or refusal to separate from a parent
  - Persistent sleep problems, including trouble falling asleep and nightmares
  - Persistent refusal to participate in normal age-related activities outside the home with peers or family members
- Frequent or persistent physical complaints without a medical basis
- Hyperactivity, fidgeting, constant movement beyond regular playing, with or without difficulty paying attention
- Persistent disobedience, fighting, or aggression, particularly involving violence or unexplainable temper tantrums
- Any threat to harm or kill oneself

GUIDELINES FOR OLDER SCHOOL-AGED CHILDREN AND ADOLESCENTS

When considering whether to seek professional help for older children or teens, keep in mind the preceding guidelines and keep an eye out for the following issues:

- Persistent inability to cope with daily activities and problems
- Marked changes in sleeping and/or eating habits, including intense fear of "becoming fat" that is unrelated to actual body weight, excessive dieting (including attempts to lose weight through vomiting and laxative use or even excessive exercise)
- Sexual acting out
- Persistent depression, as reflected by sustained, prolonged negative mood and attitude, often accompanied by poor appetite, difficulty sleeping, loss of pleasure in previously enjoyed activities, and/or thoughts of death
- Dramatic mood swings over relatively brief periods of time
- Repeated use of alcohol and/or drugs
- Threats of self-harm or harm to others, including self-injury or self-destructive behavior
- Persistent truancy, thefts, or vandalism
- Unusual thoughts, beliefs, feelings, or sensory experiences that may suggest a loss of contact with reality

HOW TO FIND A MENTAL HEALTH PROFESSIONAL

If your child needs professional assistance, look for a mental health professional such as a psychologist, a social worker, a counselor, or a psychiatrist. If your child needs help around issues that come up when they are in school, a school counselor or school psychologist can help to evaluate your child and also provide a recommendation for further help. Your family physician or a member of your local clergy also may be someone to share your concerns with, and they may be able to assist you in finding appropriate help.

Other ways of identifying an appropriate mental health professional include:

- Contact the American Psychological Association (APA) at 1-800-964-2000. The operator will use your ZIP code to locate and connect you with an appropriate referral source in your area. You can also do this online by going to the APA website at www.apa.org and clicking on *Find a Psychologist.*
- Contact the Association for Cognitive and Behavioral Therapies (ABCT) through their website (www.abct.org). On their website, under the button for *The Public* you can find useful information, such as *How to Choose a Child Therapist* (*see* http://www.abct.org/sccap/?m=sPublic&fa=pub_HowToChooseChildTherapist). The ABCT website also has a button for *Find a Therapist* that enables you to search for mental health professionals by City or State within the United States and Canada.
- A website co-sponsored by ABCT and the American Psychological Association on *Effective Child Therapy* contains descriptions of evidence-based treatments for children and adolescents and a link for finding an appropriate therapist (see http://www.effectivechildtherapy.com).

SUMMARY

This book focused on the many developmental crises that children and adolescents (and their parents) encounter in the process of growing up. In the normal course of any child's development, events will occur that are upsetting and emotionally challenging to children and their parents. The purpose of this book is to provide parents and other caregivers with practical, sound advice from seasoned experts, with specific strategies for dealing with children's predictable emotional crises. The chapters emphasize ways that parents can promote coping, resilience, and recovery in their children when such crises occur.

That being said, it is also important to recognize that this book is not a substitute for professional advice. As noted in this chapter, when problems appear extreme in nature, duration, or intensity, or when they interfere with child and family functioning, seeking professional help is an important "next step." When a child sustains serious physical injuries, parents typically seek professional medical care. Although psychological bumps and bruises may be harder to evaluate than the physical ones, we encourage parents to seek professional advice if they are worried or unsure of the extent of their child's emotional or behavioral problems, or have concerns about how to manage them.

In addition to the referral sources just discussed, we list several key websites in the section on Where to Find Out More. These websites provide scientifically sound and reputable information on a wide array of child problems. We encourage parents to use these resources, the advice outlined in this book, and, of course, their own judgment in helping their children to lead successful and emotionally balanced lives.

WHERE TO FIND OUT MORE

American Psychological Association
  http://www.apa.org

American Academy of Pediatrics
 http://www.aap.org
American Association of Child and Adolescent Psychiatry
 http://www.aacap.org/
Association for Behavioral and Cognitive Therapies
 http://www.abct.org
National Institute of Mental Health
 http://nimh.nih.gov/health/index.shtml

INDEX

Note: Page numbers followed by "*t*" denote tables.